Contents

1003178617T

Acknowledgements

The majority of the photographs have been taken by Dr Sharon Taylor. However we would like to thank the following for their photographic contribution:

Dr Andrew Bush

Dr Howard Davis
1.66

Dr Martha Dynski-Klein

Prof. Victor Dubowitz
0.14, 10.15, 10.16, 10.17

Dr Tony Lynn

Dr Simon Murch
5.21, 5.22, 5.23, 5.25, 5.28, 5.34, 5.35

Dr Chann Ng
7.40, 7.48

Prof. Andrew Redington

Dr David Leo Ruben

Dr Michael Rubens

Dr Alison Shurz

Mr Richard Stokes
5.8, 15.23

Dr Mike Thomson
5.16, 5.17, 5.18, 5.19, 5.26, 5.27
5.29, 5.30, 5.31, 5.32, 5.33, 5.45

Dr Gareth Tudor-Williams

Prof. Patrica Woo
10.37, 10.38, 10.39

We are also grateful to the following photographic departments:
Great Ormond Street
Queen Elizabeth Hospital, Hackney Road
St. Mary's Hospital (Brendan Ryan)
Lister Hospitial, Stevenage
Royal Marsden Photographic Department
The Royal Post-graduate Department, Hammersmith Hospital, Queen Elizabeth II Hospital, Welwyn Garden City.

We are very grateful to the following people who either kindly reviewed the chapters in their specialist fields or made other significant suggestions and contributions:
Dr John Wyatt, Consultant Neonatal Pediatrician, University College London Hospital Trust; Dr Karen Zwi, Former Registrar in Community Pediatrics, City and Hackney NHS Trust; Prof. Andrew Redington, Prof. of Pediatric Cardiology, Royal Brompton Hospital; Dr Andrew Bush, Senior Lecturer and Honorary Consultant, Pediatric Chest Physician, Royal Brompton Hospital; Dr Simon Murch, Consultant in Pediatric Gastroenterology, Royal Free Hospital; Dr Mike Thomson, Consultant Pediatrician in Gastroenterology and Nutrition, Royal Free Hospital; Dr Jane Deal, Consultant Pediatrician, Pediatric Nephrologist, St Mary's Hospital; Dr Michael Salman, Lecturer. Pediatric Neurosciences, Kings Hospital, London; Dr Howard Davis, Consultant Hematologist, Queen Elizabeth II Hospital, Welwyn Garden City; Prof. Charles G.D. Brook, Consultant Pediatric Endocrinolgist, The Middlesex Hospital; Prof. Patricia Woo, Prof. of Pediatric Rheumatology, University College 'Hospital, London Medical School; Dr David Atherton, Consultant Dermatologist, Great Ormond Street Hospital; Prof Michael Levin, Prof. of Pediatrics, Imperial College, School of Medicine, St Mary's Hospital; Dr Marion Miles, Consultant Community Pediatrician, St. Mary's Hospital; Mr Robert L Johnson, Senior Registrar, Ophthalmology, Moorfields Hospital; Mr Munther Haddad, Pediatric Surgeon, Chelsea and Westminster Hospital; Dr Jocelyn Brooks, Senior Registrar in Radiology, Middlesex Hospital; Dr Michael Rubens, Consultant Radiologist, Royal Brompton Hospital; Dr Rodney Franklin, Consultant Pediatric Cardiologist, Harefield Hospital; Dr David Leo Ruben, Consultant Radiologist, King Edward Hospital, South Africa; Dr Sathees Singh, Registrar in Medicine, King Edward Hospital, South Africa.

Thanks to the following hospitals and especially to their patients without whom this book would not have been possible:
St Mary's Hospital
University College Hospital
The Royal Brompton Hospital
King Edward Hospital, Durban, South Africa.
Queen Elizabeth II Hospital, Welwyn Garden City

And finally.... a special thanks to the following people for their enthusiasm, encouragement and hard work: Fiona Foley, Richard Furn, Gina Almond and Leslie Sinoway.

Preface

As the complexities of modern medicine increase exponentially there remains a need for practitioners to visually recognise important clinical features, especially with potentially fatal conditions. This requires knowledge out of proportion to previous experience. In this collection of pictures we are attempting to transfer to you some of that essential knowledge.

As teachers and students of pediatrics we are only too aware of how much knowledge one requires to be a safe practitioner and to pass examinations. We feel that this book will enhance your learning and improve your clinical acumen. If only we could identify what makes a better pediatrician, we would put this into the book too; this collection of photographs is the next best thing!

By indicating some of the more important imaging techniques, and including examples of some of the common investigations we have complemented the pictorial knowledge with clinical information. To enhance the clinical significance and educational value of many of these photographs we have also included case histories.

We extend our thanks to all those colleagues who donated slides and especially our chapter reviewers whose enthusiasm for the project kept us from desperation. Thank you also to our families who understood what we were doing every Sunday.

We have enjoyed producing this book and have learned much in its gestation. Use it to make yourself a better practitioner in whatever field of child health you choose to follow.

Dr Sharon Taylor
Dr Andrew Raffles

To the loving memory of Martha Dinski-Klein,
the inspiration behind this book.

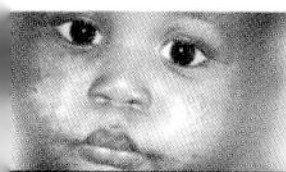

1 The newborn

Congenital Malformations

Figure 1.1 Trisomy 13 (Patau Syndrome). The scalp defects shown in **Figure 1.1** are associated with microcephaly, microphthalmia, hypotelorism, polydactyly, rocker-bottom feet and, cardiac, renal and central nervous system (CNS) abnormalities. The majority of children with this disorder die within the first year of life.

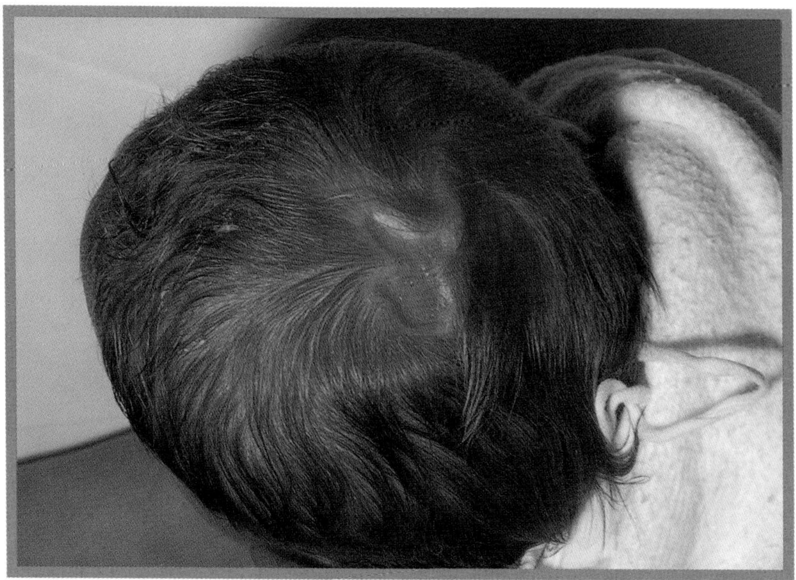

↑1.1

Figures 1.2–1.8 Trisomy 18 (Edwards Syndrome). Figure 1.2 shows typical hands, with overlapping of the second and fifth fingers over the third and fourth fingers. Note the hypoplastic nails.
Figure 1.3 shows a rocker-bottom foot with protruding calcaneum (this also occurs in Patau syndrome).

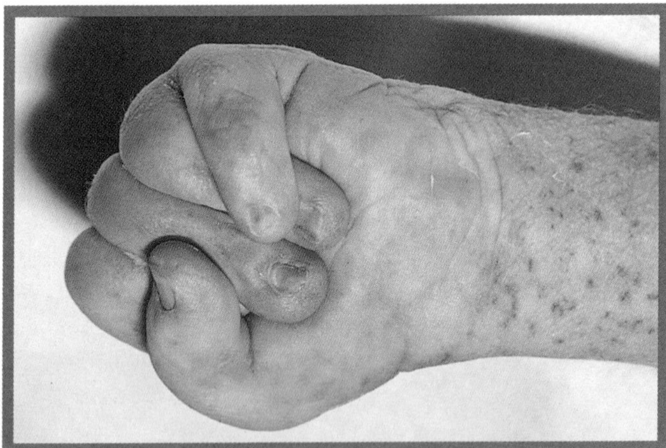

← **1.2**

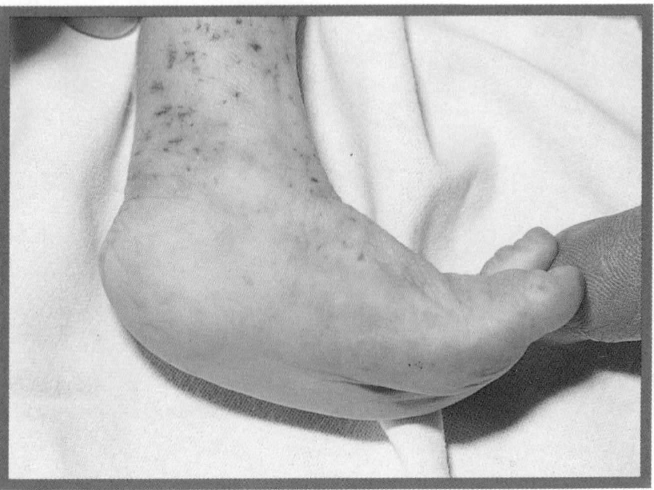

← **1.3**

1003178617

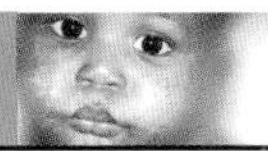

Figure 1.4 shows a cleft palate with an intact lip and alveolus.
Figures 1.5–1.7 show typical facies, with especially prominent forehead and occiput, short and upward-pointing palpebral fissures, micrognathia and low-set ears.

→ 1.4

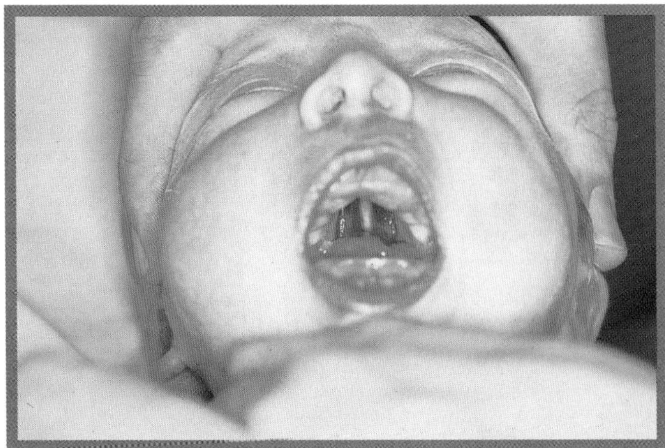

→ 1.5

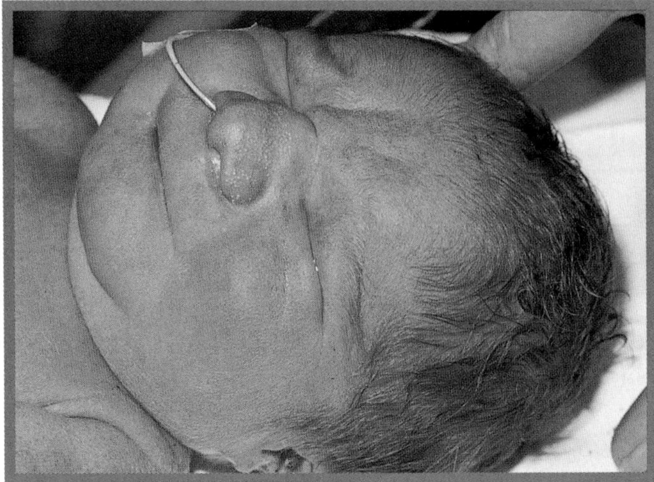

Both infants in figures 1.2 –1.7 had associated severe congenital heart disease. Both died within the first year of life, as is the case for 90% of affected infants. **Figure 1.8 Mosaic Trisomy 18.** Note the low-set dysplastic ears and repaired cleft lip.

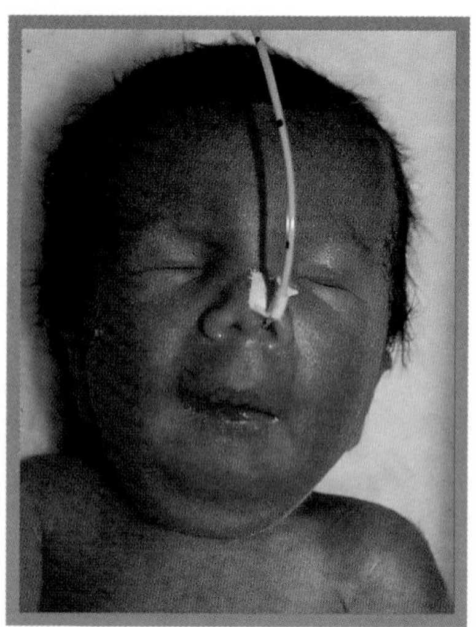

↑1.6

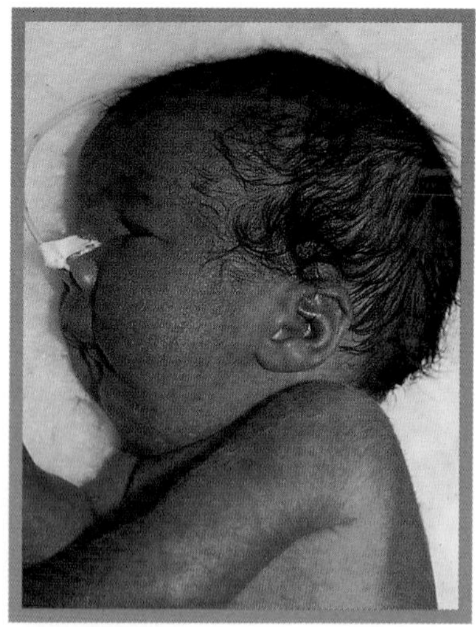

↑1.7

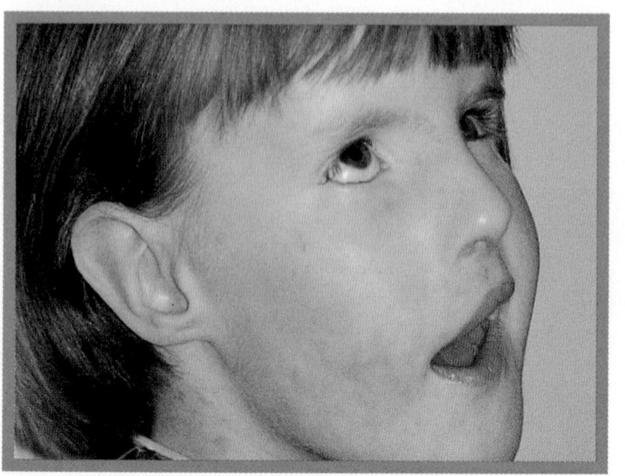

←1.8

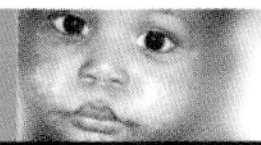

Figures 1.9–1.17 Trisomy 21 (Down Syndrome). This series of pictures shows typical facies in trisomy 21 in a variety of ethnic backgrounds. The main features are a flattened face with a mongoloid slant of the palpebral fissures,

→ **1.9**

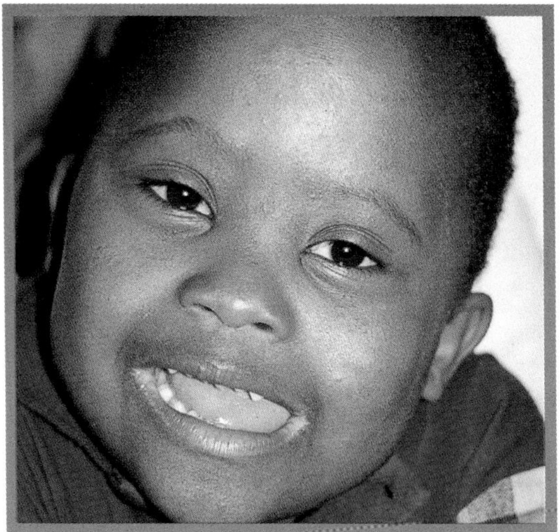

→ **1.10**

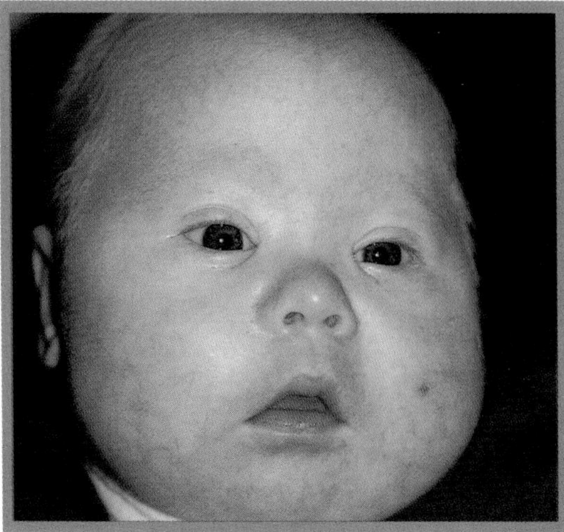

upward-slanting epicanthic folds, a low nasal root and small nose, and low-set and dysplastic ears. There is also brachycephaly with a flat occiput. The mouth is small, and the tongue appears large and is often fissured.

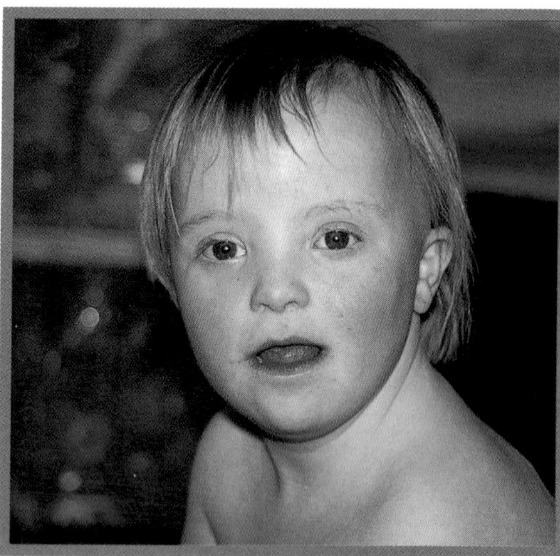

←1.11

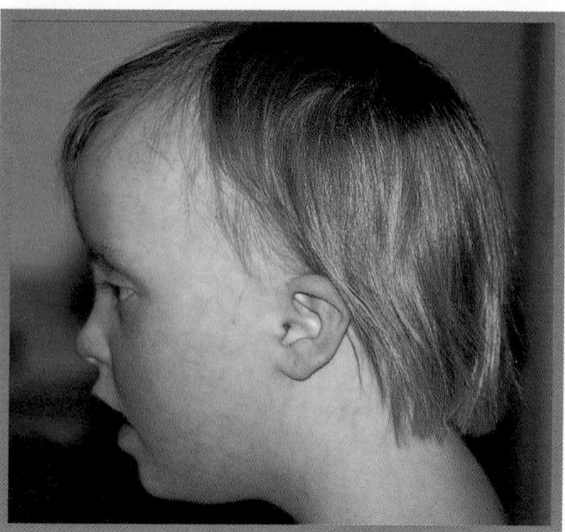

←1.12

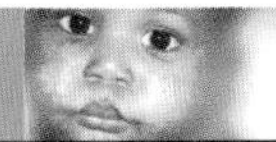

The hands show short, stubby fingers and shortened palms, with radial curvature (clinodactyly) of the fifth finger and a single palmar (simian) crease (**Figures 1.13 and 1.14**).

→1.13

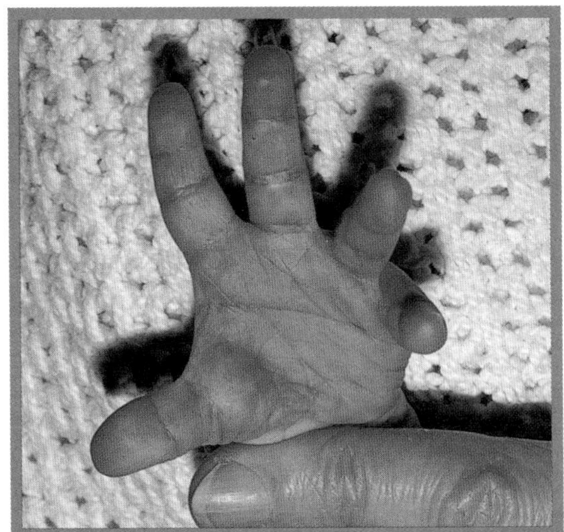

→1.14

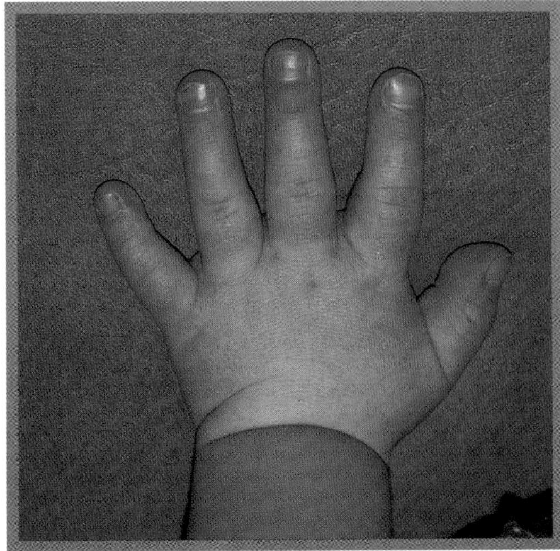

The foot shows widely spaced big and second toes (**Figure 1.15**). Eye signs include Brushfield spots (**Figure 1.16**), a squint and occasionally cataracts and myopia.

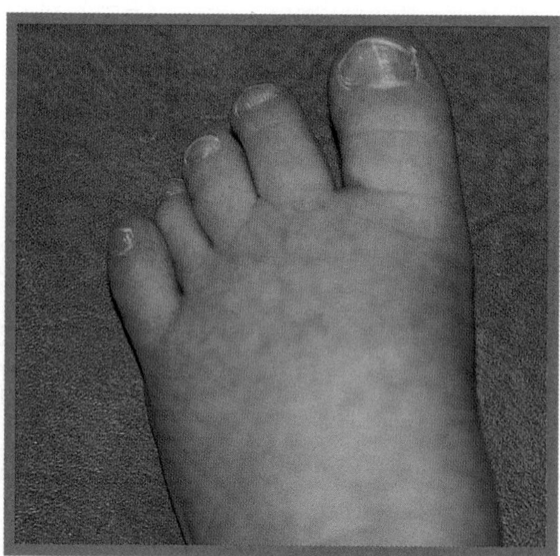

← **1.15**

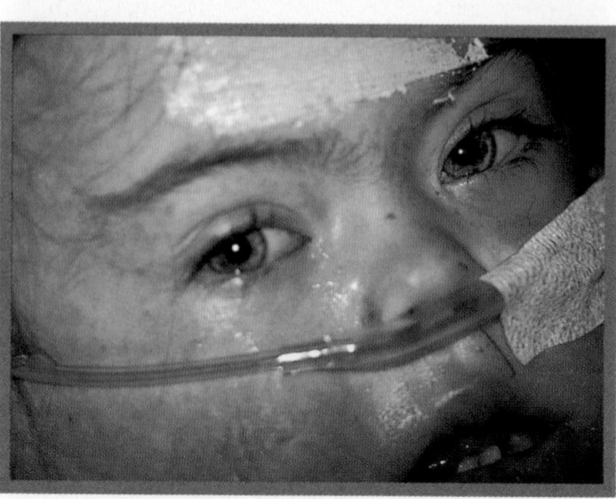

← **1.16**

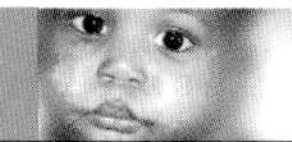

In addition, the children have hypotonia and hypermobility of the joints (**Figure 1.17**). Note the scar from recent cardiac surgery to repair an atrioventricular septal defect.

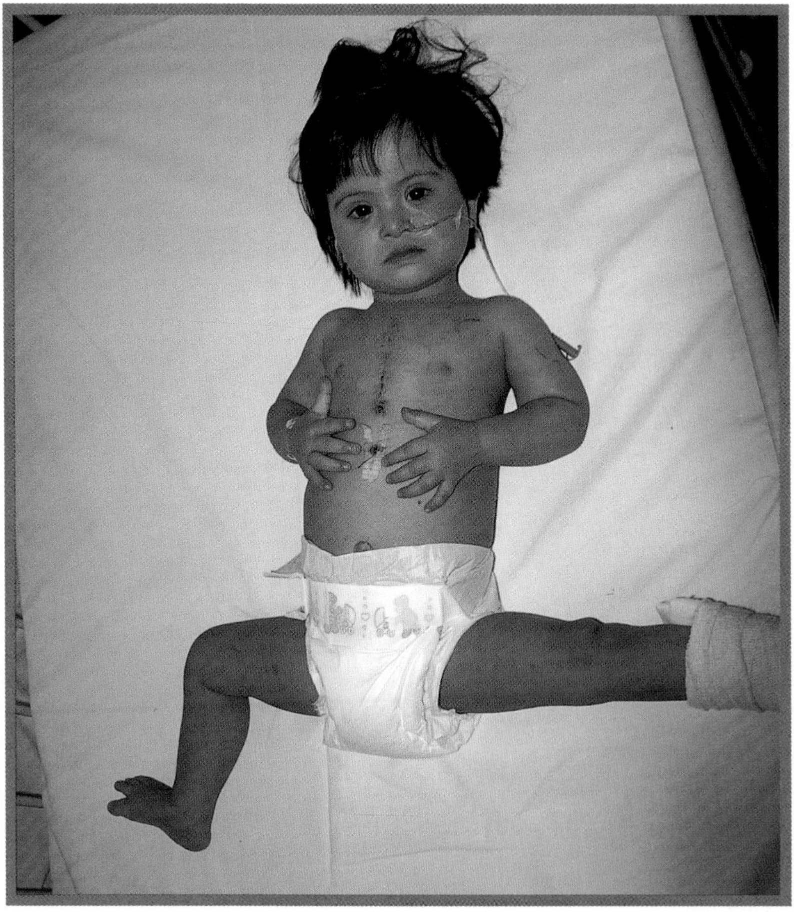

↑1.17

Figure 1.18 Cri du Chat (5p Deletion) Syndrome. This is a syndrome of typical facial features, growth failure, developmental delay, and a cat-like cry in early infancy.

The face tends to be rather round and flat, and there is hypertelorism and epicanthal folds, often with an antimongoloid slant to the palpebral fissures. The cat-like cry is usually heard only in the first few weeks of life.

Figures 1.19 and 1.20 Potter Syndrome. Potter syndrome is caused by

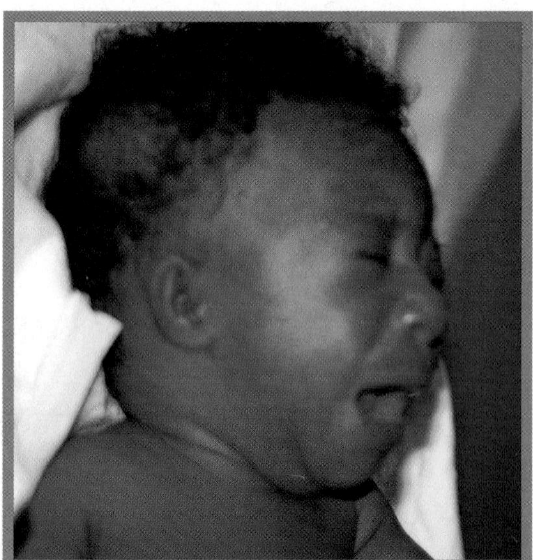

←1.18

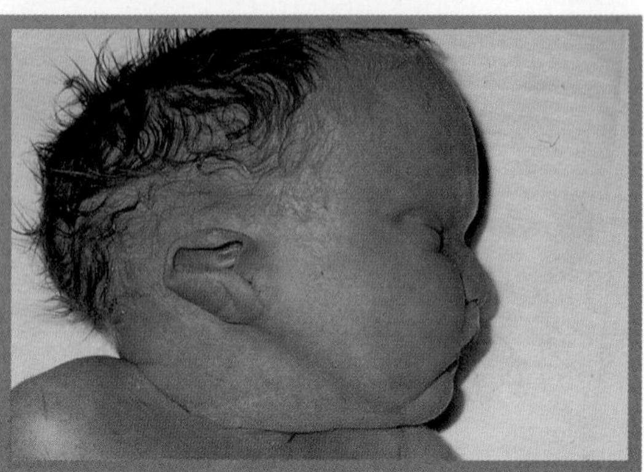

←1.19

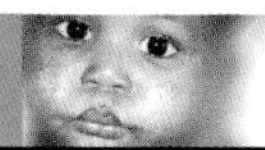

intrauterine compression due to oligohydramnios secondary to renal agenesis or dysplasia. Typical facies show marked micrognathia, dysplastic displaced ears, and compression of the skull vault. This typical infant had pulmonary hypoplasia with respiratory failure. An associated abdominal abnormality is prune belly, due to absent anterior wall musculature. This infant also demonstrates postural deformities of the upper limb, again due to compression.

Figure 1.21 Prune Belly (Eagle–Barrett) Syndrome. This is a rare disorder characterized by various degrees of deficiency of the anterior abdominal muscles, undescended testes, and urinary tract abnormalities. It probably results from urinary tract obstruction in fetal life. Prune belly syndrome is often associated with pulmonary hypoplasia.

Note the hypoplastic scrotum, small chest and laxity of the abdominal muscles in this child. This was a mild case and the child survived, although he has obstructive uropathy.

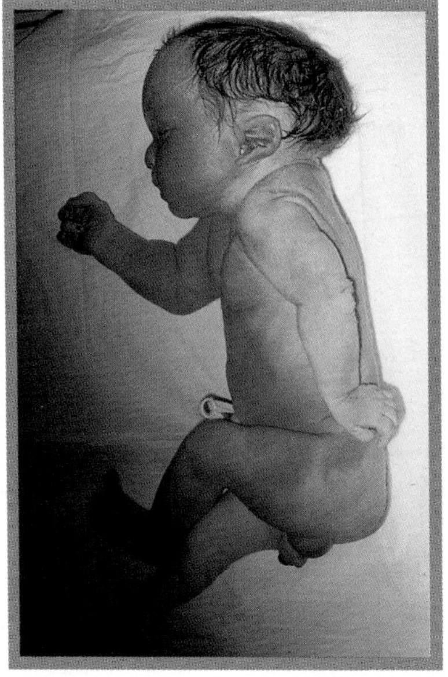

↑ 1.20

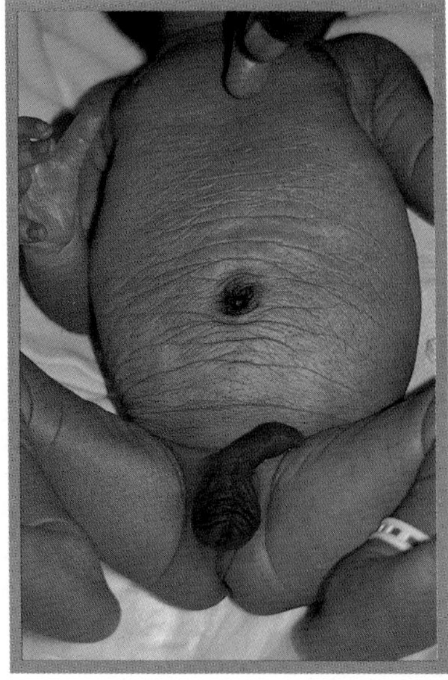

↑ 1.21

Figures 1.22 and 1.23 Turner (Ullrich–Turner) Syndrome. This is a recognized dysmorphism of female infants, and is characterized by small stature, endocrine disturbance, failure of puberty, pterygium colli (neck webbing) and lymphedema of the hands and feet. These are all due to partial or complete monosomy of the X chromosome in phenotypic females.

Puffy feet with dysplastic and hyperconvex nails are shown. Note that puffy feet can occur in normal newborns also, particularly if premature.

Figures 1.24 and 1.25 Beckwith–Wiedemann Syndrome (Exomphalos, Macroglossia, Giantism). This is a relatively frequent and very characteristic macrosomic condition. It is of practical importance because of the associated hypoglycemia and hypocalcemia in the newborn period.

Mild exomphalos is often associated with a small head and protruding occiput. Macroglossia and omphalocoele (note the wound dressing visible on the abdomen of this newborn) are also seen. There is usually also macrosomia (enlargement) of the liver, pancreas, heart and kidneys, leading to metabolic disturbance. Ear abnormalities include a variably developed slit or notch-like indentation on the dorsal edge of the helix (**Figure 1.25**).

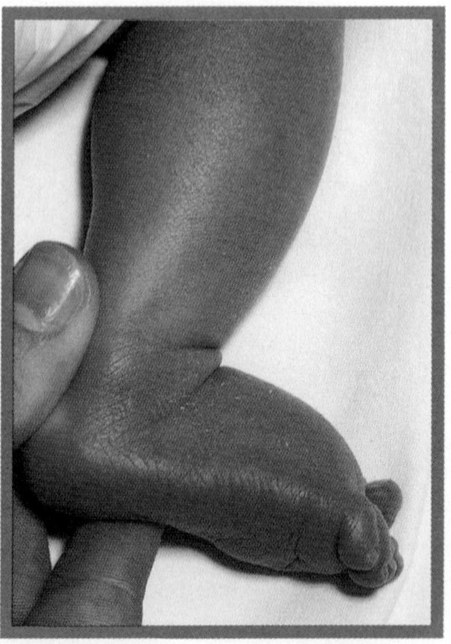

↑ 1.22

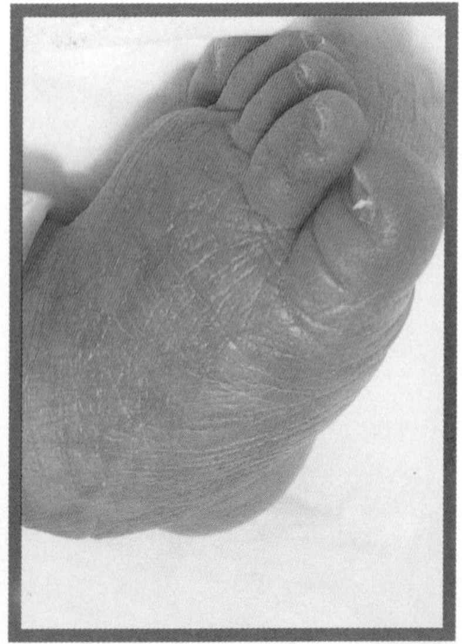

↑ 1.23

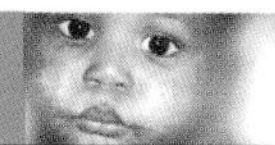

→ 1.24

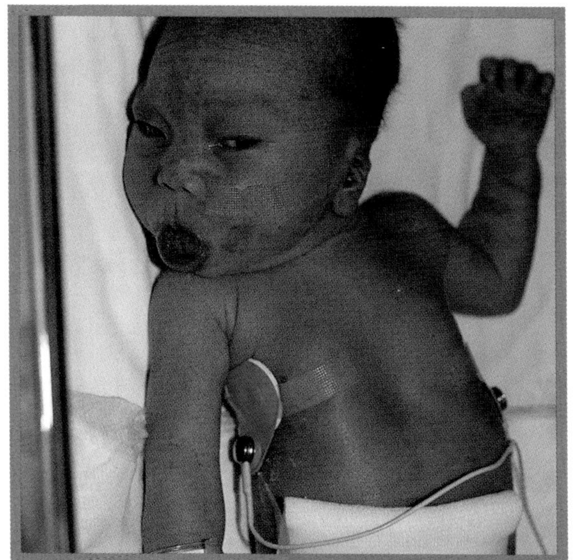

→ 1.25

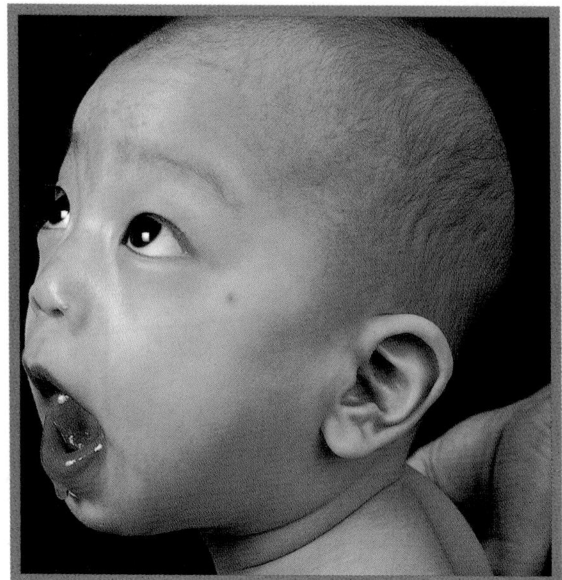

Figure 1.26 Ambiguous Genitalia. The hypoplastic scrotum and micropenis of a newborn infant are shown. This was a case of hypogonadotrophic hypogonadism. On endocrine investigation, this genotypic male was found to have a poor response to gonadotrophin releasing factor. Congenital toxoplasmosis was also found. Ultrasound of the abdomen demonstrated two testes in the inguinal canal.

There was little response to gonadotrophin treatment, but the sex of rearing was male. Investigation of ambiguous genitalia is a medical 'emergency', with the exclusion of salt-losing congenital adrenal hyperplasia being a priority.

Figure 1.27 Osteogenesis Imperfecta Type II. This figure shows a severe form of this disorder. Multiple 'congenital' fractures, limb-length reduction, frontal bossing and an achondroplastic appearance are seen. This infant died in the newborn period due to respiratory failure. Blue sclerae and wormian bones in the skull were present. This is the severe end of a spectrum of disorders.

Figures 1.28 and 1.29 Apert Syndrome (Acrocephalosyndactyly Type I). The child with acrocephalosyndactyly shown here has a short anteroposterior diameter with a high, prominent forehead and a flat occiput. The face is flat,

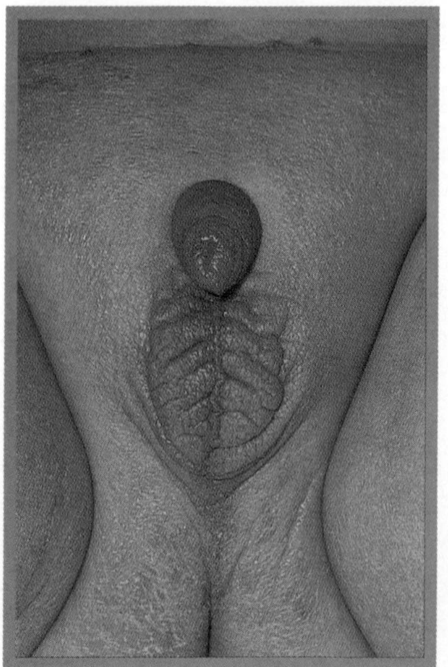

↑ 1.26

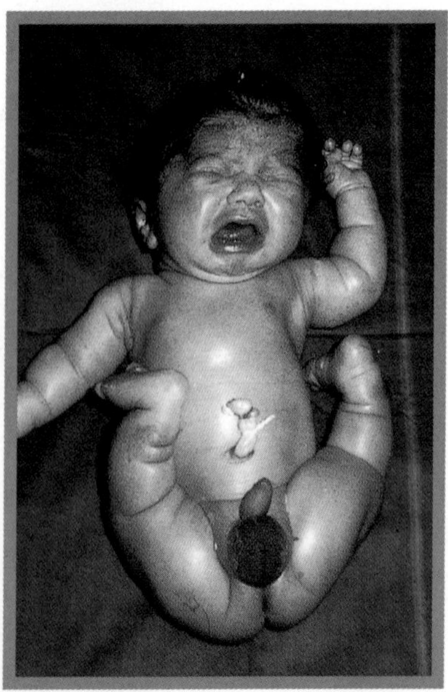

↑ 1.27

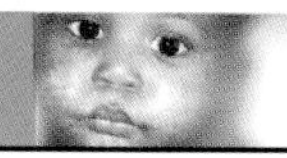

with shallow orbits, hypertelorism, downward-slanting palpebral fissures, a small nose and maxillary hypoplasia. The feet show cutaneous syndactyly and osseous syndactyly of second, third, fourth and fifth digits. The mode of inheritance is autosomal dominant, although the majority of cases spontaneously arise. Treatment of the acrocephaly is frequently required to prevent development of neurological complications.

→ 1.28

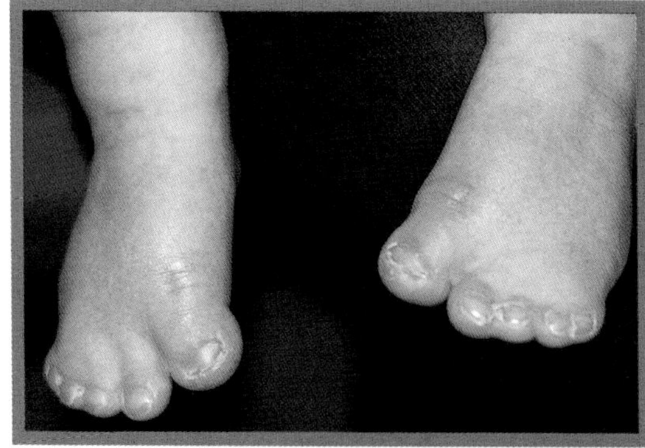

→ 1.29

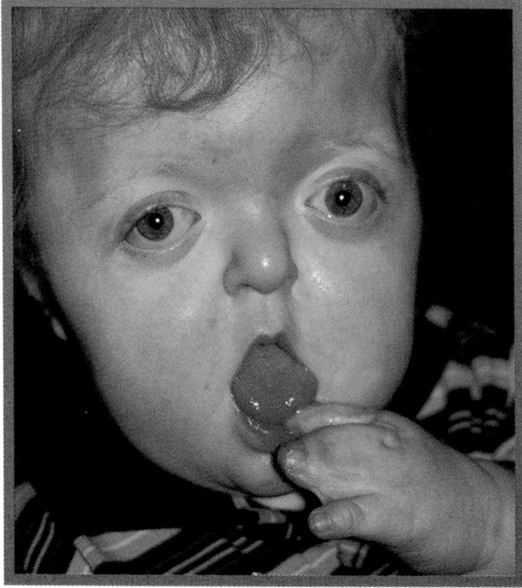

Figures 1.30 and 1.31 Cornelia De Lange Syndrome. The 15-month-old girl shown here has Cornelia de Lange syndrome. Note the short stature, short neck, limited extension of the elbow joints, small hands and feet, flexion deformity of the fingers, generalized hirsutism with synophrys and hairy ears. The nose is anteverted, flared, and there is a long filtrum and a short upper lip. She also had severe learning difficulties and irritability.

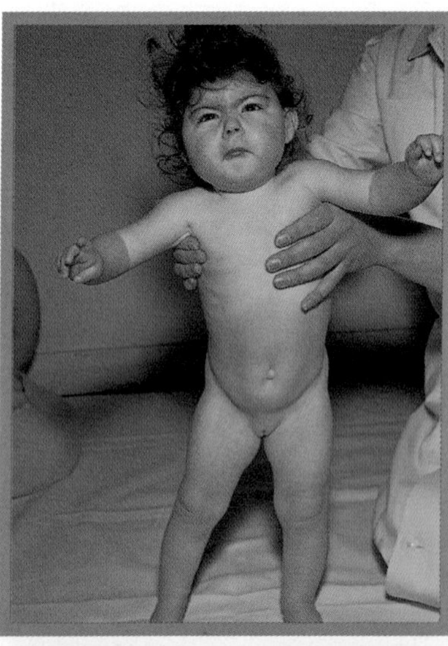

←1.30

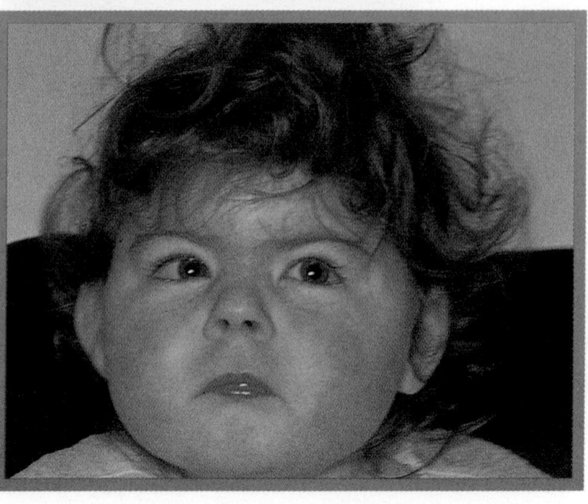

←1.31

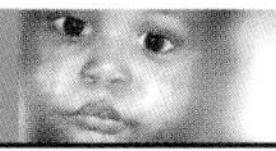

Figure 1.32 Caput Succedaneum. Edema of the scalp over the occipital region is caused by trauma during labor. The swelling crossed the suture line.
Figures 1.33 and 1.34 Parietal Hematoma and Moulding Following Birth. **Figure 1.33** shows a parietal hematoma infected due to unecessary attempts to aspirate. These hematomas can be differentiated from moulding (**Figure 1.34**) by the limitation of the edge of the hematoma to the edges of the

→1.32

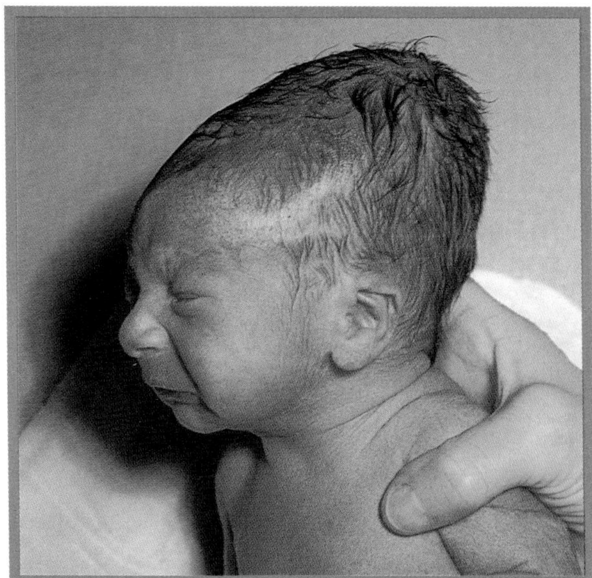

→1.33

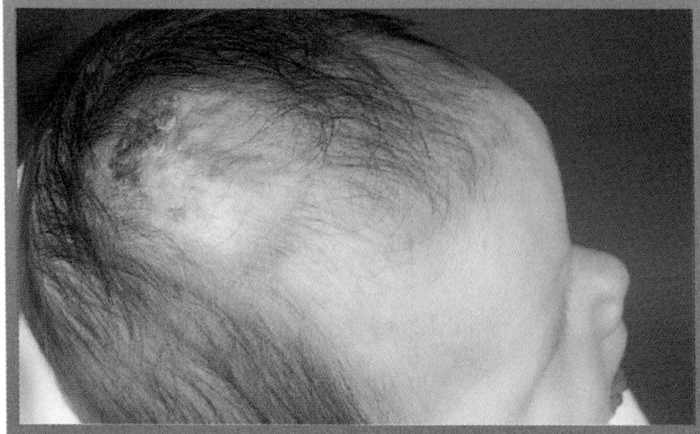

underlying bone. Such hematomas will undergo resorption after a period (up to 8 weeks after birth), and usually leave a calcified rim where the periosteum has been lifted off the underlying bone.

Figure 1.35 Scalp Defect – Ectodermal Dysplasia. Ectodermal dysplasia is relatively unimportant as it will be disguised by hair growth around, but not within, the lesion. It is not to be confused with anhydrotic ectodermal dysplasia, where aplasia of the sweat and sebaceous glands in the skin gives rise to overheating, sparse hair and dental abnormalities.

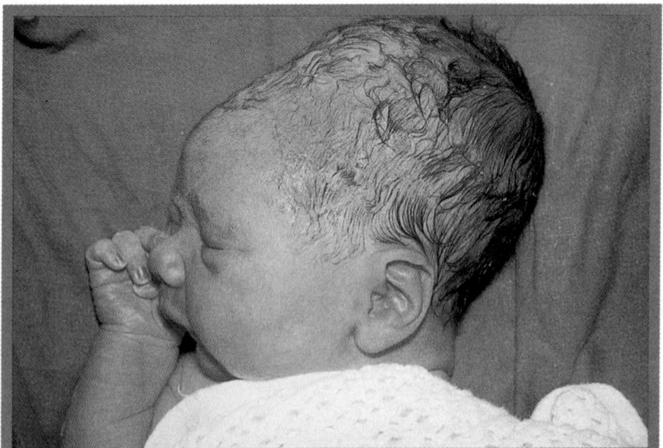

←1.34

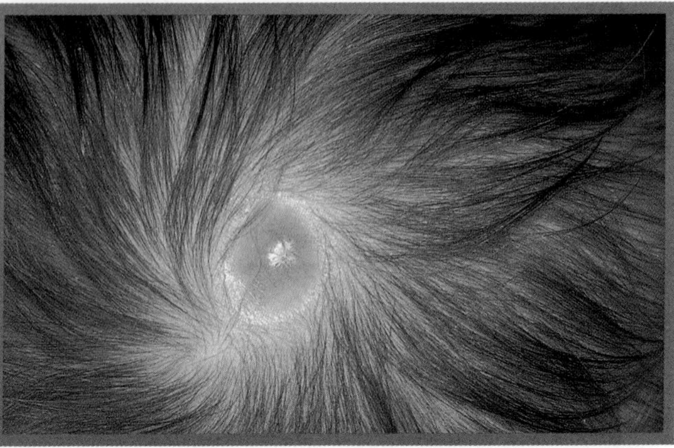

←1.35

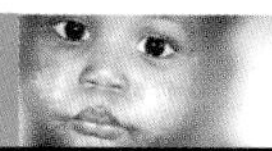

Figures 1.36–1.39 Head Shape Variation. Figures 1.36 and 1.37 show a child with scaphocephaly, which is commonly associated with prematurity due to the effect of gravity on the soft head of a premature baby.

→ 1.36

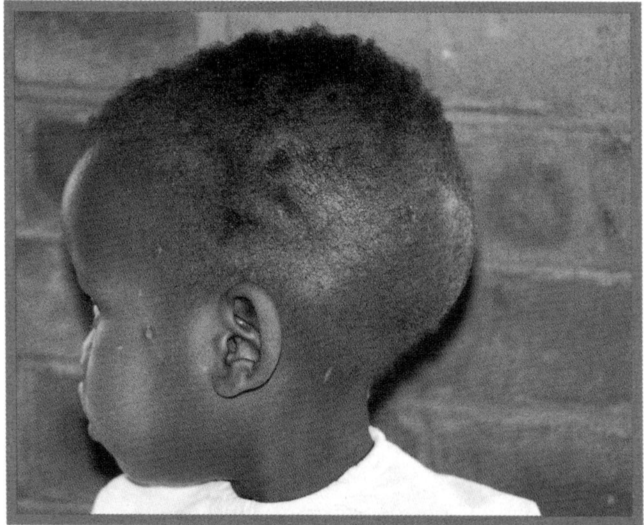

→ 1.37

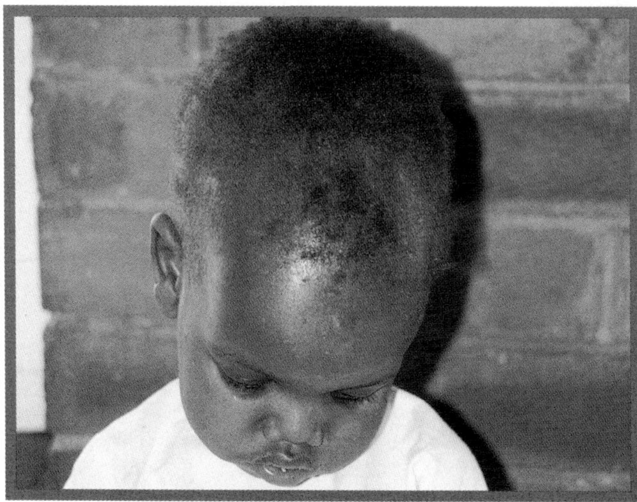

Figure 1.38 demonstrates brachiocephaly in a normal infant. This is associated in some instances with Down syndrome.
Figure 1.39 shows macrocephaly (large head), with OFC > 97th centile at birth. There is no obvious cause. Ultrasound was normal in this case, showing no evidence of enlargement of ventricles (hydrocephalus), and a diagnosis of megalencephaly was therefore made. Other causes of macrocephaly include metabolic disorders, storage disorders, and syndromes associated with macrocephaly, *e.g.*, Soto syndrome. Measurements of parental head size are essential.

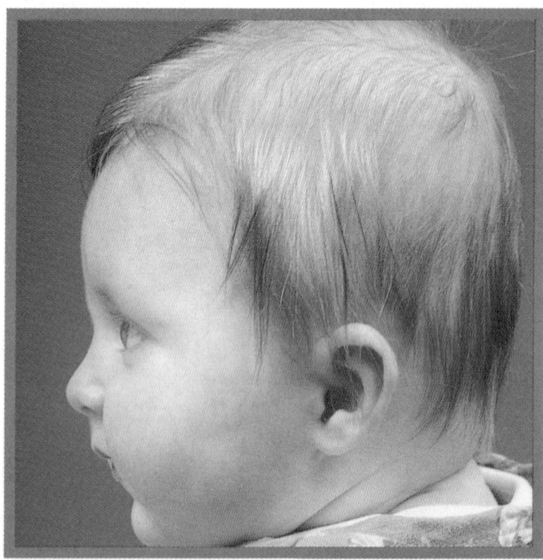

←1.38

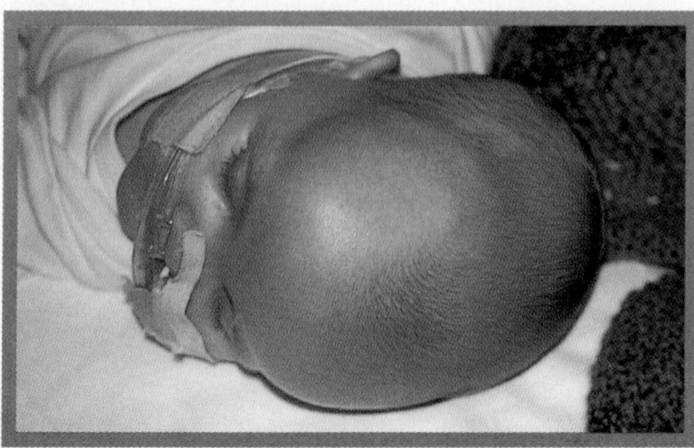

←1.39

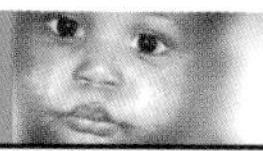

Figure 1.40 Hydranencephaly. This figure shows hydranencephaly on transillumination. The presumed cause is a cerebrovascular accident *in utero* leading to massive infarction of the cerebral hemispheres. Antenatal diagnosis is now possible by ultrasound.

Figure 1.41 Cleft Lip and Palate. This is a relatively common congenital malformation. Antenatal diagnosis is now possible, and this facilitates the provision of counselling for parents. Associated abnormalities should be looked for on delivery. Breastfeeding should be encouraged, although this may be difficult for the child. Early referral to a Cleft Lip and Palate Center is important in order to schedule operations and to involve a team including surgeons, speech therapists, orthodontists and otorhinolaryngologists.

→1.40

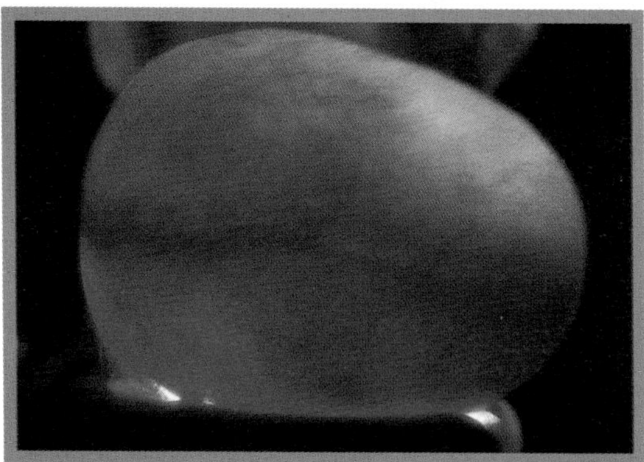

→1.41

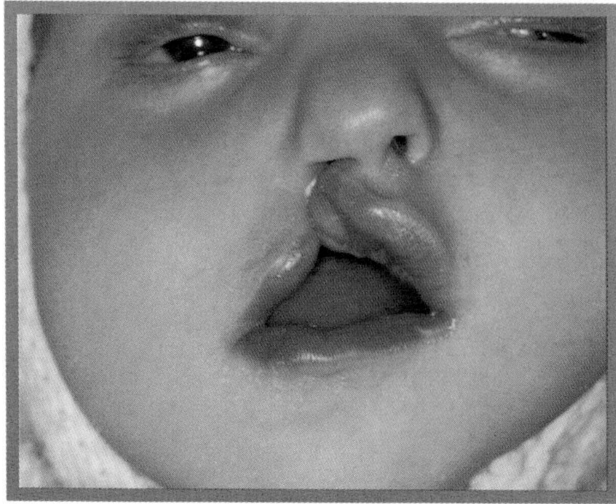

Figure 1.42 Nasal Pits. These pits are sometimes seen in the siblings of children born with a cleft palate. They may represent a very late failure of fusion of the labrum.

Figure 1.43 Milia. These are prominent sebaceous glands that appear as a crop of whiteheads over the face. They are caused by increased sebum secretion, presumably in response to either hormonal influences or trauma to the skin. No treatment is indicated.

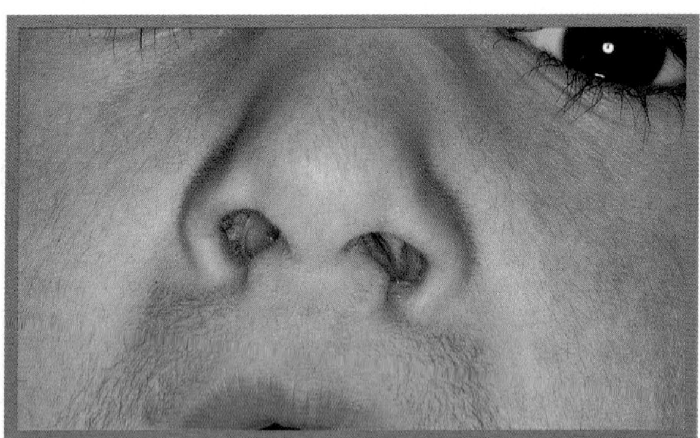

← 1.42

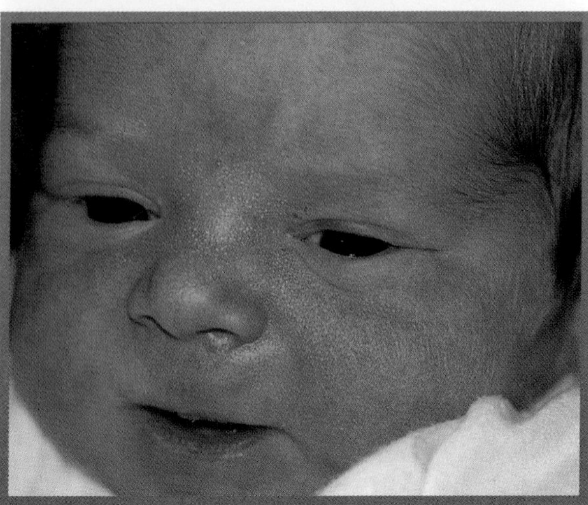

← 1.43

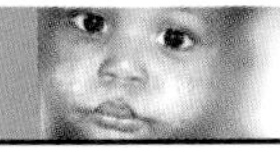

Figure 1.44–1.45 Erythema Toxicum Neonatorum. This is a very common skin condition. It is a benign, self-limiting disorder and occurs in up to 50% of term infants. The eruptions are papular, with a yellow/white center. They reach maximum intensity at about 36 hours of age, and then fade. Reassurance only is required.

Differential diagnosis includes staphylococcal pustules. Staphylococcus pustules are larger than those of erythema toxicum neonatorum and are creamier in color and occur in skin creases – particularly in the axillae, neck and groin.

→ **1.44**

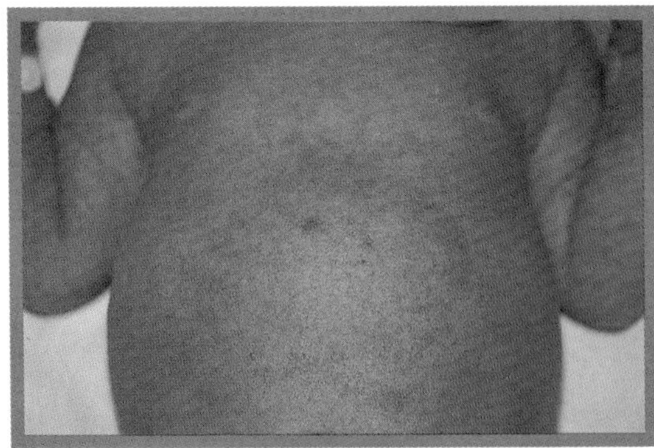

→ **1.45**

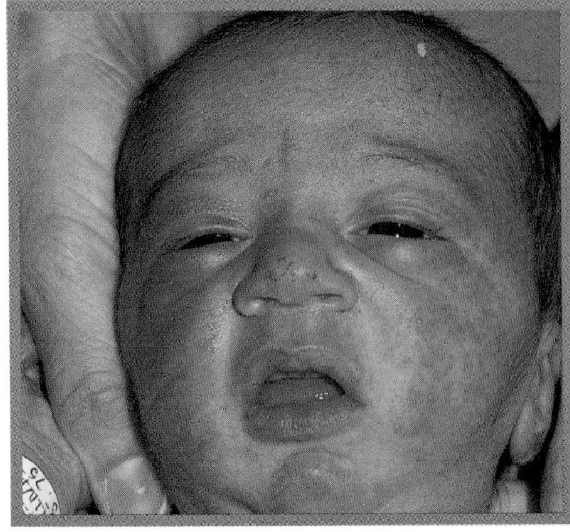

Figure 1.46 Purpura is shown here affecting the periorbital region. It is usually secondary to minor birth trauma and of little significance. However, in thrombocytopenia, purpura may be significant, and may require treatment with immunoglobulin infusion in cases of allo-immune thrombocytopenic purpura.
Figure 1.47 Accessory Nipples. These are relatively common and are often initially thought to be a pigmented nevus or hemangioma; on close inspection there is an areola and nipple present. They lie in the milk ridge and are usually insignificant.

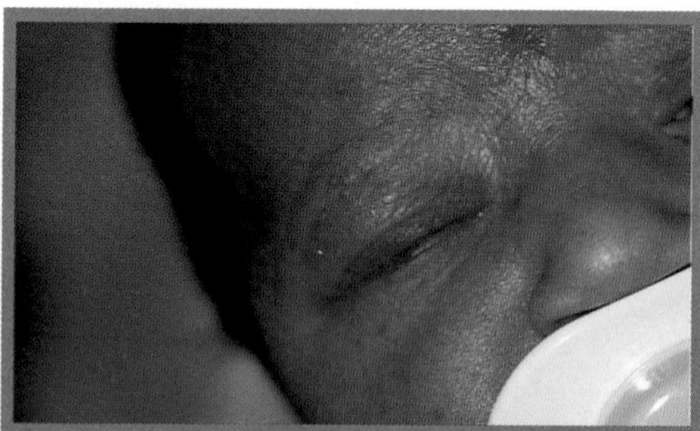

← 1.46

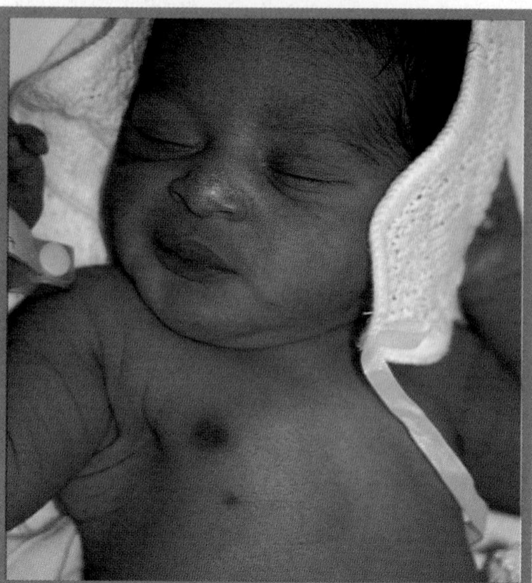

← 1.47

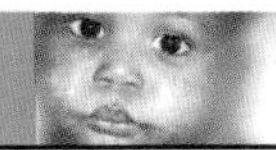

Figure 1.48 Galactorrhea. Galactorrhea, so-called witch's milk in a newborn, is usually transient and reflects maternal hormone influence on the infant's breast tissue. It is occasionally complicated by infection, leading to neonatal mastitis. It is rarely caused by an endocrinopathy, and usually resolves spontaneously.

Figures 1.49–1.51 Pneumothorax and Pneumomediastinum. Figures 1.49 and 1.50 demonstrate transillumination in a neonate with massive air leaks. Figure 1.49 shows tranillumination of a pneumothorax.

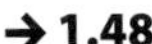

→1.48

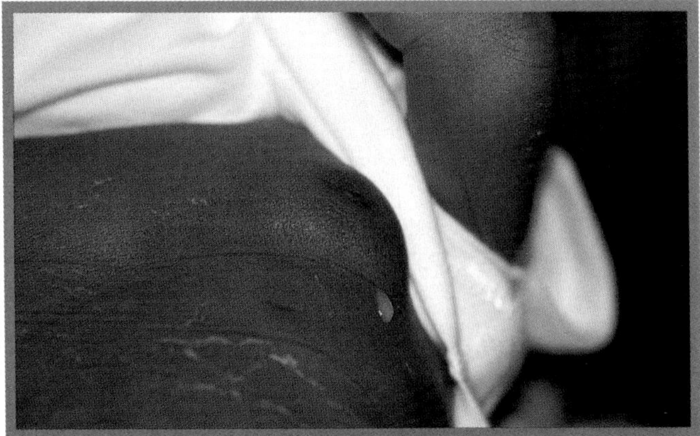

→1.49

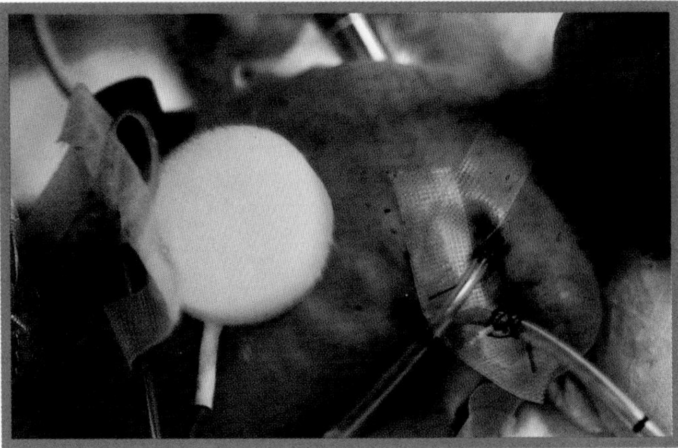

Figure 1.50 shows transillumination of pneumoperitoneum. The accompanying X-ray (**Figure 1.51**) demonstrates free air not only in the chest and abdomen, but also in the great vessels and heart causing catastrophic loss of cardiac output.

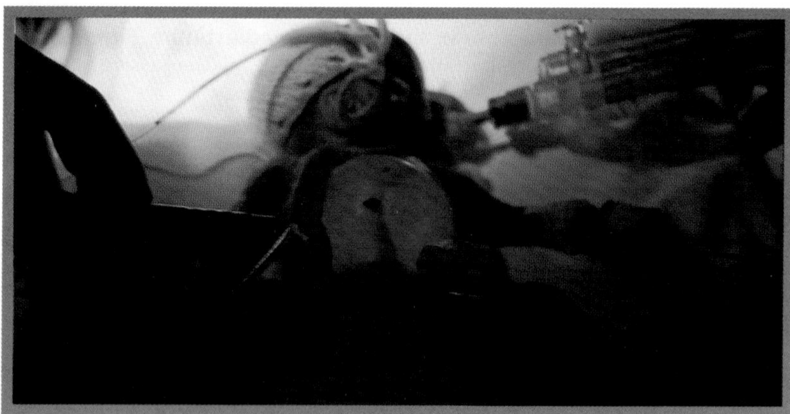

↑ **1.50**

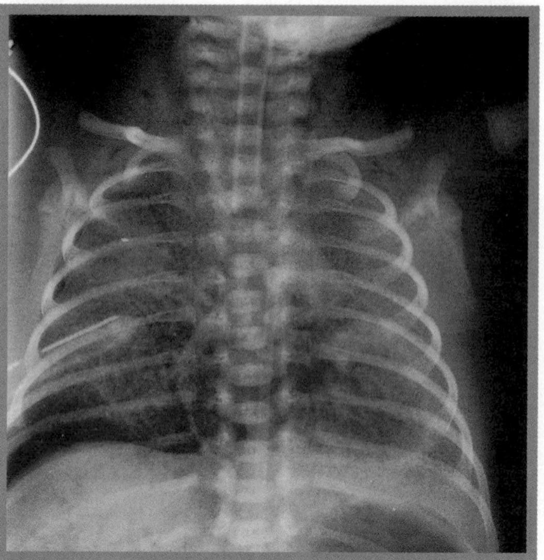

← **1.51**

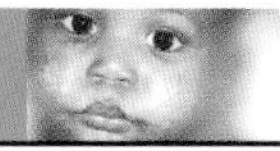

Figure 1.52 Collapse of the Left Lung and Right Upper Lobe. This chest X-ray shows an endotracheal tube in the right mainstem bronchus with associated collapse of the left lung and right upper lobe. Also shown is an umbilical arterial oximeter *in situ* in the descending aorta.

Figure 1.53 Bilateral Consolidation with Partial Collapse Secondary to Streptococcal Infection. This figure shows pneumonia in a neonate. The differential diagnosis is hyaline membrane disease.

→ 1.52

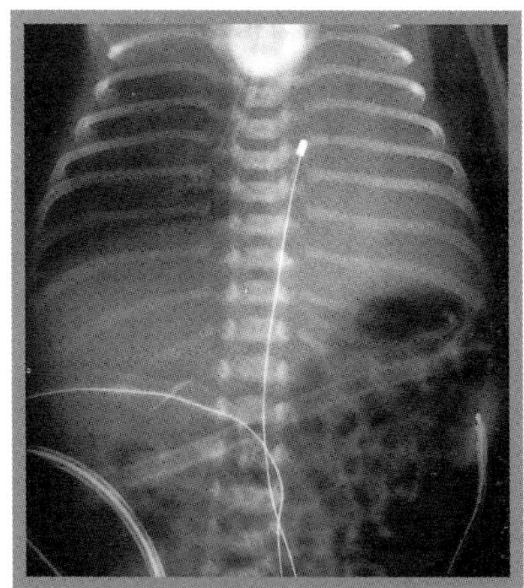

→ 1.53

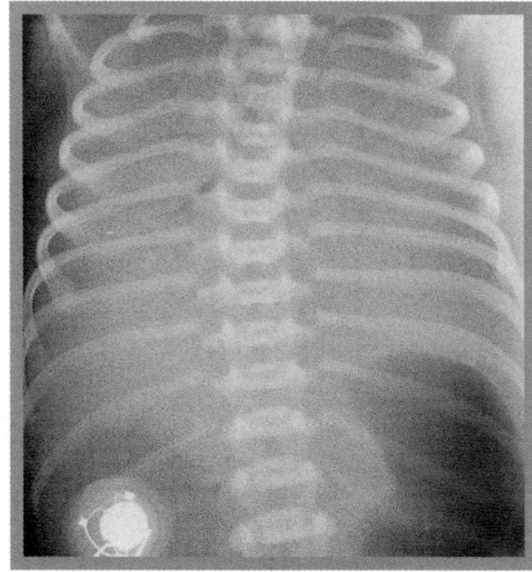

Figure 1.54 Bilateral Ground-Glass Appearance. This bilateral ground-glass appearance is seen in an infant with surfactant-deficient respiratory distress. The figure shows air bronchograms bilaterally.

Figure 1.55 Pulmonary Interstitial Emphysema in a Ventilated Infant. Coarse, granular, bilateral shadowing is seen with a low diaphragm and narrowing of the mediastinum. Note the chest drain in the right chest. High-pressure ventilation associated with infection may predispose to this condition. Treatment consists of the judicious use of ventilation and chest-tube drainage. Modern techniques of ventilation, *e.g.*, high-frequency oscillation and surfactant use, have helped make this condition less common and have facilitated treatment.

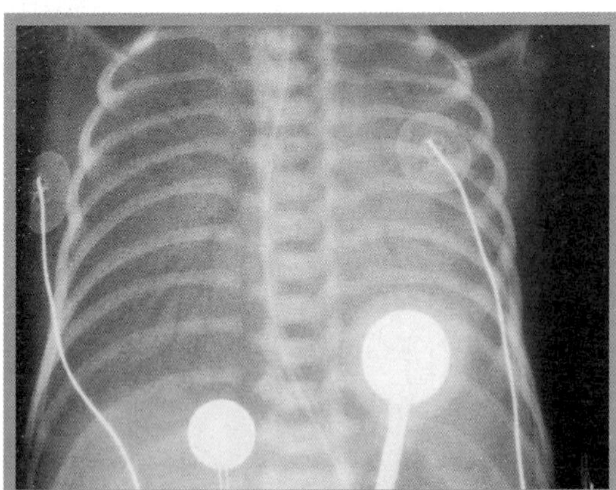

←1.54

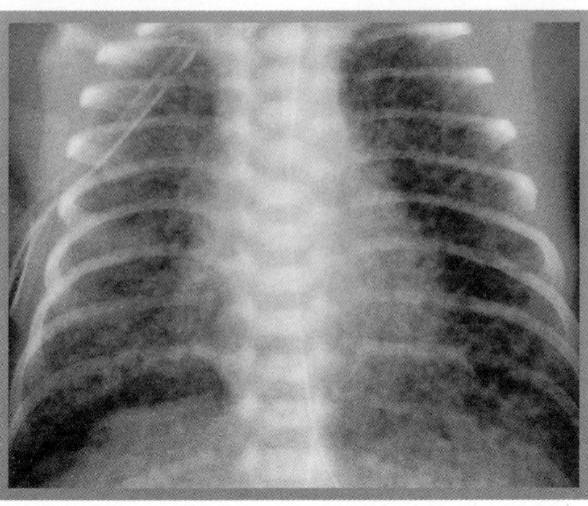

←1.55

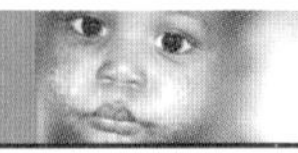

Figure 1.56 Changes of Chronic Lung Disease. There is patchy collapse and consolidation with areas of hyperlucency.

Figure 1.57 Chronic Lung Disease with Prolonged Ventilation. Note the areas of collapse and consolidation as well as the areas of hyperlucency in this figure. A mismatch of ventilation and perfusion contribute to the intrapulmonary shunting and the persisting oxygen requirement.

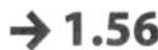
→1.56

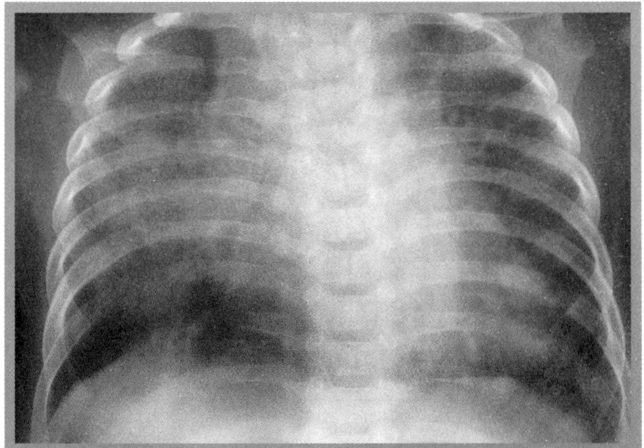

→1.57

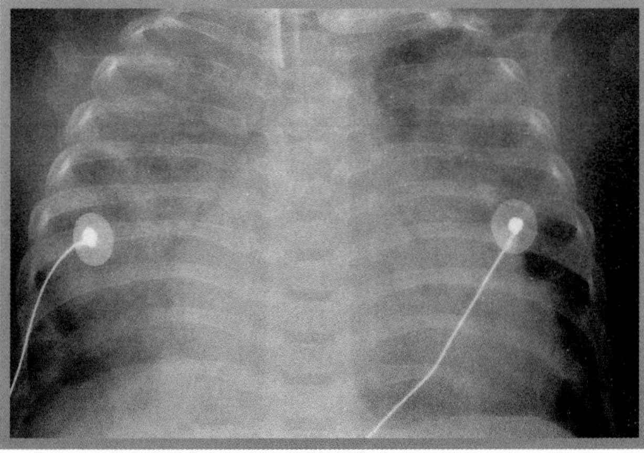

Figure 1.58 Ex-premature Baby in Low-Flow Oxygen through Nasal Cannulae with Marked Changes of Chronic Lung Disease. Note the Harrison sulcus, intercostal recession and scaphocephaly in this figure. These infants are susceptible to infection, and reventilation is often required. The 9-month-old infant with chronic lung disease shown here developed RSV-positive bronchiolitis.

Figure 1.59 Neonatal Intensive Care. A ventilated, preterm (24 weeks'gestation) infant is shown. Note the frog-like posture, endotracheal tube *in situ*, umbilical arterial catheter, and ECG leads obscuring much of the chest.

Figure 1.60 Continuous Positive Airway Pressure (CPAP) Driver. The development of these devices allows some infants with respiratory distress to avoid intubation.

Figure 1.61 Continuous Pressure and Oxygen Delivery via Specialized Nasal Prongs.

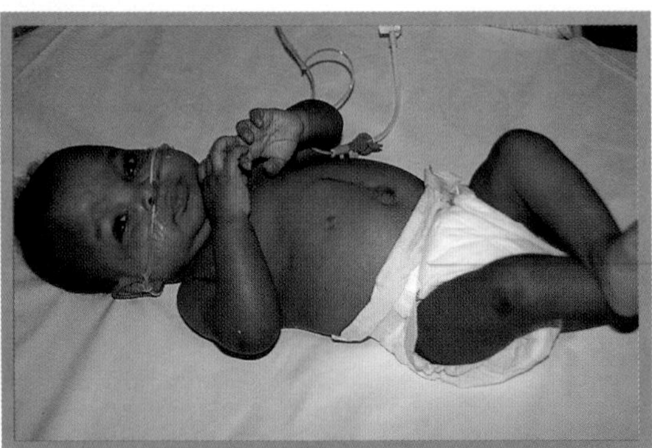

← 1.58

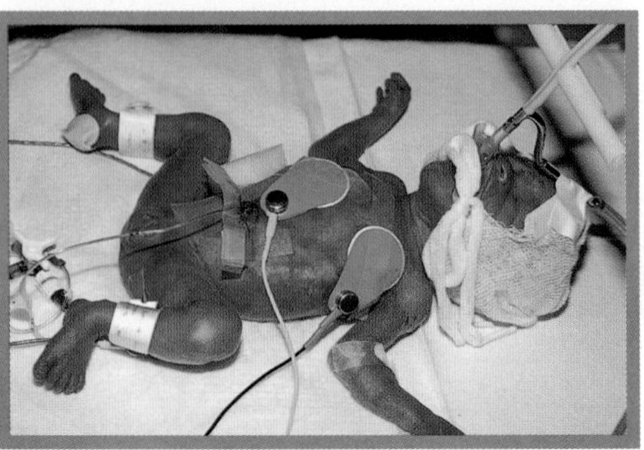

← 1.59

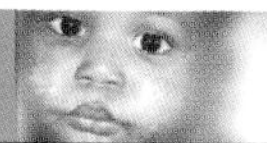

→1.60

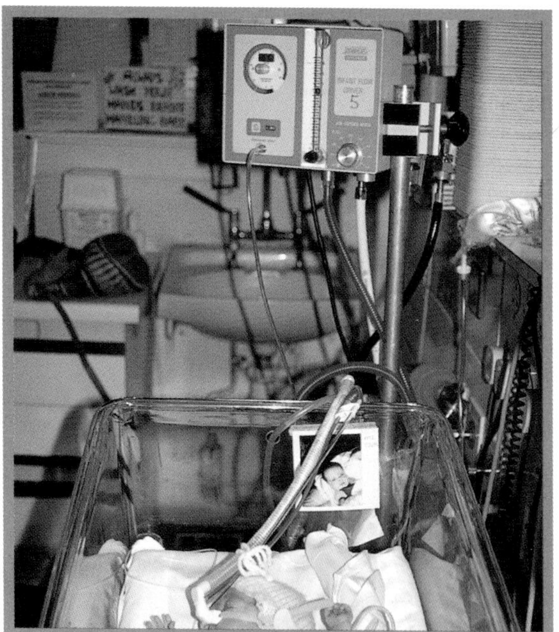

→1.61

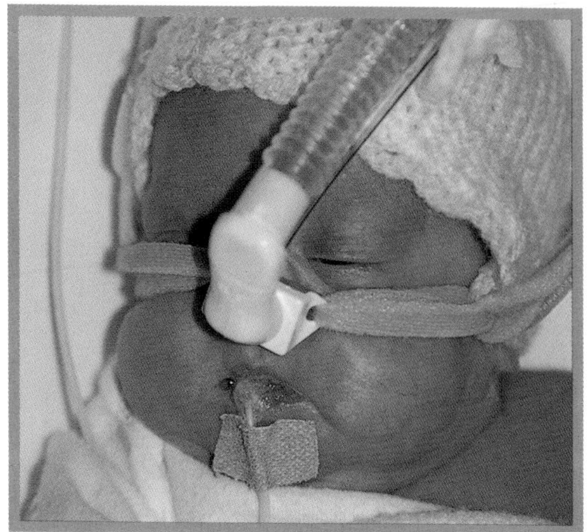

Figures 1.62 and 1.63 Phototherapy Systems for High Bilirubin Levels. Bilirubin in the skin absorbs light energy in the blue part of the spectrum (not the ultraviolet part), converting toxic, insoluble unconjugated bilirubin into a soluble, unconjugated photoisomer. This is excreted in the bile and, to a lesser extent, in the urine. A conventional overhead light source is shown turned off (**Figure 1.62**) and in use (**Figure 1.63**). The infant's eyes need to be protected, and in this case an orange-colored headbox is being used. An alternative method of protection is the use of eye patches, which can, however, slip and traumatize the cornea.

Figure 1.64 A Bilirubin Blanket in use. Light of the correct wavelength is delivered to the infant via a fiber-optic blanket. This allows the infant to remain dressed, and the blanket can even be used at home. The blanket is shown illuminated, and is used by placing the blanket adjacent to the infant's skin, under the clothes.

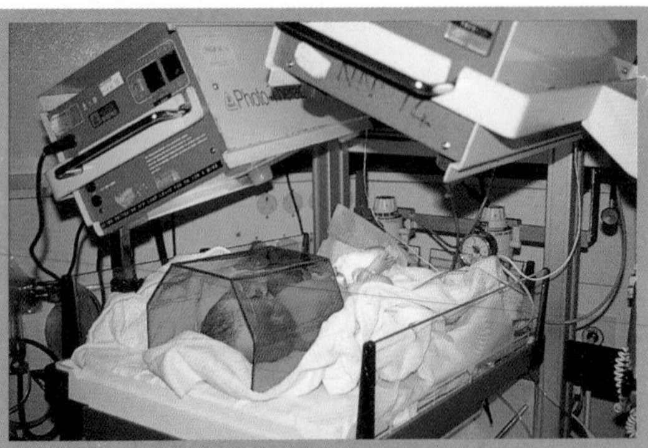

← 1.62

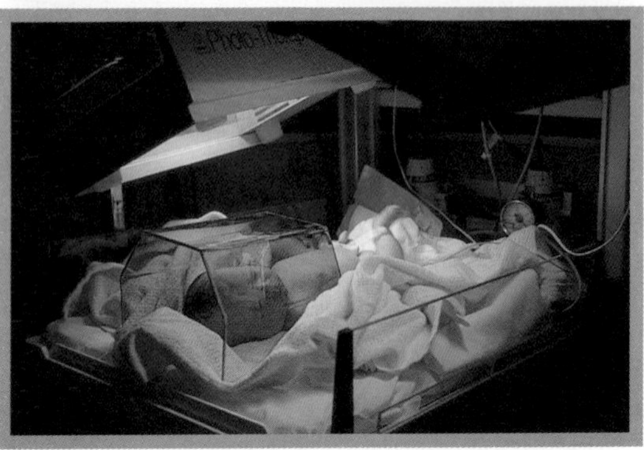

← 1.63

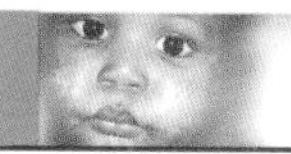

Figure 1.65 Jaundiced Term Infant. The infant shown here had an unconjugated hyperbilirubinemia that failed to respond to phototherapy. Thyroid function tests showed a very high thyroid stimulating hormone level and a low thyroxine level. The jaundice responded well to thyroid replacement treatment.

→1.64

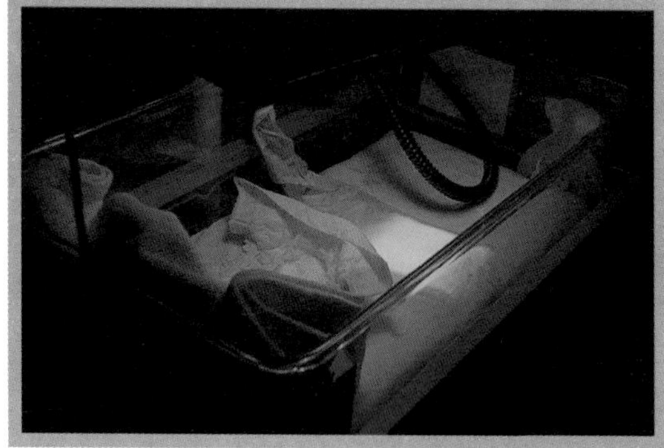

→1.65

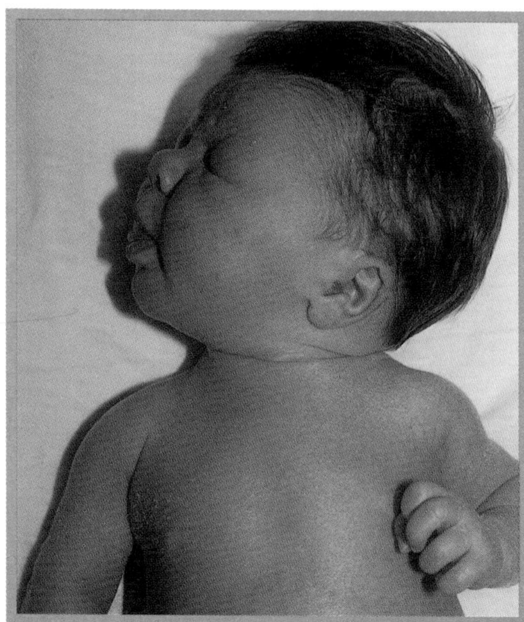

GROWTH RETARDATION

Figure 1.66 Growth Retardation in Term Twins. The smaller of these twins had marked growth retardation and suffered from profound hypoglycemia and poor temperature control. The other twin was well. There was also a twin-to-twin transfusion.

Figures 1.67–1.70 These figures show the effects of growth retardation at advancing levels of maturity. **Figures 1.67 and 1.68** demonstrate growth retardation occuring relatively early in pregnancy. Note the relatively large head suggestive of brain sparing. **Figure 1.69** show a term infant with moderate growth retardation. Note the peeling skin of the extremities, the alert facies and the loss of subcutaneous fat causing laxity in the skin of the upper thighs.

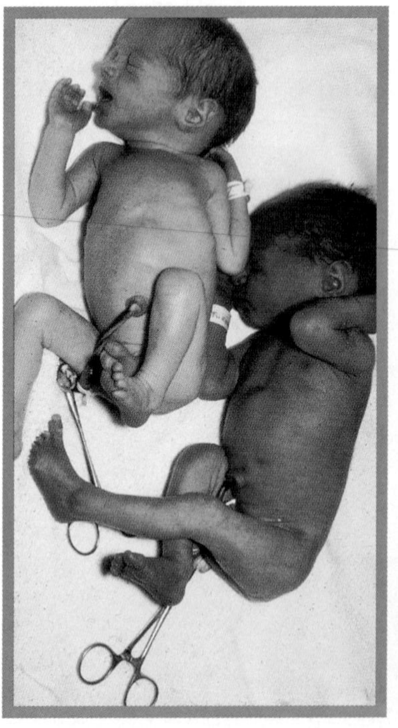

↑ 1.66

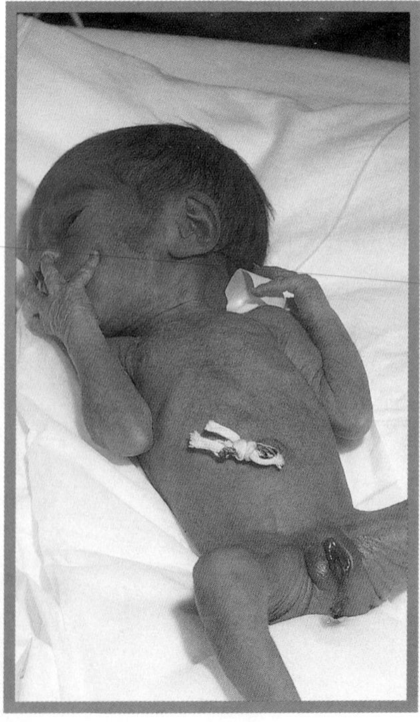

↑ 1.67

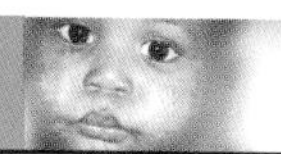

→ 1.68

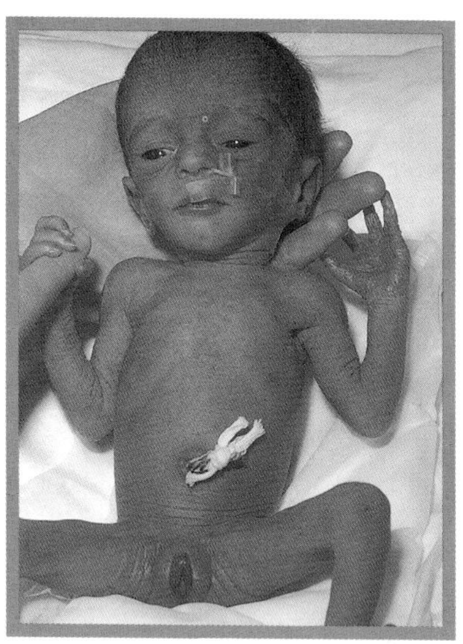

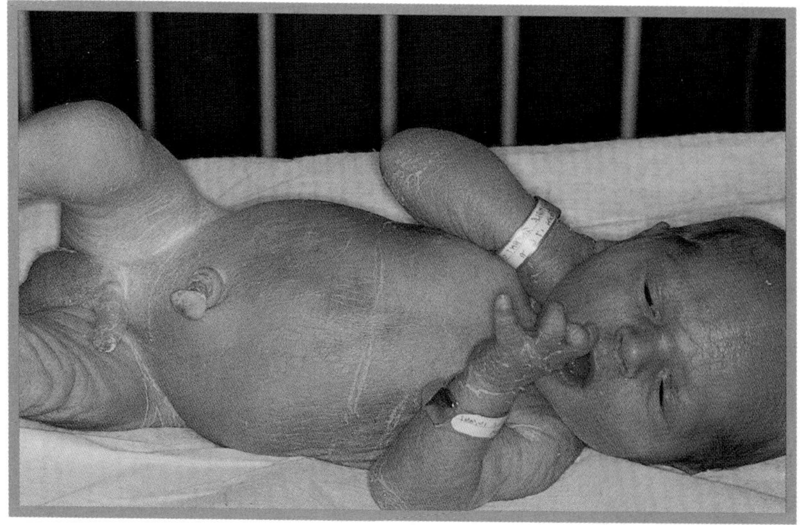

↑ 1.69

Figure 1.70 shows an infant born at 43 weeks' gestation (post mature). Note the peeling dry skin, wasted buttocks, and reduced subcutaneous tissue. There may also be meconium staining of skin, cord and nails.

Figure 1.71 Infant of an Insulin-Dependent Diabetic. This figure shows the excess adipose tissue laid down as a result of hyperglycemia in pregnancy. Typical 'cherubic facies' are seen. Maternal hyperglycemia results in prenatal hyperinsulinemia, which may result in hypoglycemia after birth. Other metabolic consequences include a high incidence of intrauterine death from 36 weeks onwards.

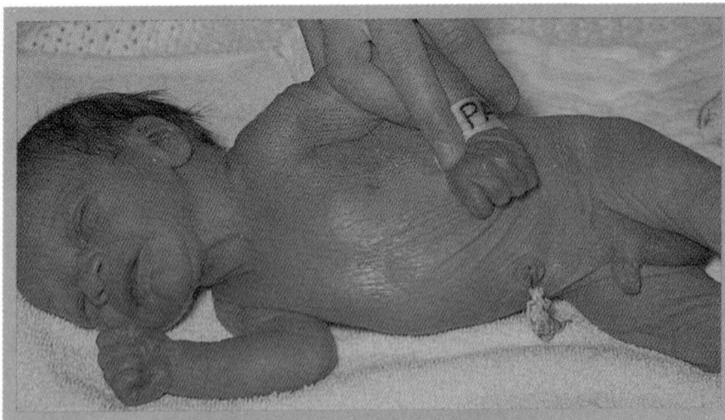

←1.70

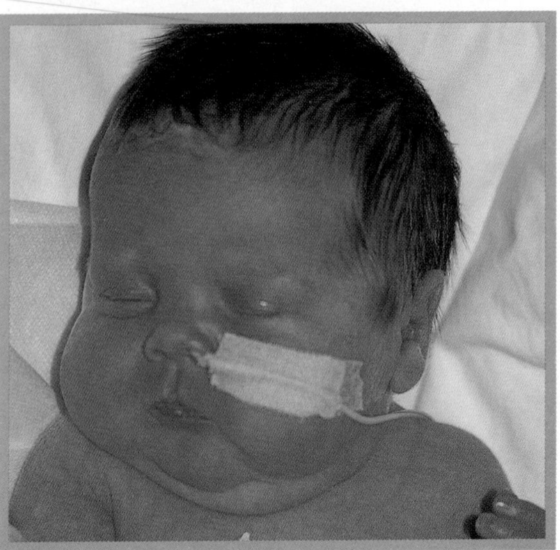

←1.71

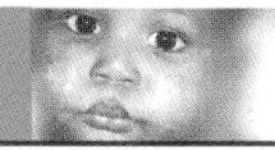

Figure 1.72 Floppy Infant. This is the typical posture of a floppy newborn when held in ventral suspension. The significance of the floppiness depends upon the length of the gestation (preterm infants are usually floppy), generalized effects of sepsis, and neurological illness.

Figures 1.73 and 1.74 Brachial Plexus Injury. These figures show the effect of brachial root injury. Note that the injury is on the right in **Figure 1.73** and on the left in **Figure 1.74**. Such injury may occur in macrosomic infants or if lateral traction is applied to the head and neck during a difficult delivery. A breech delivery with arms extended or shoulder dystocia may be associated causally in many cases.

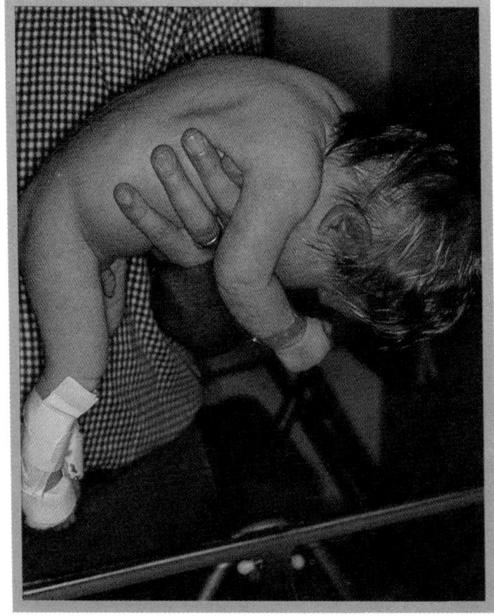

↑ 1.72

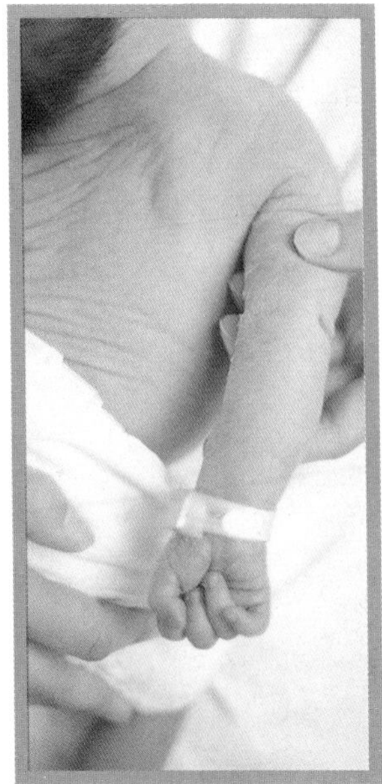

↑ 1.73

Erb (Erb–Duchenne) palsy is also illustrated. This palsy involves the higher roots (the fifth and sixth cervical nerves). The infant has lost the ability to abduct at the shoulder, to rotate externally and to supinate at the elbow. Power in the forearm and hand are maintained and the presence of normal palmar grasp is a favorable prognostic sign.

Klumpke paralysis is much less common. This is a lesion of the lowermost roots and may involve the sympathetic chain if nerves of the first thoracic root are involved. The signs of this disorder are a weak or paralysed hand, ipsilateral ptosis and myosis (Horner syndrome).

Figure 1.75 Talipes Equinovarus (Club Foot) in a Newborn. Talipes is one of the most commonly observed congenital postural abnormalities. It is usually not associated with any other significant abnormality. The outlook is excellent in the majority of cases. Most cases result from intrauterine moulding, but other causes should be considered. Neuromuscular diseases may predispose to talipes and in these cases treatment of the underlying disease must be the priority.

Treatment consists of manipulation and strapping. Occasionally, surgery is an option if more conservative methods have not worked.

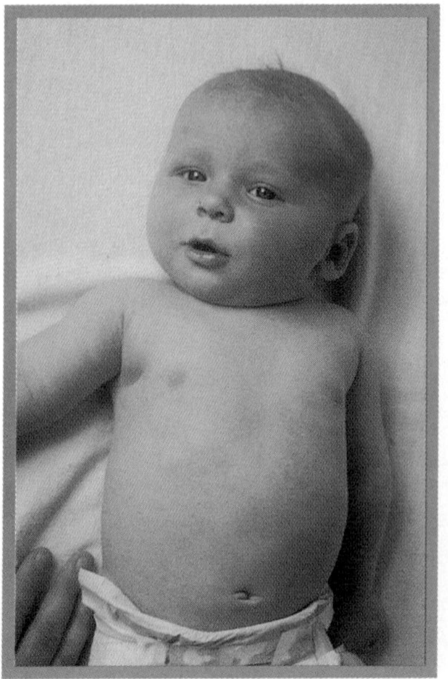

↑ 1.74

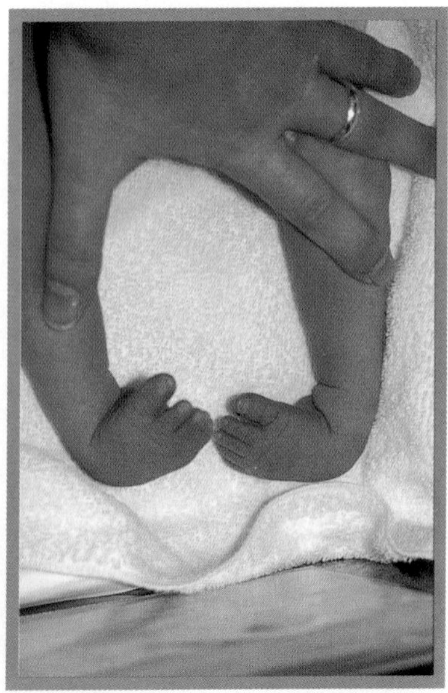

↑ 1.75

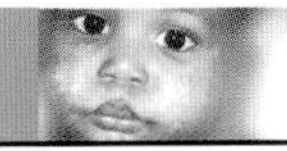

Figure 1.76 Accessory Digits. Accessory digits are commonly found, and are most common in black infants. They may be familial. They are usually isolated occurrences, but may occur as a result of a syndrome. The usual treatment consists in surgical excision, especially in female infants. Tying of the pedicle may be effective, but can give poor cosmetic results.

Figures 1.77 and 1.78 Abnormalities of the Digits in a Newborn Infant. Disruption of the digits as shown usually occurs when there is destruction of a previously normally formed part. If an amniotic band is involved, the digits may become entangled and tearing or amputation may occur. Infarction due to vascular accident will lead to resorption and necrosis of the affected part. Teratogens , of which the best known is thalidomide, can cause a wide range of abnormalities and sequences of abnormalities. Genetic factors play a limited role in this type of disruption of development.

→ 1.76

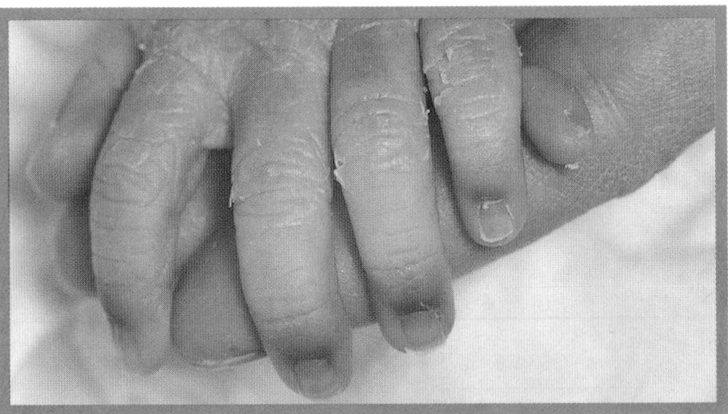

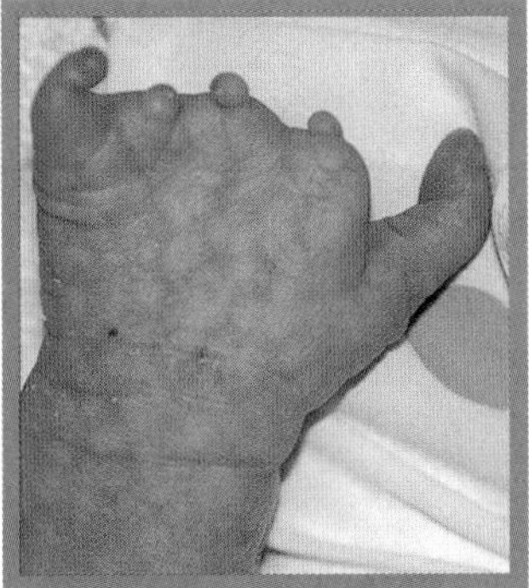

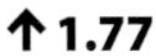

↑ 1.77

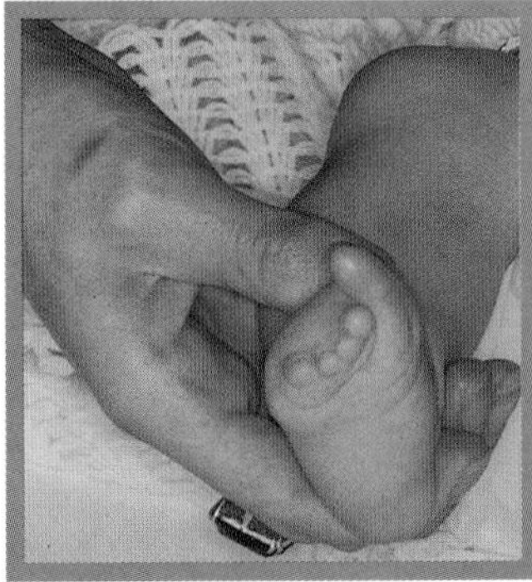

↑ 1.78

Figure 1.79 Collodion Baby. This is caused by a disorder of keratinization, and is one of the ichthyotic conditions. It is characterized clinically by a variety of patterns of scaliness, and by different patterns of inheritance. The precise diagnosis is based upon the clinical, histopathological and genetic patterns. A newborn is shown affected by a parchment-like membrane. In this infant the collodion-type skin split and peeled, leaving an ichthyotic base that was kept soft and pliable by the use of emollient. Subsequently a histopathological diagnosis of lamellar ichthyosis was made. The eyes may need protection if ectropion occurs.

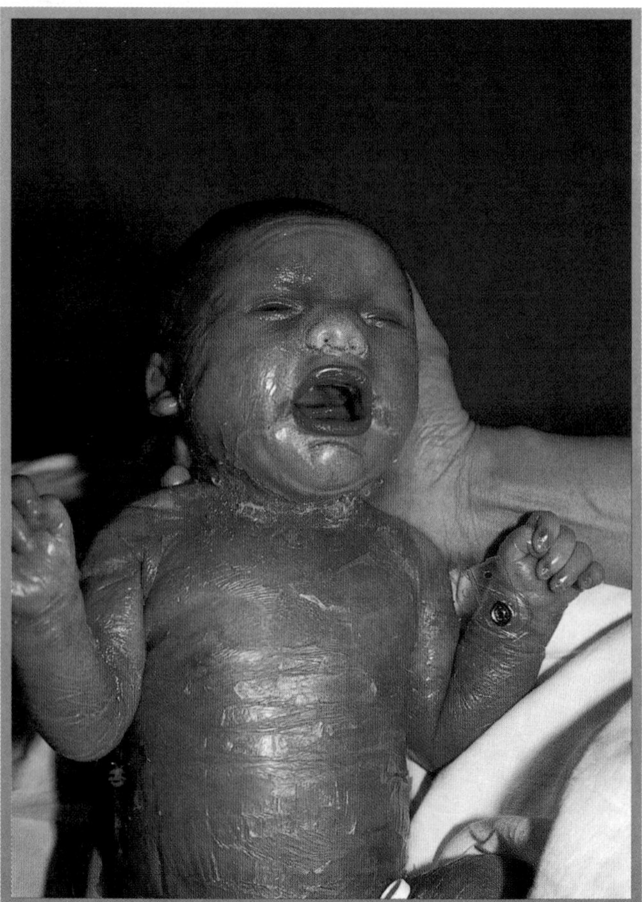

←1.79

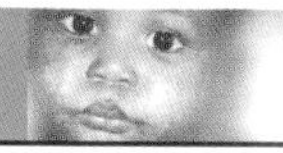

Figure 1.80 Ammoniacal Dermatitis (Diaper or Nappy Rash). This is due to the irritant effect of a wet diaper rubbing against the surface of the bottom. Note the sparing of the intertriginous regions. Differential diagnosis includes perianal dermatitis, seborrheic dermatitis, and candidiasis. Treatment consists in erradication of infection and use of barrier creams. Exposure of the region allows drying and improves the condition.

Figure 1.81 Seborrheic Dermatitis. This has a similar distribution to ammoniacal dermatitis (see **Figure 1.80**) but is less irritating. The distribution is along the areas of the seborrheic glands. The disease usually occurs in the first year and predominantly affects the scalp (cradle cap). It may coexist with atopic dermatitis (eczema). It responds to topical steroids and descaling preparations.

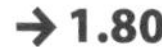

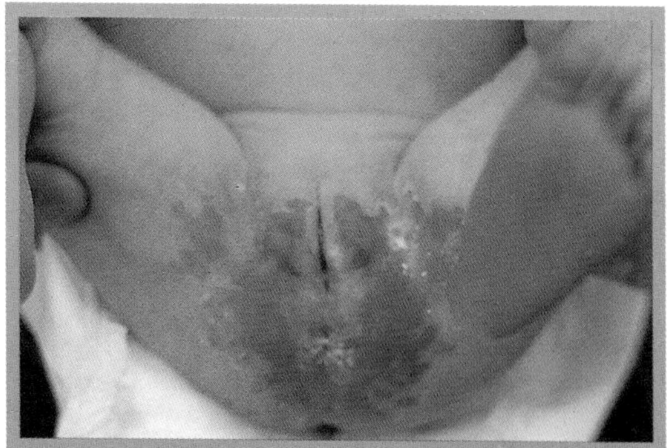

→ 1.81

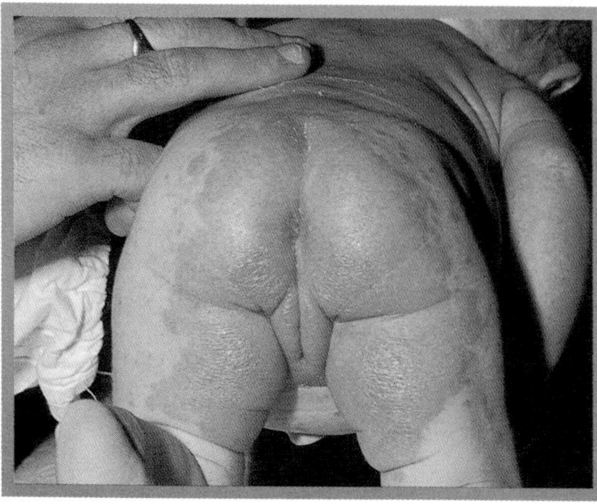

Figure 1.82 Candidal Nappy Rash. This extensive rash occurs in the nappy area and has satellite lesions. It is intensely irritating and itchy. This case responded well to topical and systemic antifungals. Note the degree of erythema and involvement of the intertriginous areas.

Figure 1.83 Staphylococcal Scalded Skin (Ritter Disease) in a Newborn. The newborn infant discussed here presented at 3 days with stripping of the superficial dermis and a florid, red, macular rash. The infant was irritable and febrile. These symptoms were caused by phage type 2 staphylococci. The effects can be extensive and can cause a necrotizing fasciitis.

Ritter disease is caused by a toxin rather than by direct invasion and infection. It responds to antibiotic treatment and recovery may be rapid. Multisystem failure may occur and shock may be severe.

This condition is intensely infectious and can cause epidemics in nurseries; therefore the child should be isolated.

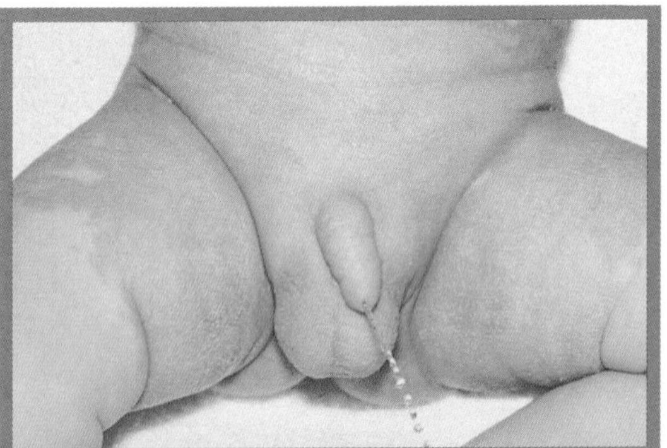

← 1.82

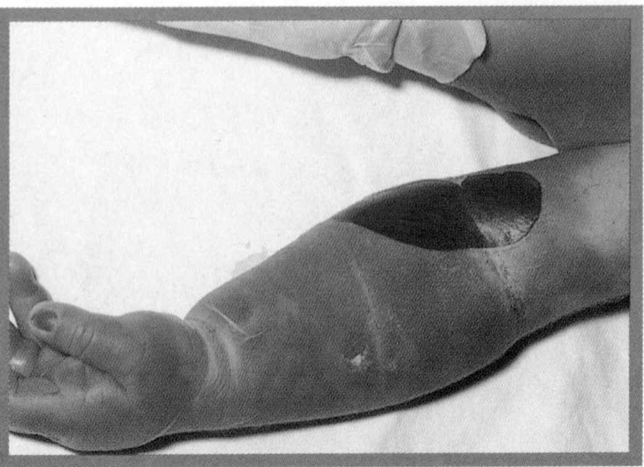

← 1.83

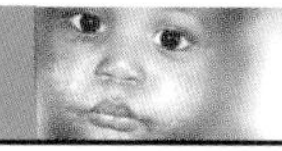

Figure 1.84 Congenital Chickenpox (Herpes Varicella–Zoster). The newborn infant shown here displays typical scarring (cicatrix) affecting the dermatome supplied by the ophthalmic division of the fifth cranial nerve. The mother contracted chickenpox at the beginning of the third trimester. The infant was otherwise normal and at 1 year of age is developing normally. A baby with neonatal shingles is infectious to non-immune babies. The treatment consists of administration of intravenous acyclovir.

Figure 1.85 Neonatal Chickenpox. The 7-day-old infant shown here developed this typical rash 5 days after delivery. The mother developed a similar rash at the same time. This is neonatal (not congenital) chickenpox. It is often a very severe disease for both the mother and infant. This infant had no protective varicella–zoster antibody. Treatment involves using intravenous antiviral agents, and the use of hyperimmune immunoglobulin and antibiotic for super-added infection.

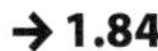

→1.84

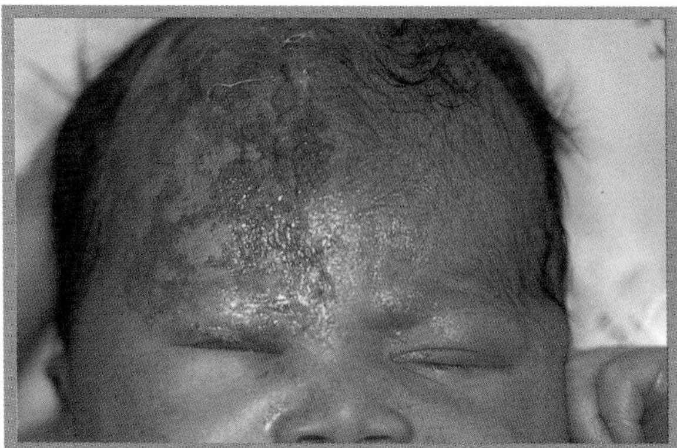

→1.85

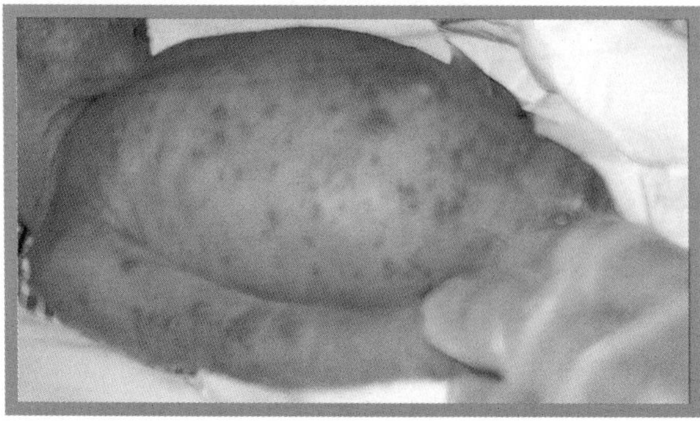

Figure 1.86 Mongolian Blue Spot. This is a common, pigmented nevus usually found over the lower back and buttocks. It is more common in darker-skinned infants but is still often seen in caucasians. It may be confused with bruising, triggering child protection investigations. Mongolian blue spots are slate-gray in color, are not tender, and fade over a period of months to years, whereas the purple color of a bruise progresses through a sequence of color changes over a period of days.

Figure 1.87 Extensive Chemical Burns to the Skin of a 25-Week Premature Infant. The baby shown here had been prepared for an umbilical artery catheterization, and povidone iodine in spirit had been used to prepare the site. The infant had lain in a pool of the fluid and sustained the chemical burn. This eventually healed with scarring.

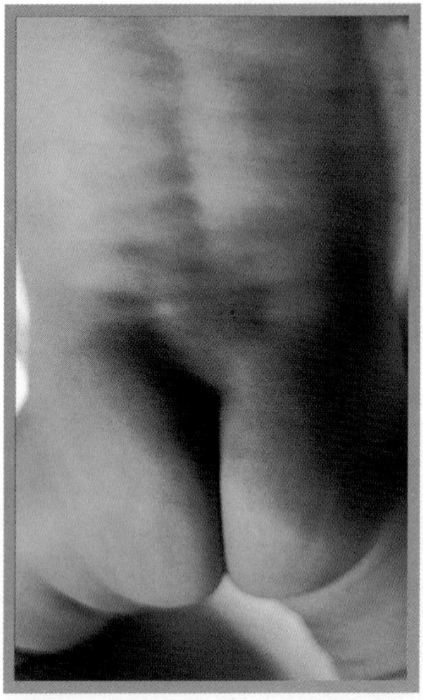

↑ **1.86**

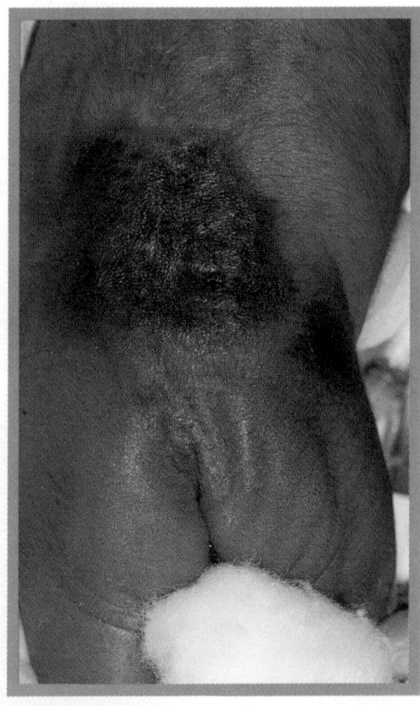

↑ **1.87**

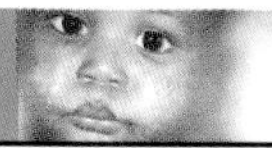

Figure 1.88 Scrotal Edema in a Newborn Infant. This edema was related to a breech delivery. Neonatal torsion will present with similar edema, but is unilateral, tender and one can feel the swollen testicle.
Figure 1.89 Vulval Edema in a Breech Delivery. This edema resolved over a period of 3 days. Note the vaginal mucosal tag resulting from maternal estrogens acting on the vaginal mucosa; such tags often protrude between the labia majora.

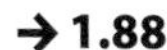

1.88

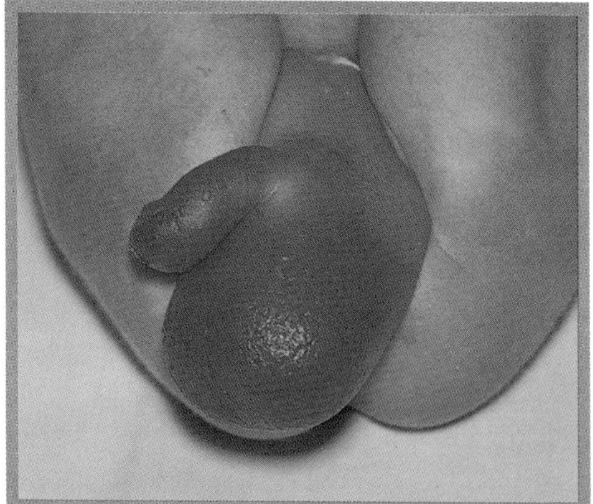

→ 1.89

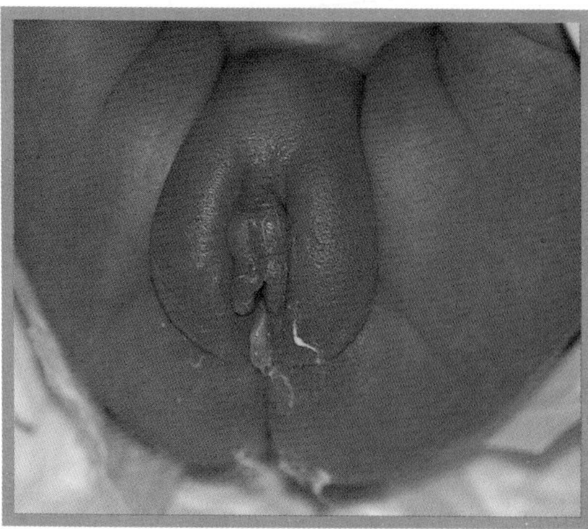

Figure 1.90 Skin Lesion. This lesion was caused by the application of a ventouse suction device to the buttocks of an unsuspected breech delivery.
Figure 1.91 Hydrops Fetalis. Hydrops was diagnosed antenatally in this preterm infant (born at 28 weeks' gestation).
Fetal blood sampling confirmed severe anemia and Doppler studies showed high-output cardiac failure. Intrauterine transfusions were administered, but gross edema developed with pleural and peritoneal effusions.

At delivery, ascites and pleural effusions were drained and the infant was ventilated. Supportive transfusion and parenteral nutrition were initiated and the infant survived intact. No obvious cause was found.

There are multiple causes of hydrops, and they can be categorized as follows:

1. Hematological: Rh and other incompatibilities.
2. Infections: parvovirus, toxoplasmosis, leptospirosis.
3. Cardiovascular: congenital heart disease, arteriovenous malformations, SVT.
4. Pulmonary: congenital lung cysts, diaphragmatic hernia.
5. Neoplasia: neuroblastoma, hemangioma of the cord or placenta.

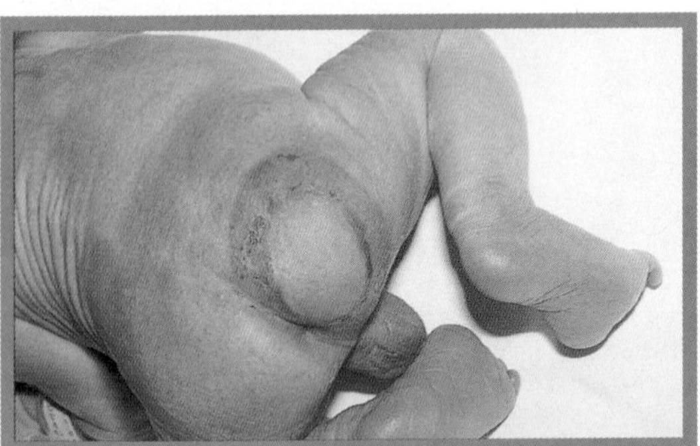

←1.90

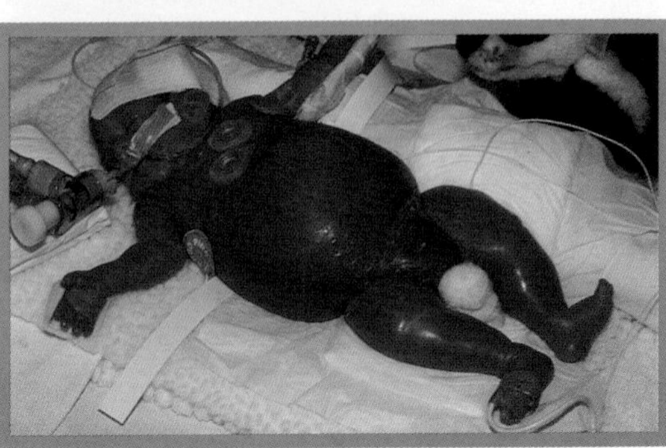

←1.91

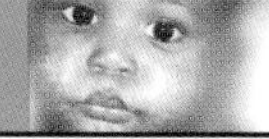

6. Hepatic: hepatitis.
7. Renal: urethral valves.
8. Gastrointestinal tract: cystic fibrosis.
9. Metabolic disorders: maternal diabetes.
10. Syndromes: Noonan sydrome, any trisomy, Turner syndrome.
11. Idiopathic.

Figures 1.92–1.95 Necrotizing Enterocolitis (NEC). Figure 1.93 shows gross abdominal distension in an infant with necrotizing enterocolitis. Note the shiny, edematous, anterior abdominal wall with distended vessels. **Figure 1.93** shows another infant who had been ventilated prior to laparotomy.

→1.92

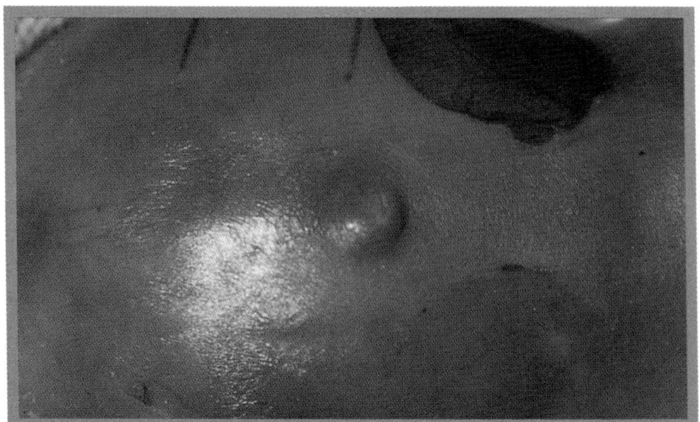

→1.93

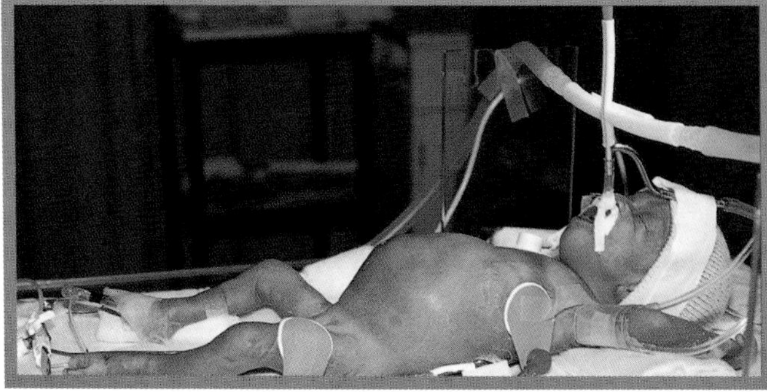

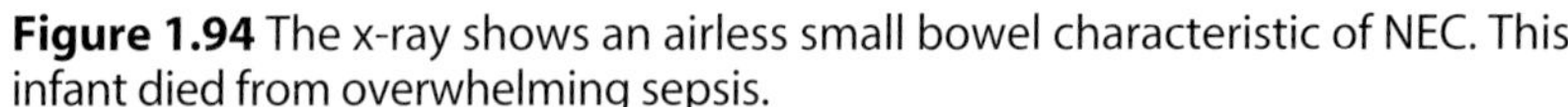

Figure 1.94 The x-ray shows an airless small bowel characteristic of NEC. This infant died from overwhelming sepsis.
Figure 1.95 shows a classic X-ray of necrotizing enterocolitis (NEC). Free intraperitoneal and intramural air is shown in the large bowel. There is no intrahepatic air.

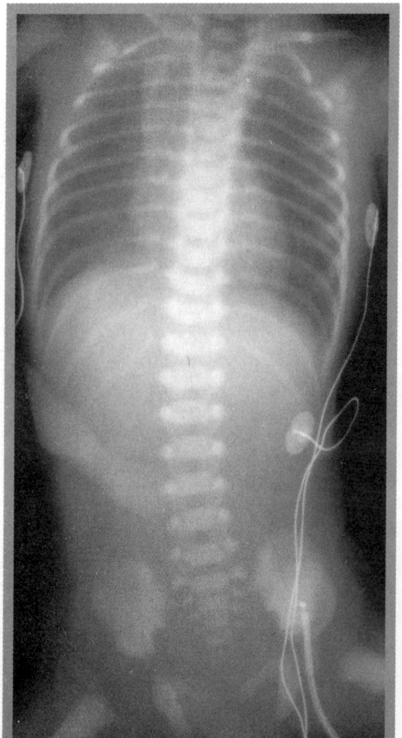

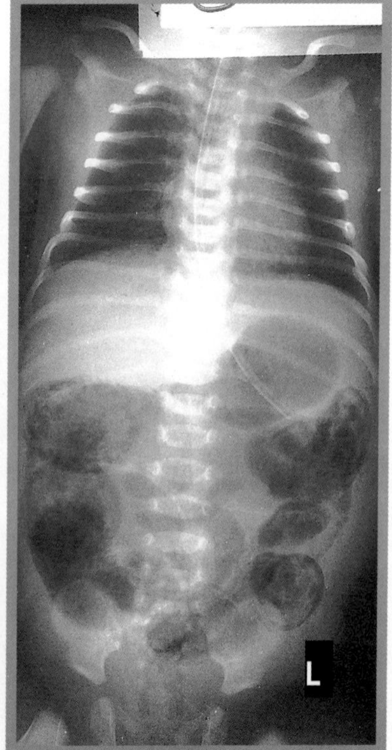

↑ 1.94

↑ 1.95

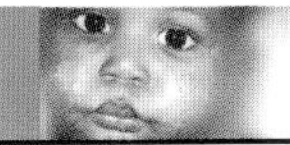

Figures 1.96 and 1.97 Exomphalos. Exomphalos was diagnosed antenatally in this term infant. Note the abdominal contents extending into the cord.

Management consists of two phases. First, the infant is resuscitated if in shock and the gastric contents drained with a nasogastric tube. Fluid loss may be reduced by the application of plastic film. Saline packs should not be used as they will cool the baby. The second phase consists in surgical reconstruction. Frequently, replacement of the bowel into the abdomen has to be delayed as there is initially inadequate space. **Figure 1.97** shows the same child as in **Figure 1.96** but at a later stage, following restoration of bowel to abdomen. The application of mercurichrome to the umbilical tissues encourages epithelialization. This reduces fluid losses. In exomphalos the abdominal contents pass through the umbilicus, with the result that sparing of the umbilicus never occurs.

→ 1.96

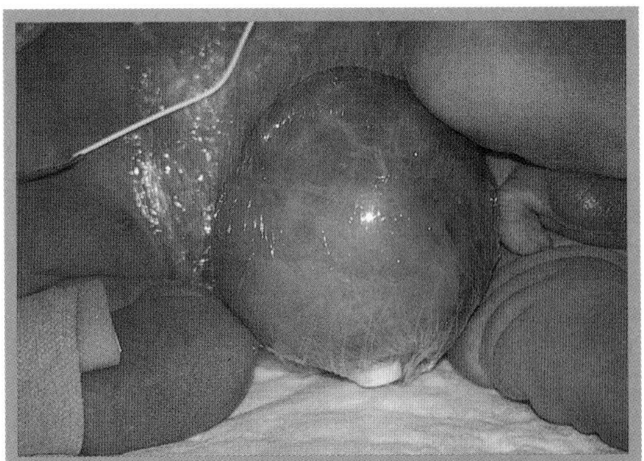

→ 1.97

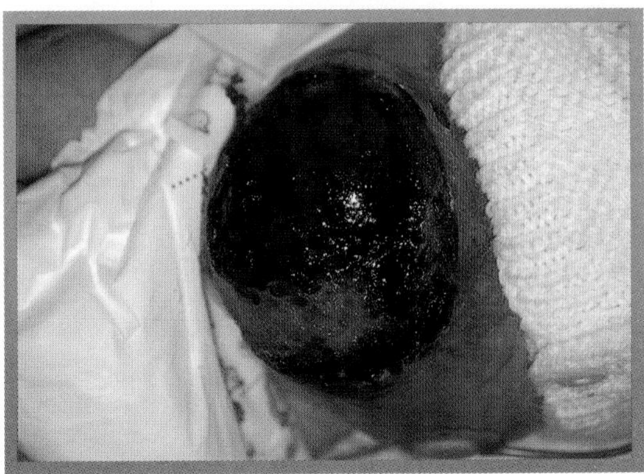

Figure 1.98 Gastroschisis Repair. This figure shows the results of repair of gastroschisis. Note that the umbilicus is spared. Malrotation needs to be excluded prior to surgical closure. Frequently, there are gastric motility problems postoperatively.

Figure 1.99 Left Diaphragmatic Hernia. This chest and abdominal X-ray shows bowel gas in the left hemithorax. This is due to herniation of the bowel through the foramen of Bochdalek, which is posterolateral. This infant was diagnosed antenatally. Labor and delivery were preterm, and at delivery the infant was noted to have a scaphoid abdomen. Resuscitation was provided by intubation and positive-pressure ventilation in an attempt to prevent distension of the bowel with air.The hernia was subsequently repaired.

Mortality is high (40–50%), and is usually due to pulmonary hypoplasia, a condition present in all cases to a greater or lesser extent.

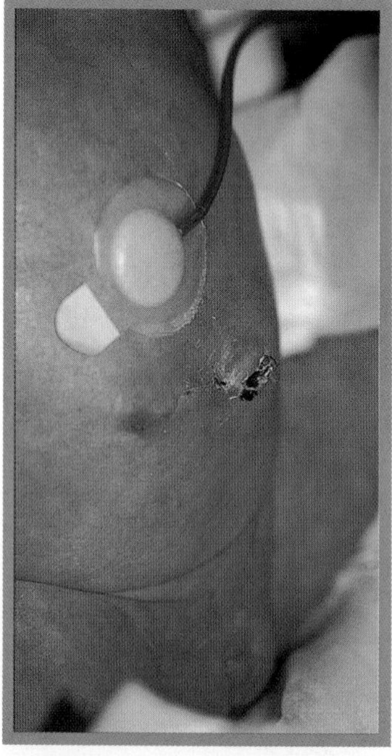

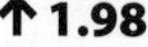

↑1.98

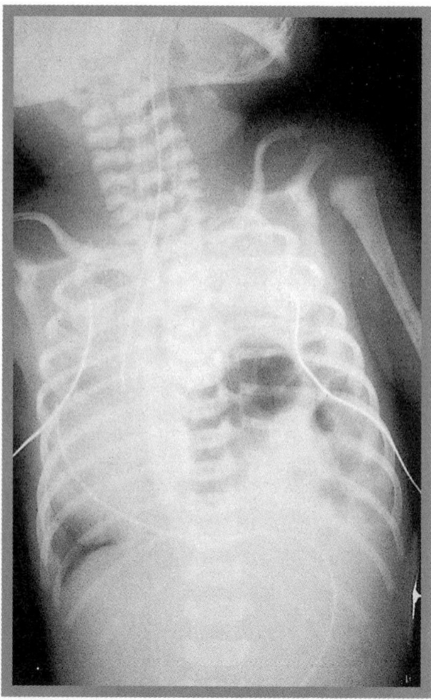

↑1.99

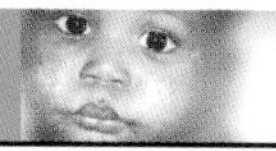

Figure 1.100 Umbilical Granuloma. This is a common clinical problem. After separation of the cord the raw surface usually becomes covered by epithelium. This occasionally fails to occur and the granulation tissue is exposed. The cord weeps and may develop a low-grade infection. Simple treatment with silver nitrate or isopropyl alcohol sterilizes the stump and encourages epithelium to grow.

Figure 1.101 Umbilical Polyp. Differential diagnosis of an umbilical granuloma (see **Figure 1.100**) includes an umbilical polyp, which is a remnant of either the vitelline duct or the urachus. This may be differentiated from a granuloma by the presence of feces or urine at the site of the polyp. Treatment consists of complete excision.

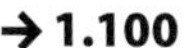

→ 1.100

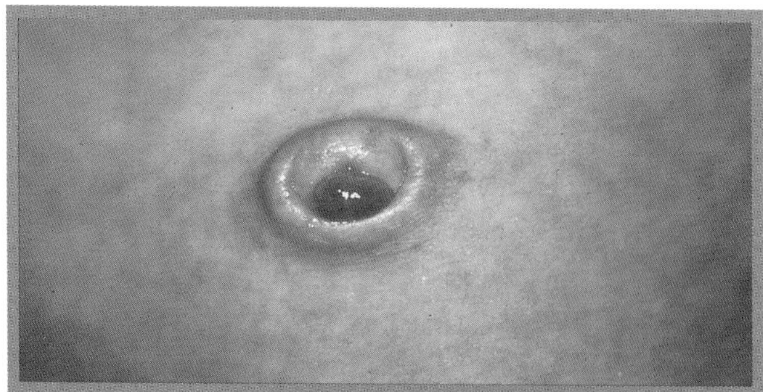

→ 1.101

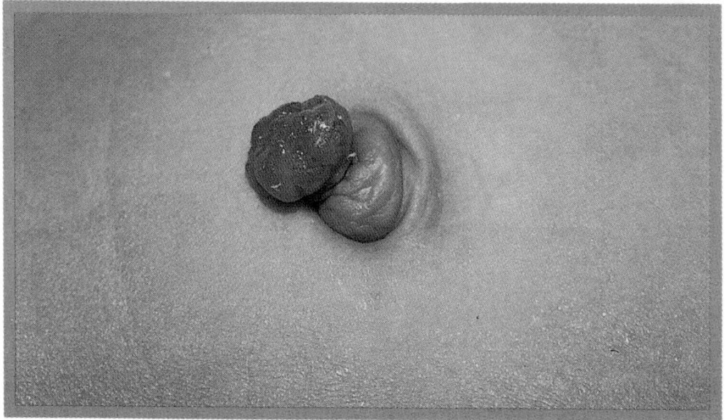

Figure 1.102 Umbilical Hernia. This otherwise healthy child was noted to have a swelling at the umbilicus. The child had occasional episodes of screaming but was otherwise well.

Such hernias are common and very rarely obstructive as they have a wide neck. They are more common in preterm and small-for-dates infants, afro-caribbean infants and female infants.

Most of these hernias appear before the age of 1 year and disappear spontaneously by 4–6 years of age. Surgery is occasionally carried out if the hernia shows no sign of resolution by the age 4 years, or if the hernia becomes larger after the age of 1 year.

Figures 1.103 and 1.104 Lipomeningocele. This large mass was diagnosed antenatally. Delivery was by cesarian section because of malpresentation. At birth, a large solid mass was noted. This mass arose from the sacrum and extended posteriorly down over the buttocks. There was a full range of movements at the hips, but the leg was held flexed at the hip and internally rotated.

Figure 1.104. The X-ray shows widening of the spinal canal and spina bifida. There was widening of the intervertebral spaces of the lumbar vertebrae. At operation, the lipoma was found to arise from the spinal cord. Postoperatively there was residual lower motor deficit affecting the lower limbs, bladder and bowels. Neurogenic bladder persists as a long-term problem.

Figure 1.105 Hypoplastic Scrotum and Bilateral Undescended Testes in a Neonate. This type of problem needs relatively urgent investigation as, although the penis appears well formed, there may be a degree of genital ambiguity and one must consider the possibility of a virilized female. Karyotype tests, ultrasound of the abdomen to identify gonads, and endocrine investigation are all required.

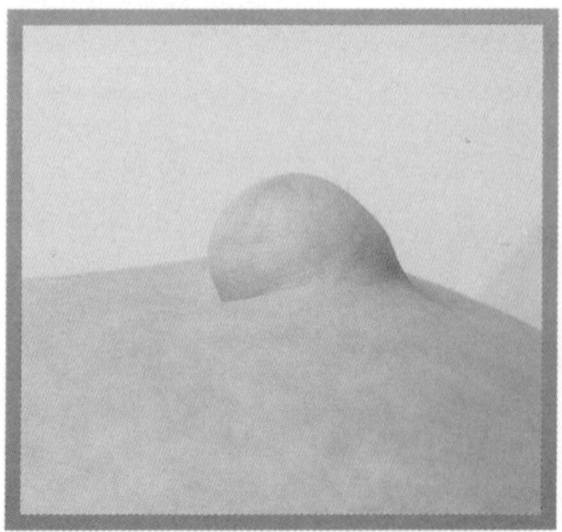

↑ 1.102

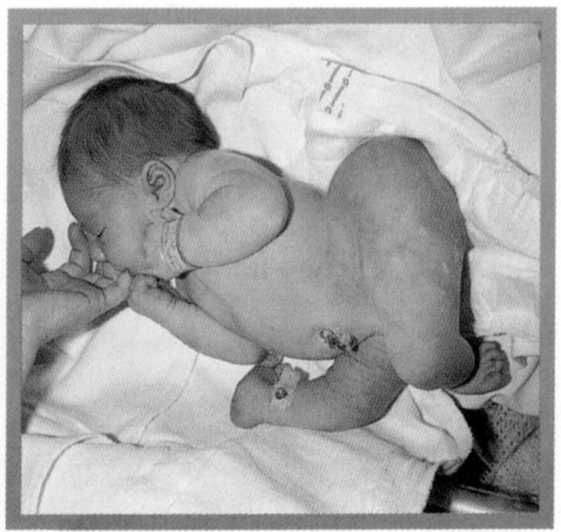

↑ 1.103

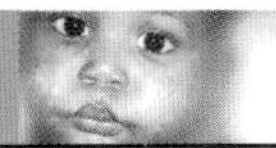

→ 1.104

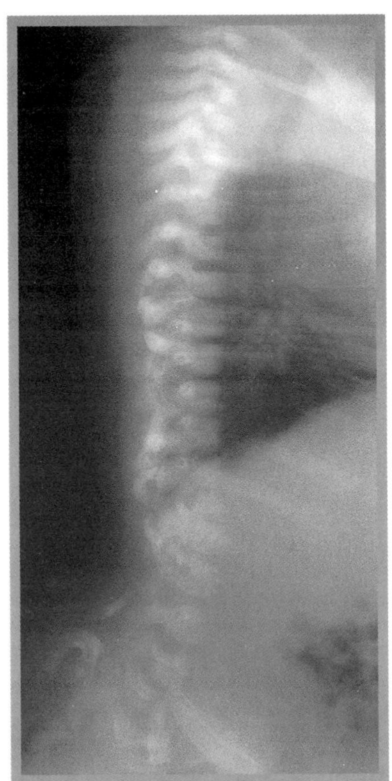

→ 1.105

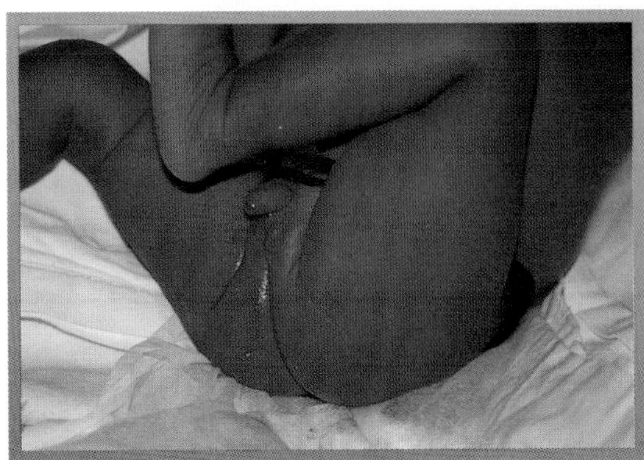

Figure 1.106 Abdominal X-ray. The X-ray shows a 'double bubble' and the remaining abdomen to be airless associated with high, small-bowel atresia. The neonate discussed here presented in the first 3 days of life with bile-stained vomiting and abdominal distension. At laparotomy an annular pancreas was noted. Malrotation was also found. Any bile-stained vomiting in the neonatal period must be investigated and managed as if resulting from a surgical cause until proven otherwise.

Figure 1.107 Ultrasound of Intraventricular Hemorrhage. Echodense material can be seen in the left lateral ventricle, and there is ventricular dilatation on the right.

Figure 1.108 Left Porencephalic Cyst. This figure shows a porencephalic cyst in an ex-premature child following an intraparenchymal hemorrhage. The child developed a contralateral hemiplegia.

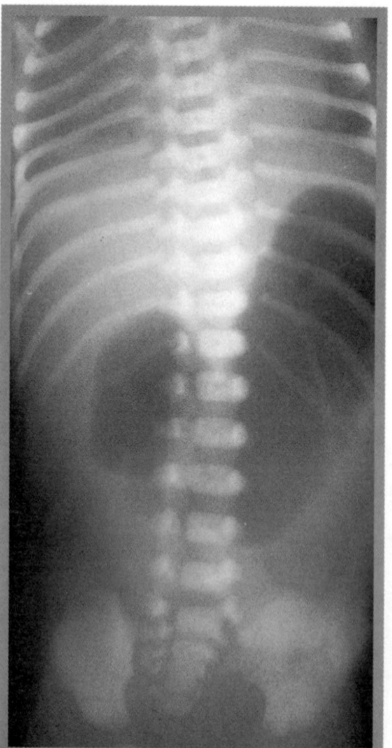

↑ **1.106**

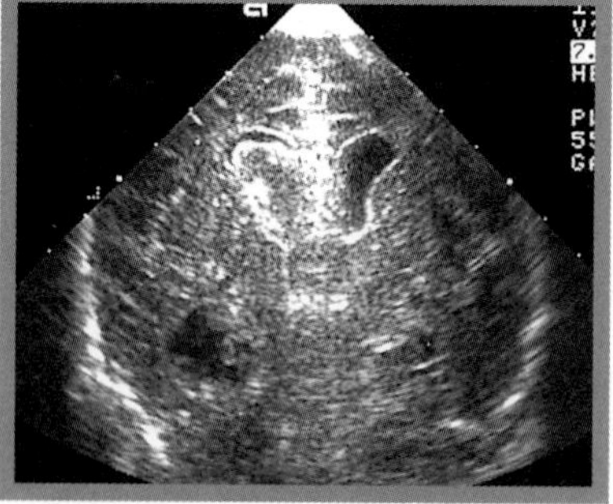

↑ **1.107**

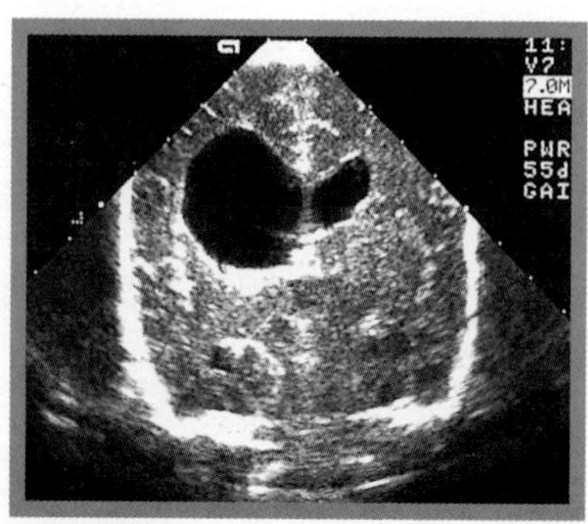

↑ **1.108**

2 Development in the first year of life

This chapter charts the development of one male child, Jacob over the first year of his life. It must, however, be remembered that the range of normal development varies considerably between children.

At each assessment the following five categories should be considered:

1. Gross motor.
2. Vision and fine motor.
3. Hearing and speech.
4. Social interaction.

With special thanks to Karen and Jacob Zwi Söderlund.

NEWBORN

Gross Motor and Posture

Figure 2.1 Prone. The head is shown turned to the side, and the arms are close to the chest with the elbows fully flexed. The hips and knees are flexed under the buttocks. Note that the hands are tightly closed.

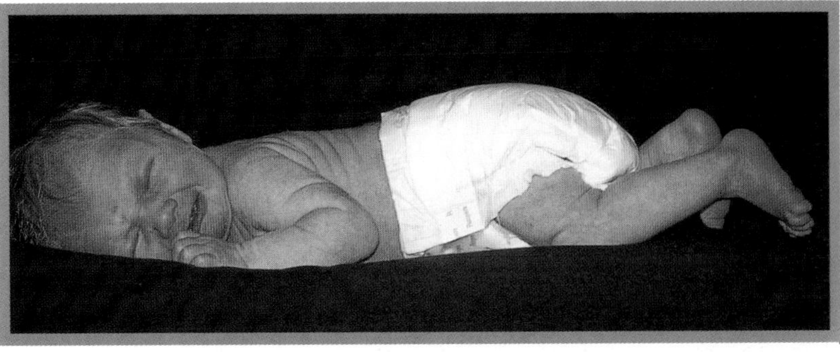

↑2.1

Figure 2.2 Supine. The baby is lying in a flexed position, and the hands are now open. Continual fisting at this age is always abnormal.
Figure 2.3 Ventral Suspension. The head droops below the plane of the body, the hips are fully flexed and the limbs hang down.

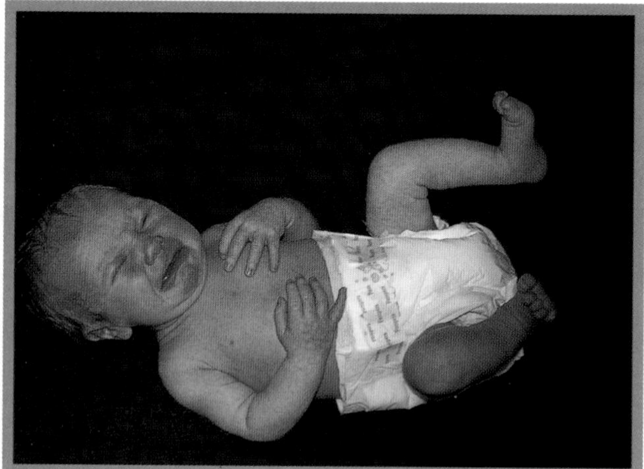

←2.2

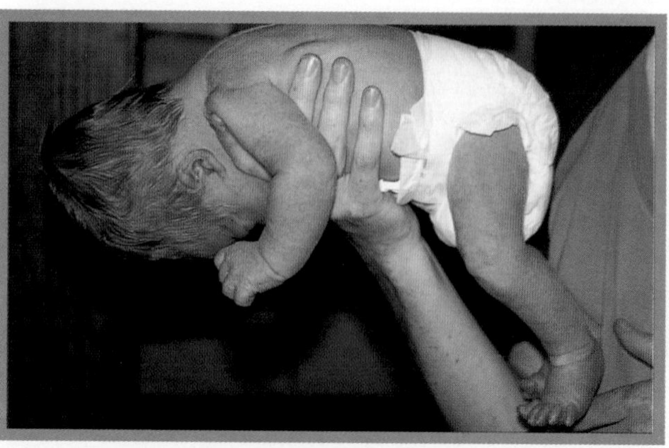

←2.3

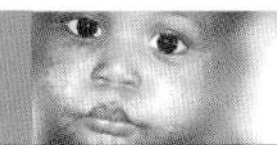

Figure 2.4 Pulled to sit. The baby is shown at 10 days. Note the marked head lag, which is normal.

Vision and Fine Motor

Figure 2.5 Vision. The baby is shown fixating on the mother's face.

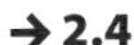

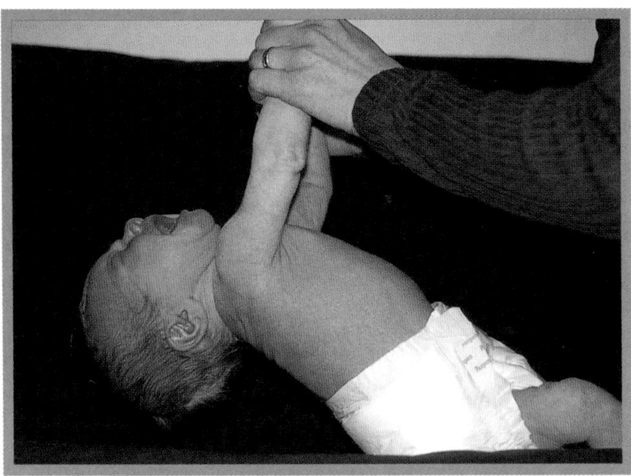

→2.5

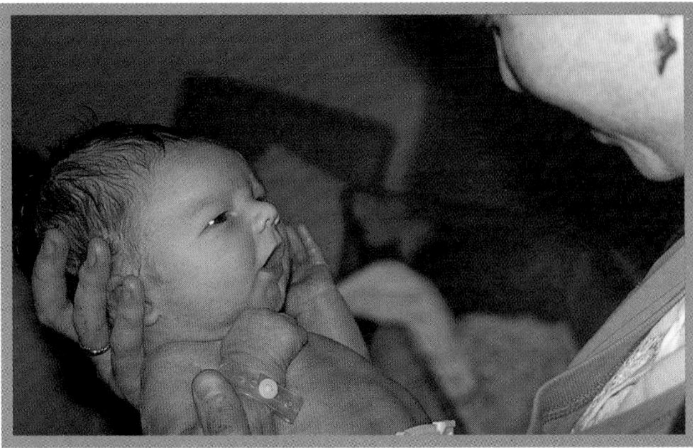

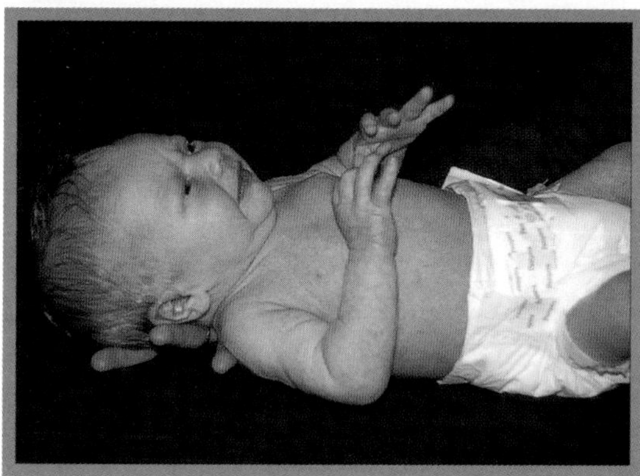

←2.6

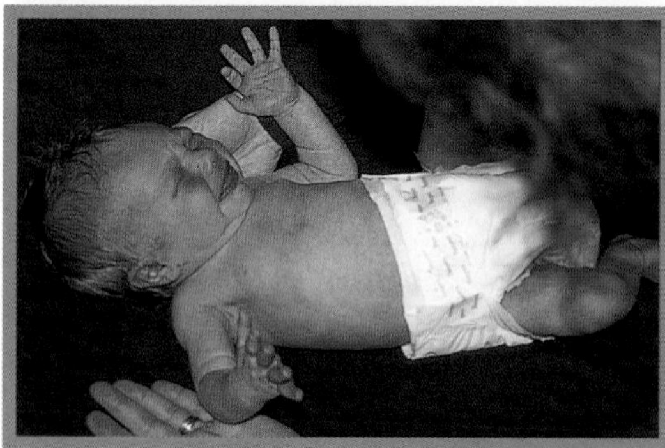

←2.7

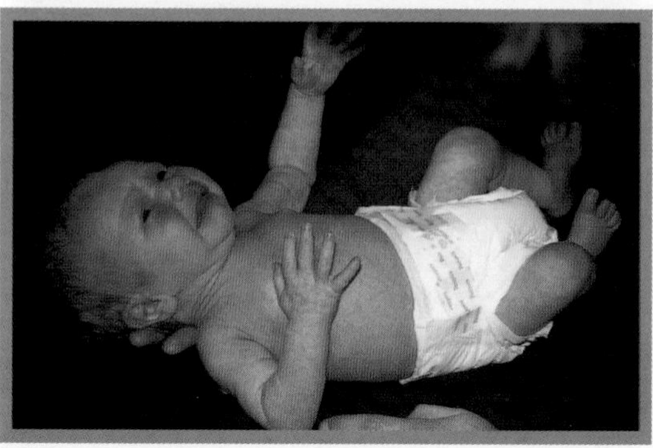

←2.8

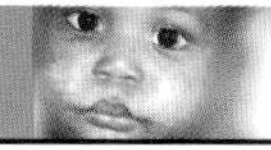

Figures 2.6–2.8 Moro Reflex. In this series of slides the Moro reflex is demonstrated. While the head is held in the examiner's hands, a sudden extension of the neck results in abduction and extension of the arms with extension of the fingers, and subsequent flexion of the fingers and arms, which are then adducted. The symmetric Moro reflex requires the head to lie in the midline

6–8 WEEKS

Gross Motor and Posture

Figure 2.9 Prone. The pelvis is flat, and the arms are flexed with the elbows away from the body. The hips are more extended than previously, and the chin is off the couch.

Figure 2.10 Supine. The baby's arms are slightly flexed, the knees are apart, and the soles of the feet are facing upward. Note that there is no asymmetry.

→2.9

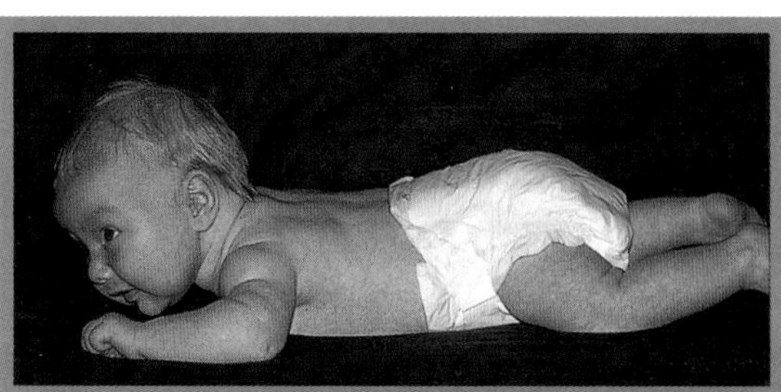

→2.10

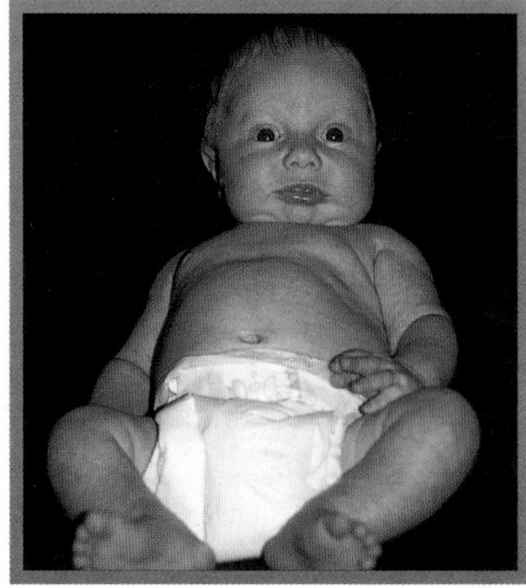

Figure 2.11 Ventral Suspension. The head is in same plane as the body, and the hips are extended.

Figure 2.12 Standing. The baby is shown standing with his body straightened. Note the position of the extended legs, with the weight on the feet and no scissoring (adductor spasm).

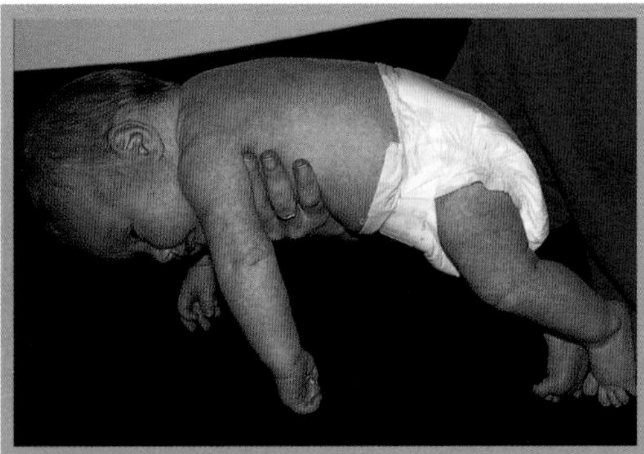

←2.11

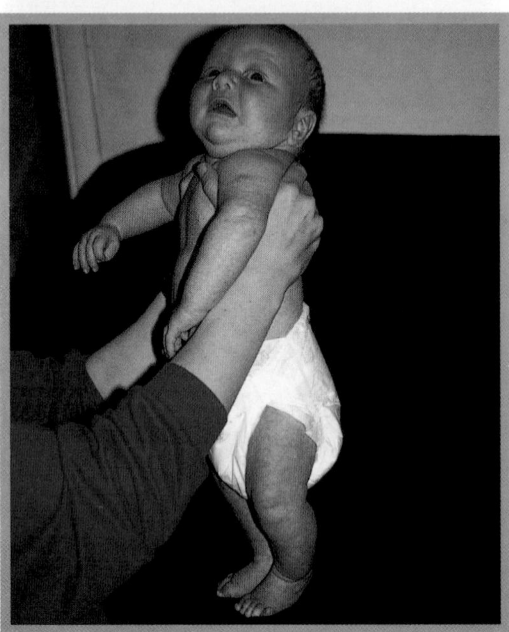

←2.12

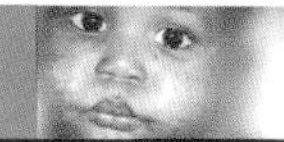

Primitive Reflexes

Figures 2.13 and 2.14 Rooting Reflex. Gentle stimulation of the cheek (top) causes the baby to turn to suck. The lower figure shows two important features: a good sucking response and a red retinal reflex (which is checked by using an ophthalmoscope on +1 to +3 at 30 cms from the eye).

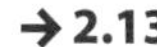

→2.13

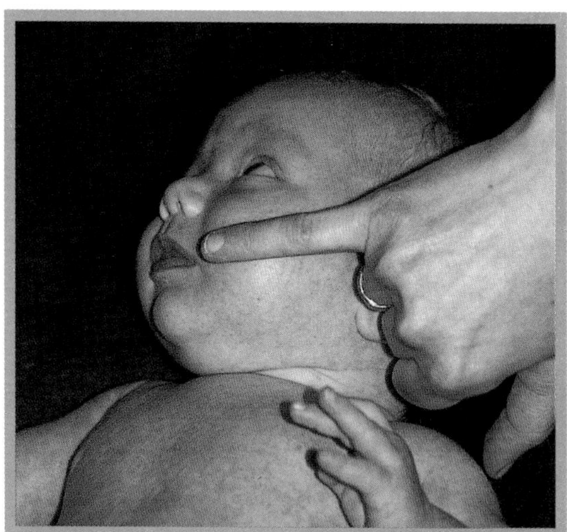

→2.14

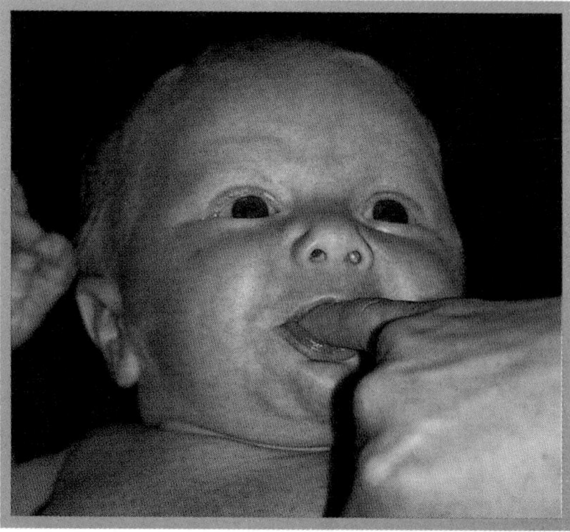

Figure 2.15 Grasp Reflex. The grasp reflex may be elicited in the hands or the feet. Note the strength of the grip.

Figure 2.16 Asymmetric Tonic Neck Reflexes (ATNR). Lateral turning of the head results in extension of the arm on the same side, with flexion of the limbs on the opposite side ('fencing' position). Persistence of this reflex beyond 4 months is abnormal. Occasionally, the reflex is absent at birth but is usually present by the end of the first month.

Figure 2.17 Walking Reflex. Stimulation of the dorsal aspect of the foot results in walking movements.

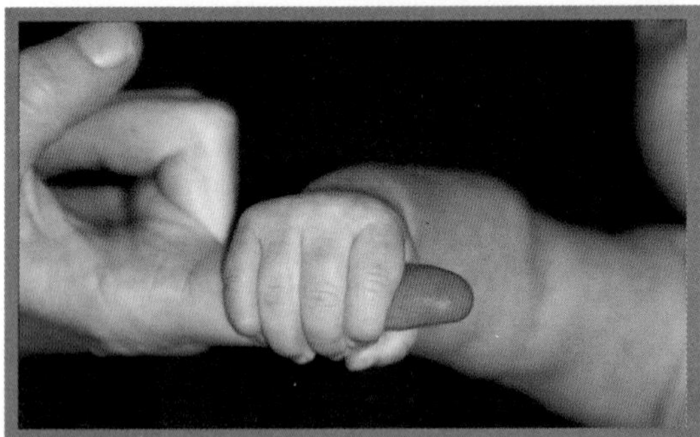

←2.15

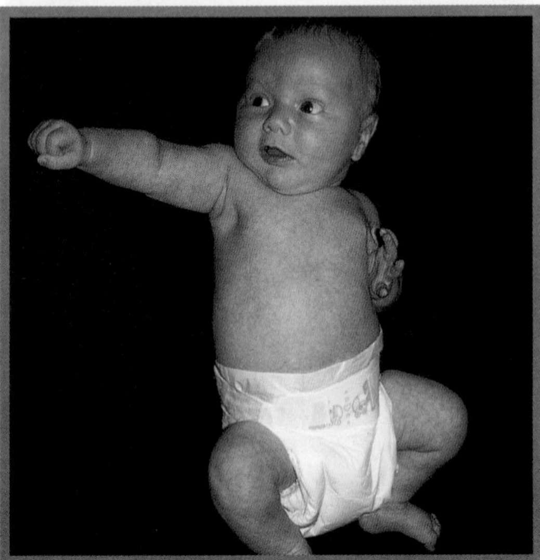

←2.16

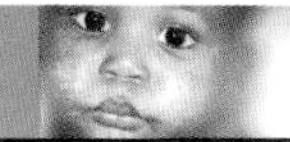

Vision and Fine Motor

Figure 2.18 Vision. In the supine position, the baby fixes on and follows the movement of a toy horizontally through an angle of 180°. To elicit this response, use a bright red ball held 50 cm from the baby's eyes.

Hearing may be assessed by parental questionnaire. At-risk babies should be referred for expert audiological opinion.

Social interaction is observed as consolability and smiling, which is nearly always present by six weeks.

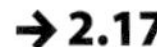

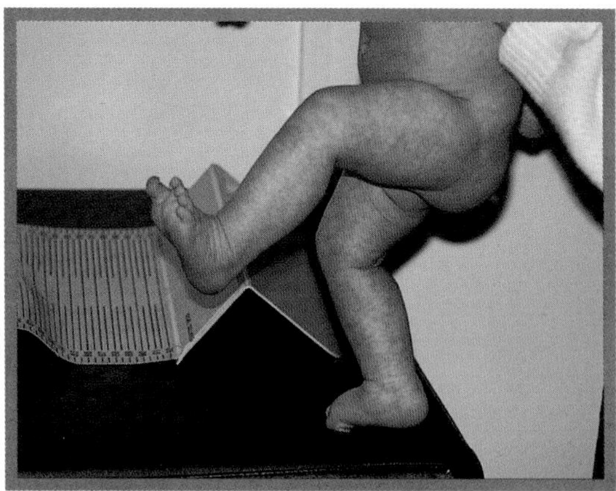

→2.18

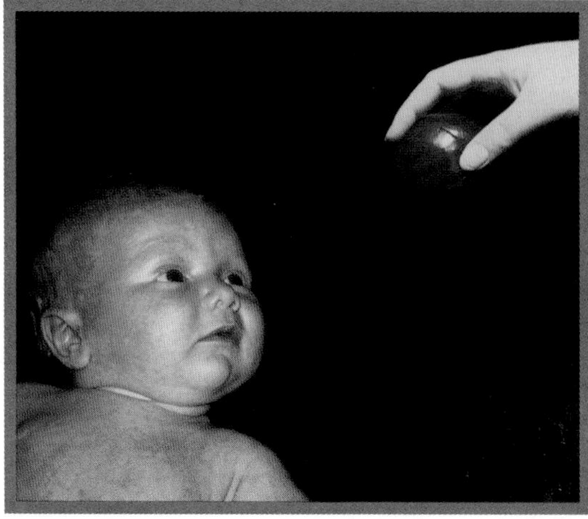

3 MONTHS

Gross Motor and Posture

Figure 2.19 Prone. The baby holds his head and shoulders off the surface, using flexed forearms as support. When he is held in ventral suspension (see **6–8 Weeks**) the head should also be in the same plane as the body.

Figures 2.20 and 2.21 Sitting. In **Figure 2.20** the baby has been pulled up to sit, and there is little head lag. Note the interaction with the mother.

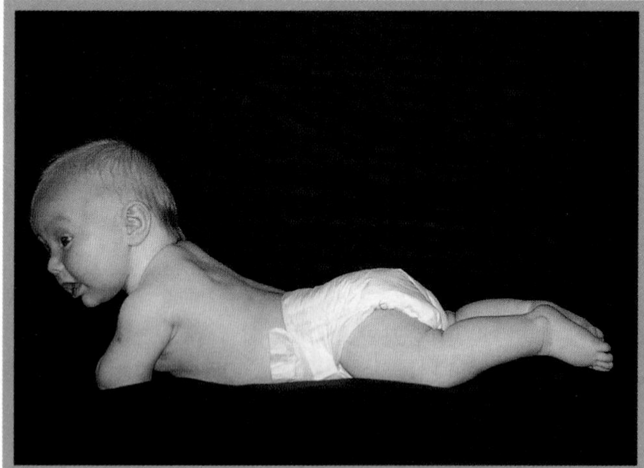

←2.19

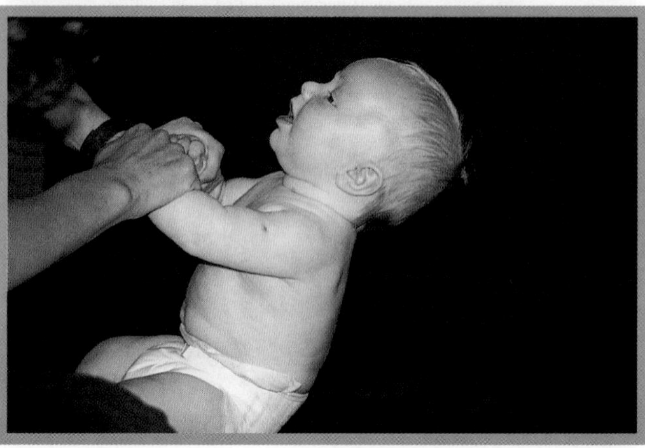

←2.20

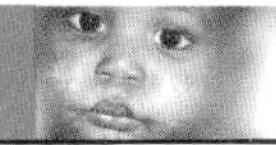

Figure 2.21 shows supported sitting,in which a lumbar curve is present and the head is held up momentarily. Note the BCG scar on the upper left arm.
Figure 2.22 Grasp. The baby grasps toys when they are placed in his hand.

→ **2.21**

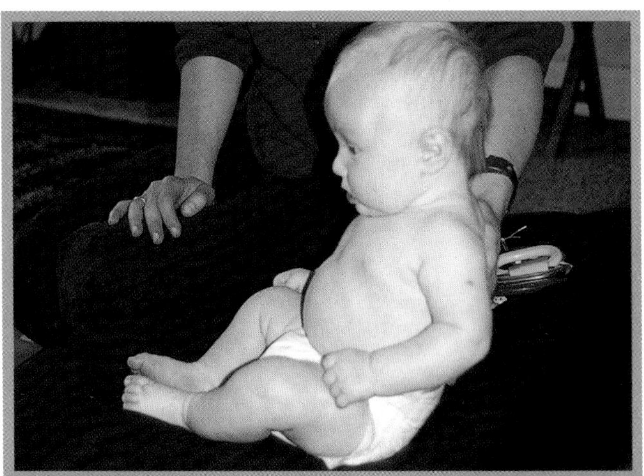

→ **2.22**

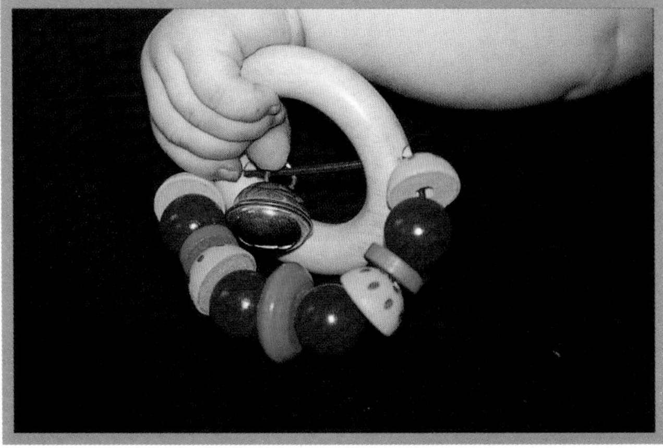

Vision and Fine Motor

Figures 2.23 and 2.24 Vision. The baby prefers faces, although will follow a red ball through 180°. He follows vertically (**Figure 2.23**), and horizontally(**Figure 2.24**), with converging eyes, and in a circle. Note that the hands are held mostly open.

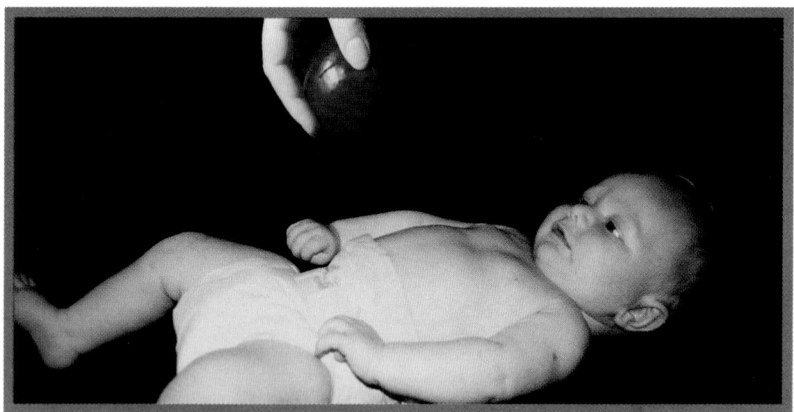

↑ 2.23

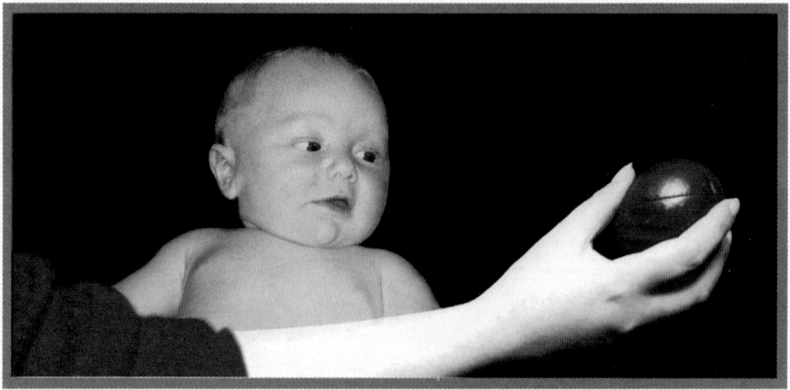

↑ 2.24

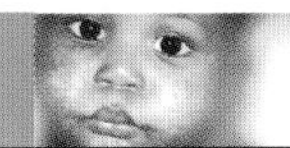

6–7 MONTHS

Gross Motor and Posture

Figure 2.25 Prone. The head, chest and upper abdomen are shown supported on the extended arms. The baby anticipates moving forward.
Figure 2.26 Supine. The baby is shown with his legs lifted, and his feet in a grasping position.

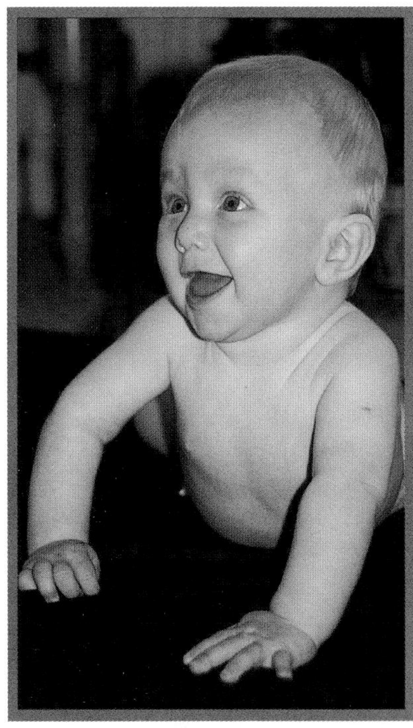

↑ 2.25

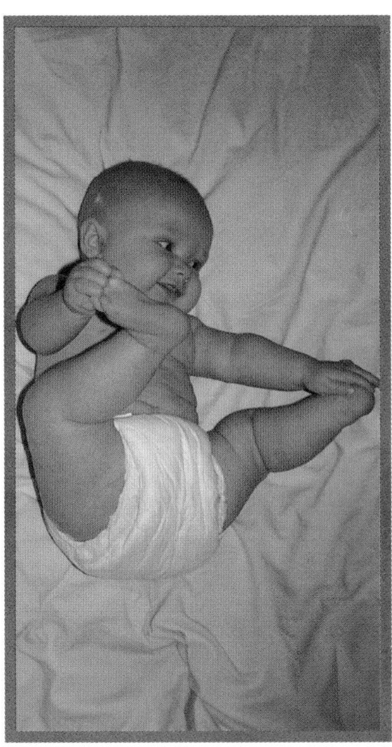

↑ 2.26

Figure 2.27 Rolling. The baby rolls from front to back, and then from back to front.
Figures 2.28 and 2.29 Sitting. The baby sits unsupported with a straight back by 10 months old (**Figure 2.29**). Independent sitting is dependent on the righting

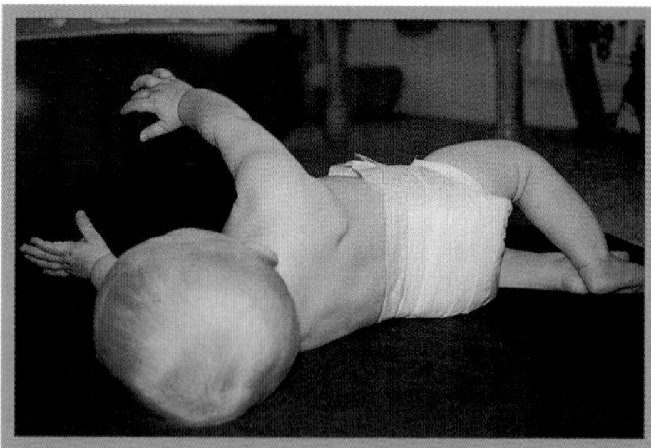

←2.27

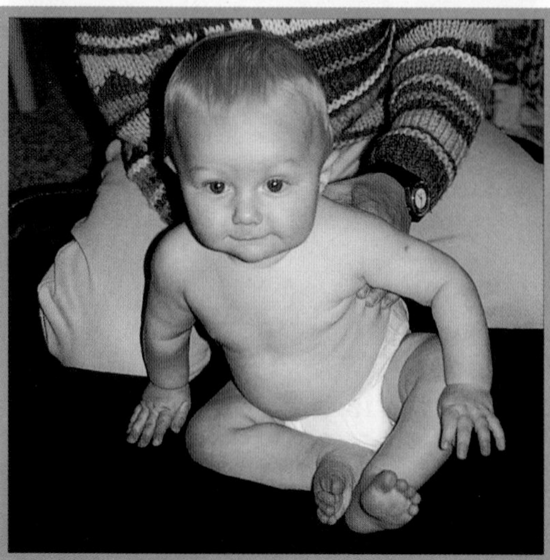

←2.28

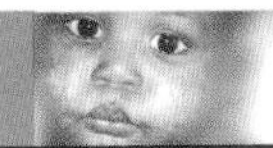

reflex (**Figure 2.28**). When the body is tilted to either side while in a sitting position the arm is extended to prevent falling.

Figure 2.30 Standing. When held standing, the baby bears the greater part of his weight.

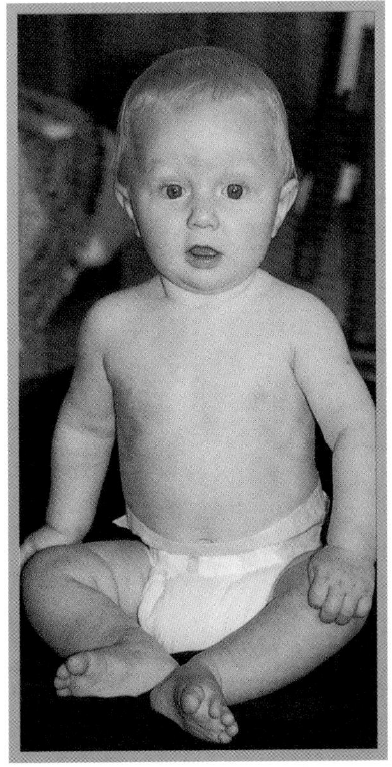

↑ **2.29**

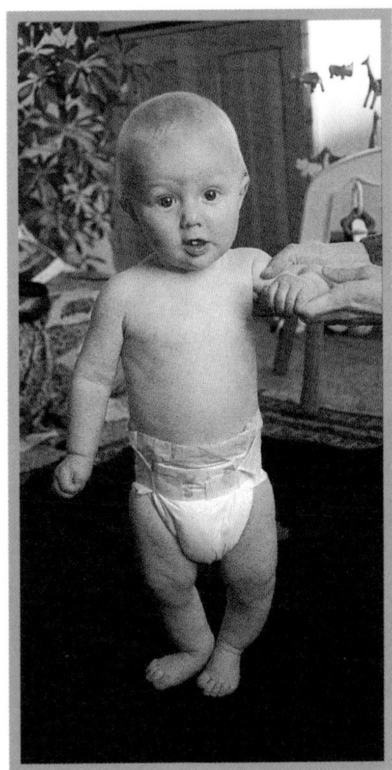

↑ **2.30**

Figure 2.31 Reflexes. Downward parachute: sudden, downward movement causes symmetrical extension of the legs.

Vision and Fine Motor

F**igure 2.32** The baby shows a palmar grasp and mouthing of objects.

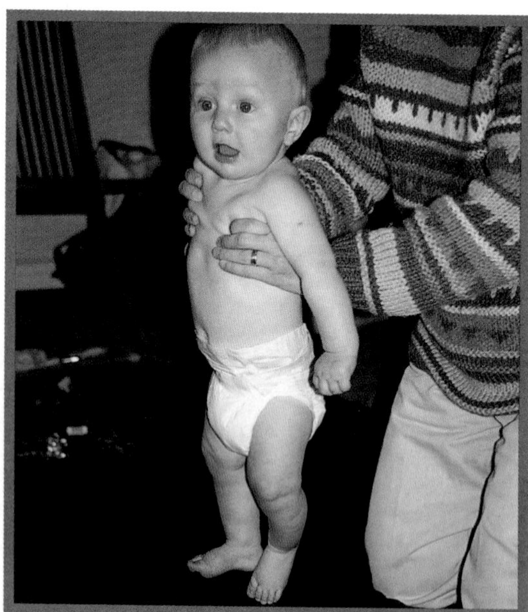

←2.31

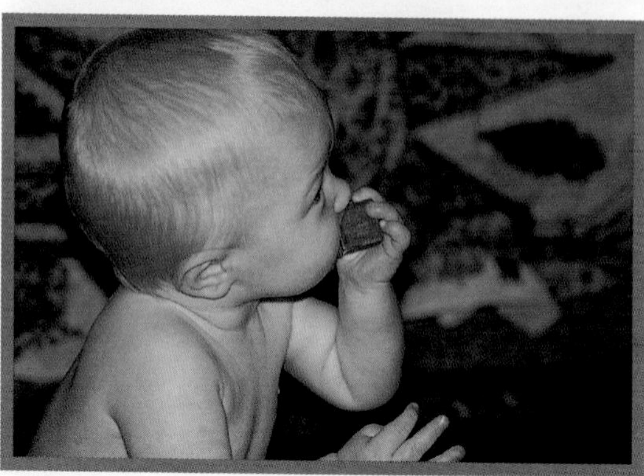

←2.32

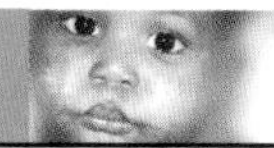

Figure 2.33 When a second cube is offered, the first cube is retained.

Figure 2.34 Hearing. The tester, mother, observer and baby are shown during distraction testing. This is used as a screening test of hearing at a time when independent sitting is present and before object permanence has developed. Meticulous technique is needed to avoid a false-positive result. Refer to standard textbooks of audiology for detailed information.

→2.33

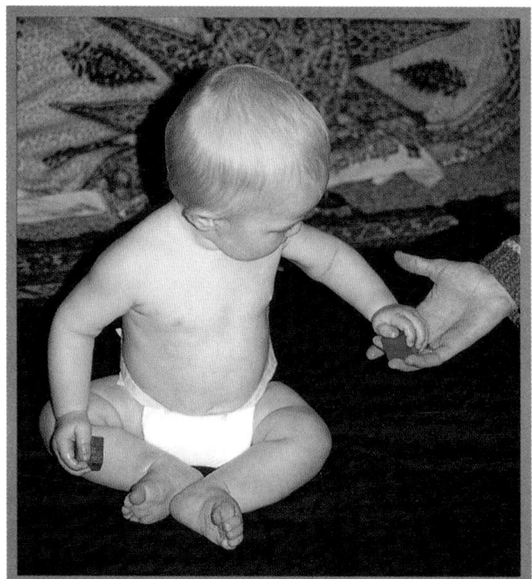

→2.34

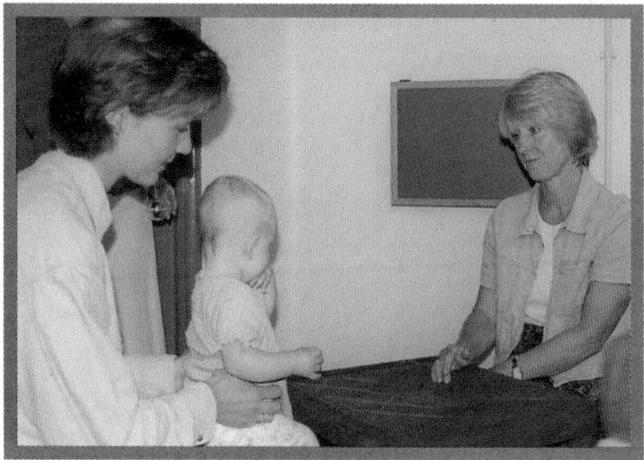

Social Interaction

Figure 2.35 The baby smiles and vocalizes at his mirror image.
Figure 2.36 The baby loves to play and crumple paper, and he is able to play in a sitting position.

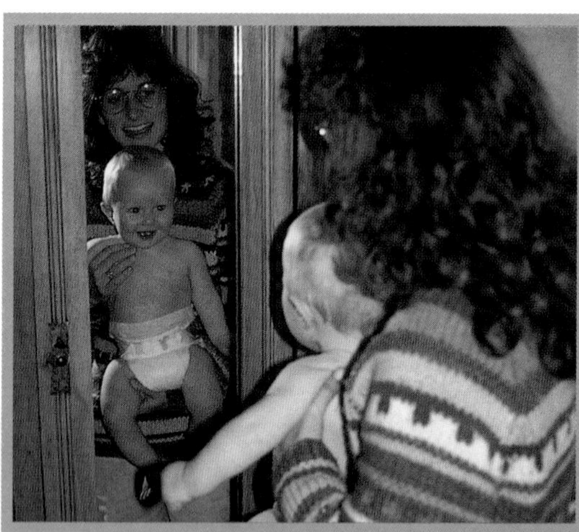

←2.35

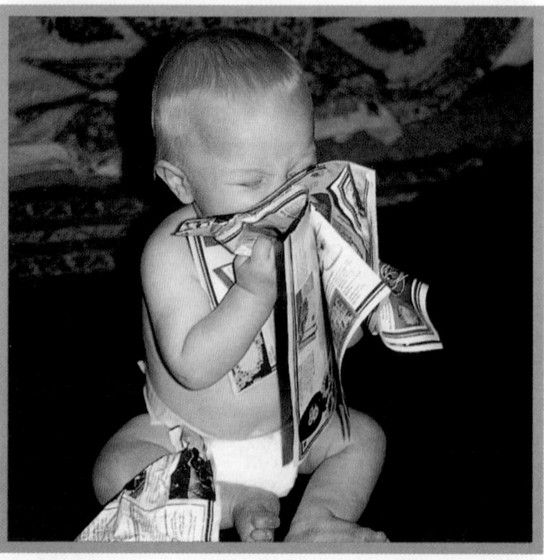

←2.36

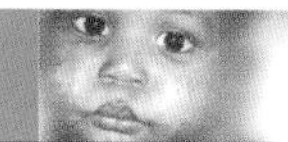

9 MONTHS

Gross Motor and Posture

Figure 2.37 Sitting. The baby sits alone, and can lean forward to pick up a dangling toy without losing his balance.

Figure 2.38 Crawling. The baby is beginning to crawl on his knees, using his hands for support.

→2.37

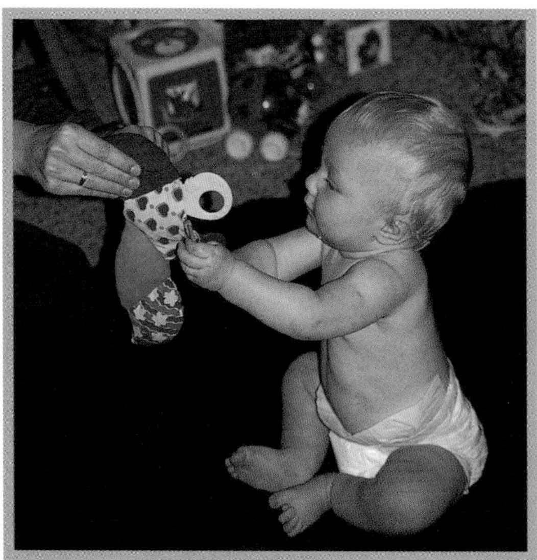

→2.38

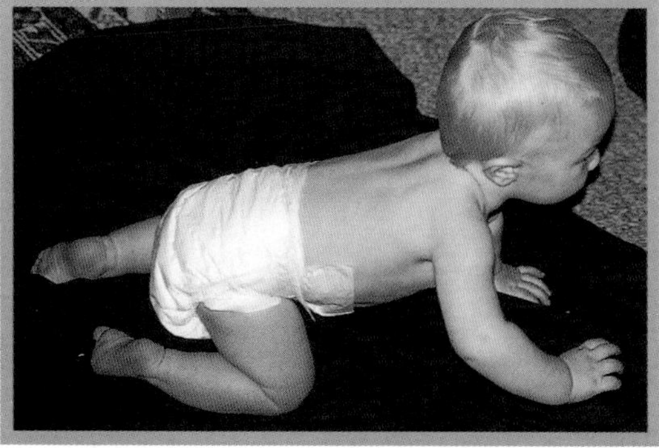

Figures 2.39 Pull to stand. The baby is shown attempting to pull himself to a standing position

Figure 2.40 Standing. At 10 months. Standing with one hand held.

Fine Motor and Vision

Figures 2.41 and 2.42 Grasp. The baby reaches out for small objects (**Figure 2.41**). Between 9 and 12 months he will develop a pincer grasp, between index finger and thumb. He pulls a toy, grasping the string (**Figure 2.42**).

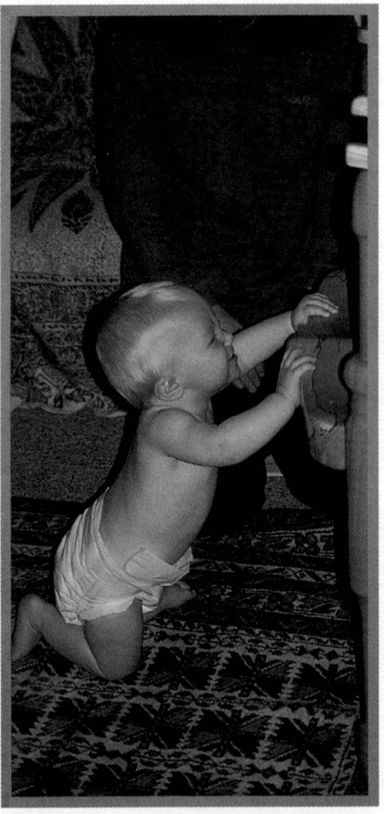

↑2.39

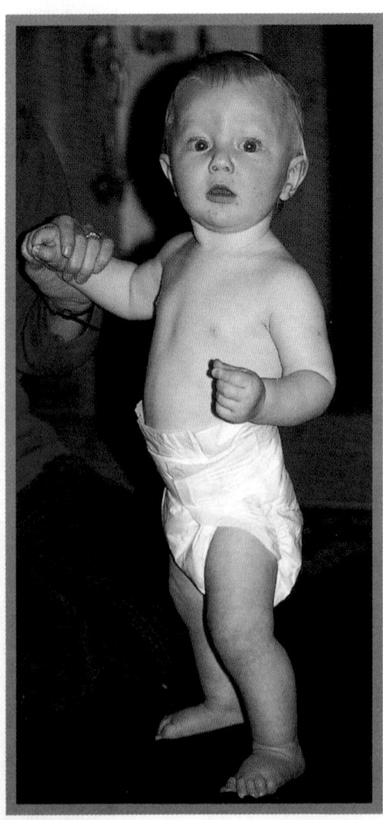

↑2.40

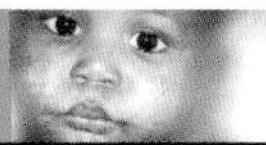

→ 2.41

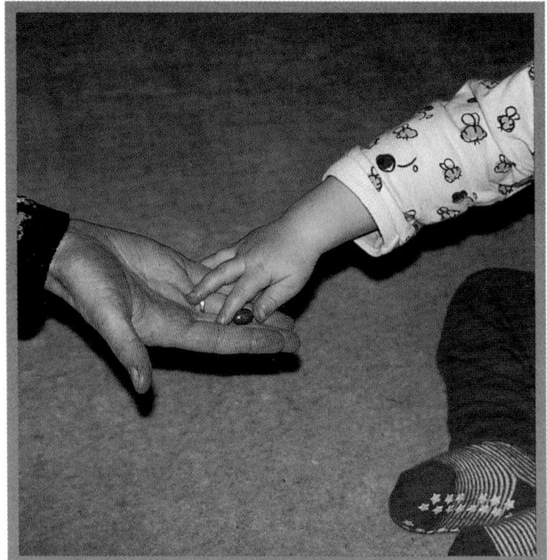

→ 2.42

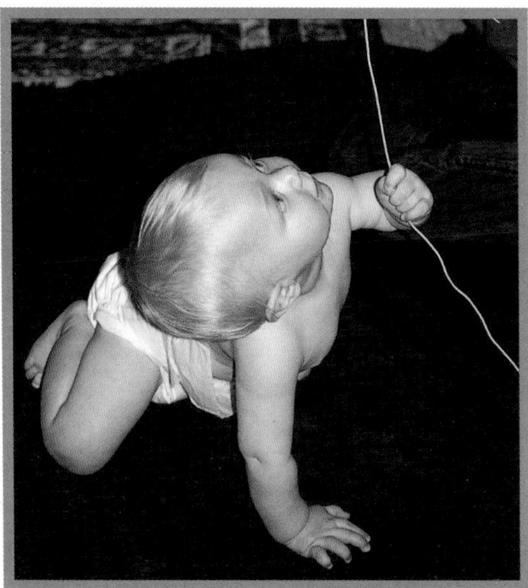

Social Behavior and Play

Figure 2.43 Finger feeding. The baby holds, bites, and chews a bread stick, and plays peek-a-boo.

Figure 2.44. **Social development** at this age includes an understanding of object permanence. In this picture the infant is watching his mother leave the cot side. Separation anxiety appears at this age.

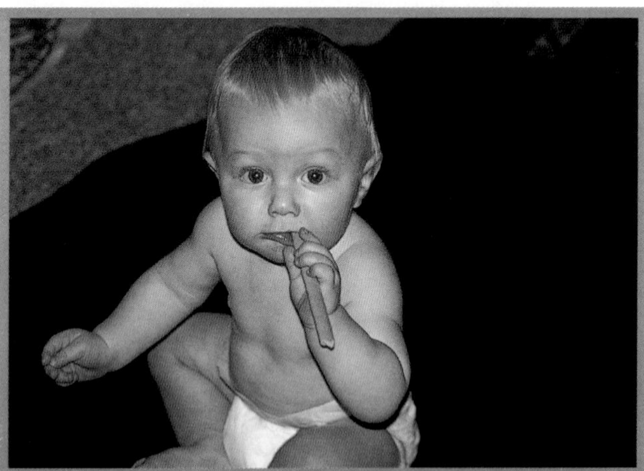

←2.43

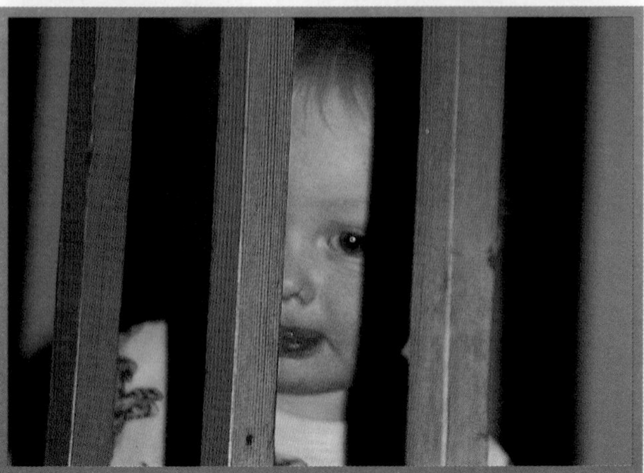

←2.44

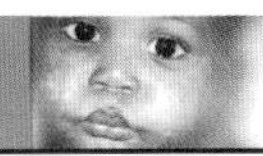

Figure 2.45 Reflexes. Forward parachute: the boy is held prone and then suddenly lowered toward the floor. This is useful in detecting asymmetry in motor function.

1 YEAR

Gross Motor and Posture

Figure 2.46 The child stands alone.

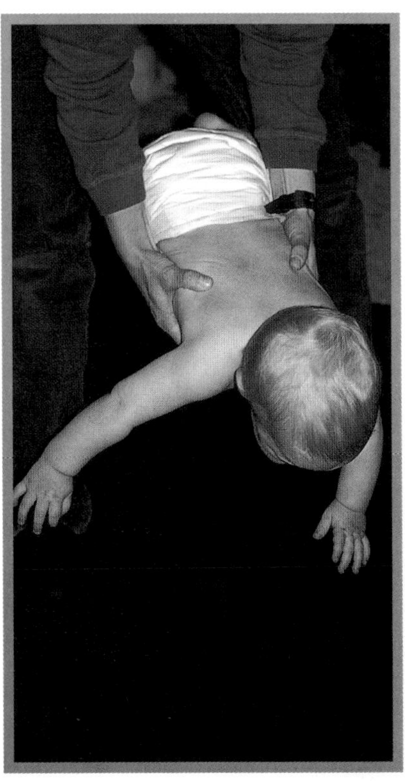

↑ 2.45

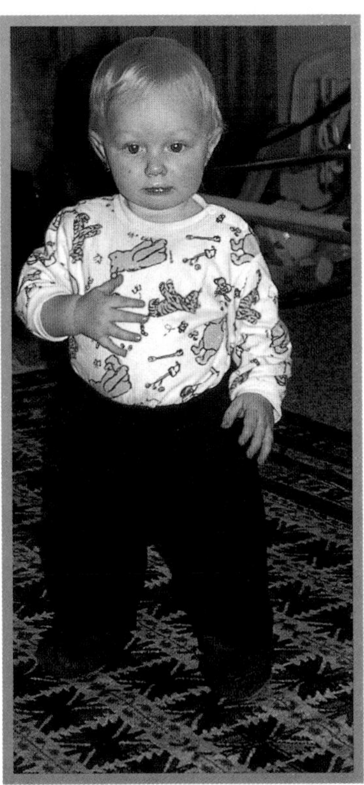

↑ 2.46

Figures 2.47–2.51 Walking. At 11 months, Jacob can walk by holding on to furniture (cruising) (**Figure 2.47**), or with one hand held (**Figure 2.48**). **Figure 2.49** The child begins to take his first steps with a broad-base gait. **Figure 2.50** A few children at this age may crawl upstairs.

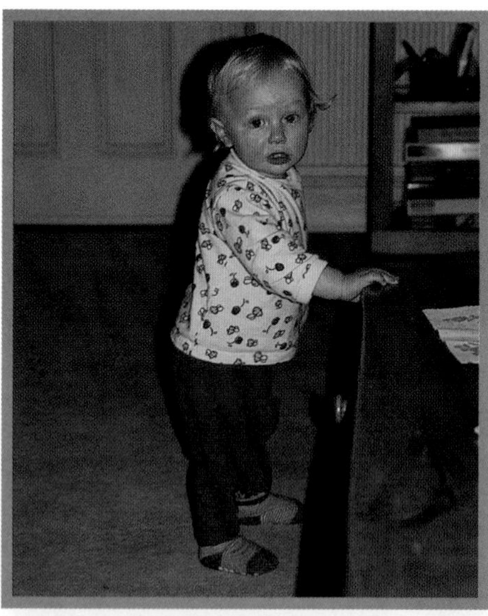

←**2.47**

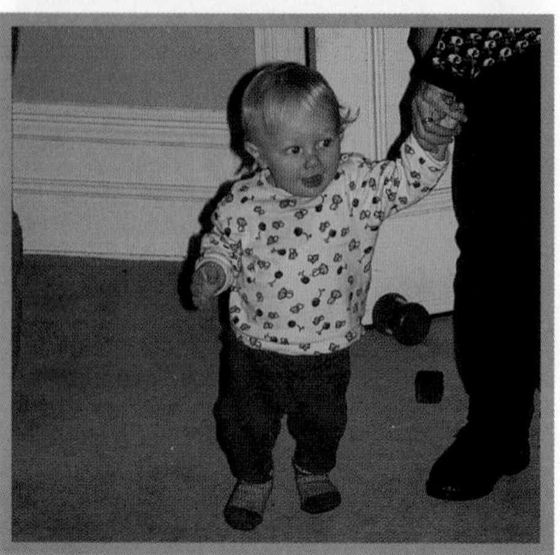

←**2.48**

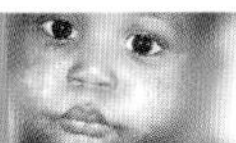

→2.49

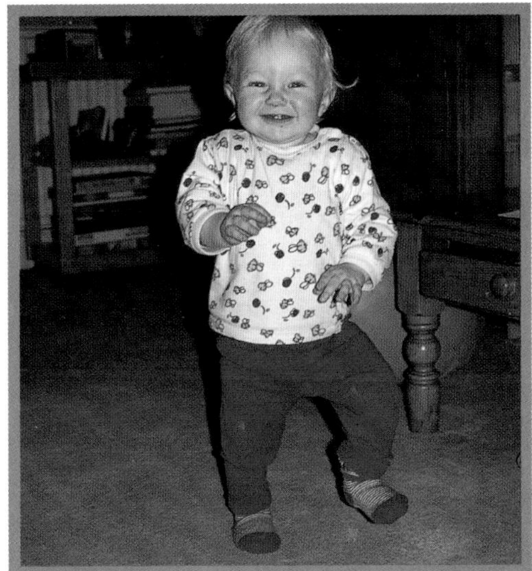

→2.50

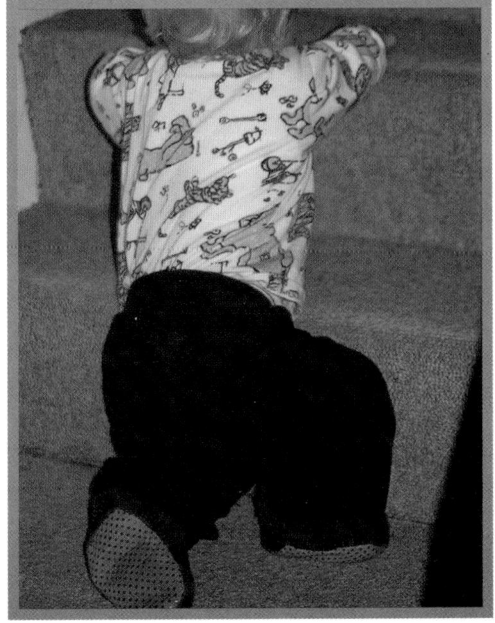

Figure 2.51 A few children at this age may pick up objects from a standing position.

Vision and Fine Motor

Figure 2.52 A mature pincer grasp is used to pick up a raisin.

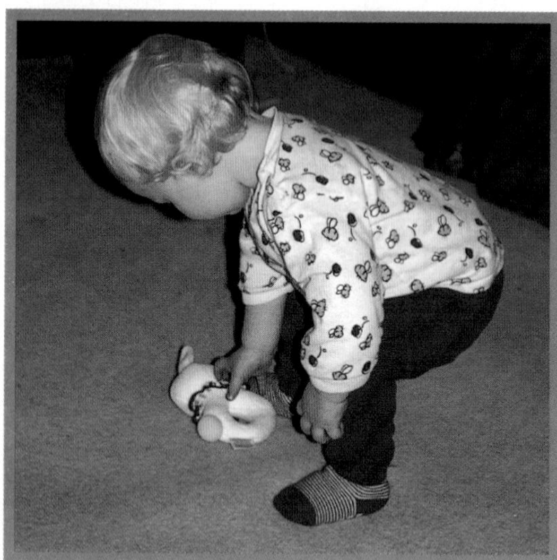

←2.51

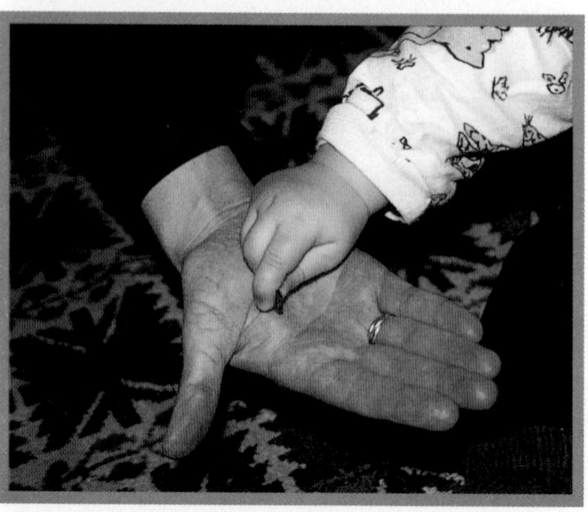

←2.52

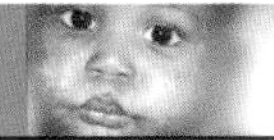

Figure 2.53 'Hundreds and thousands' (tiny objects) are pointed at with the index finger.
Figure 2.54 Two cubes are banged together.

→2.53

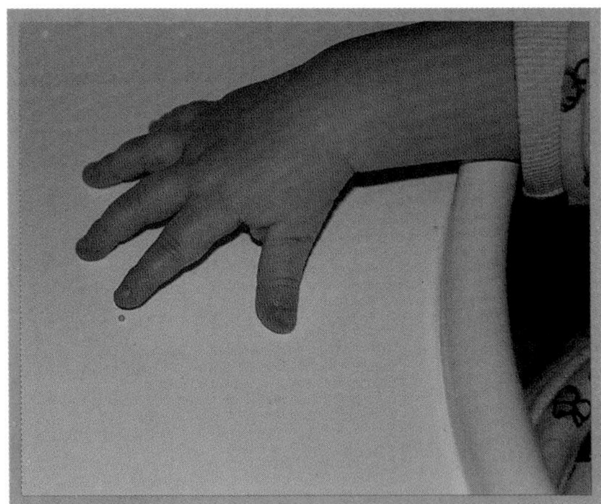

→2.54

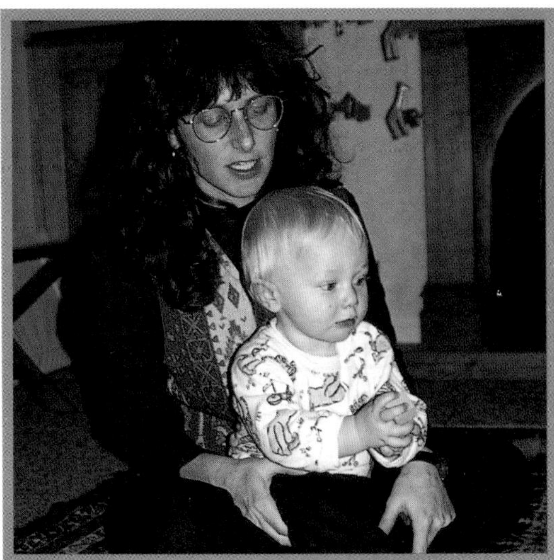

Figure 2.55 Attempts are made to mark paper with a pencil.
Figure 2.56 The child plays pat-a-cake (imitates hand clapping).

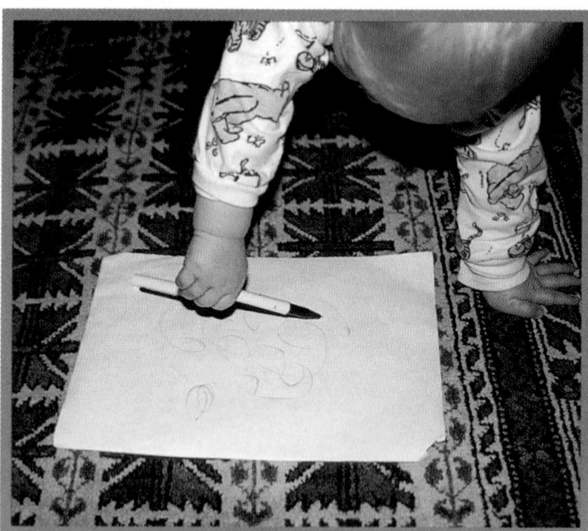

←2.55

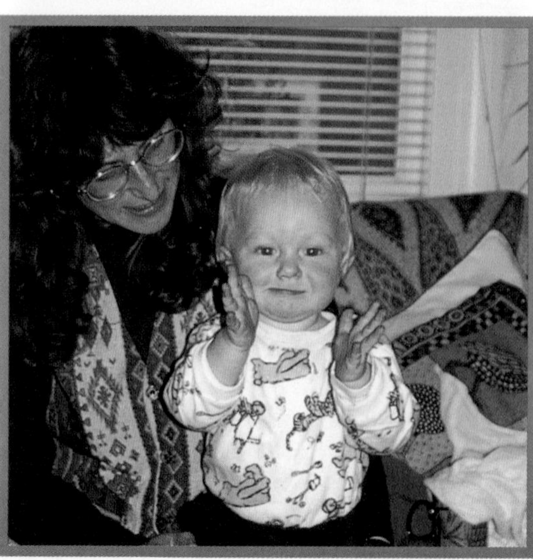

←2.56

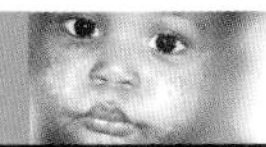

Social Interaction and Play

Figure 2.57 Objects are given by the child on request.

Figures 2.58 and 2.59

A dropped object is sought object permanence has developed.

→ 2.57

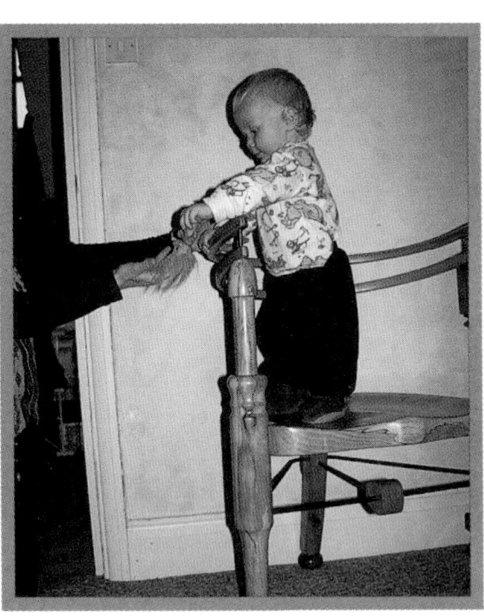

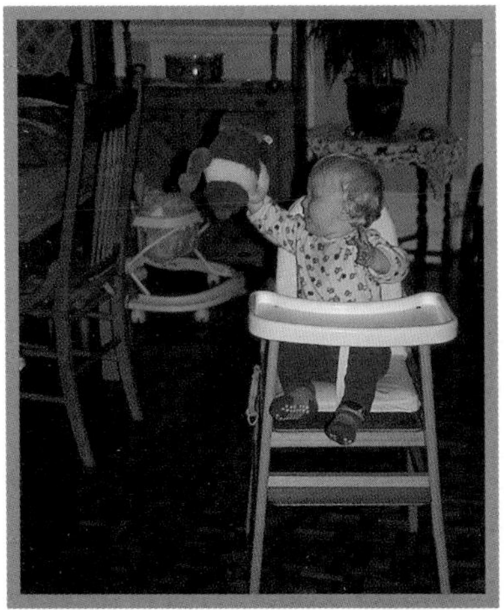

↑ 2.58

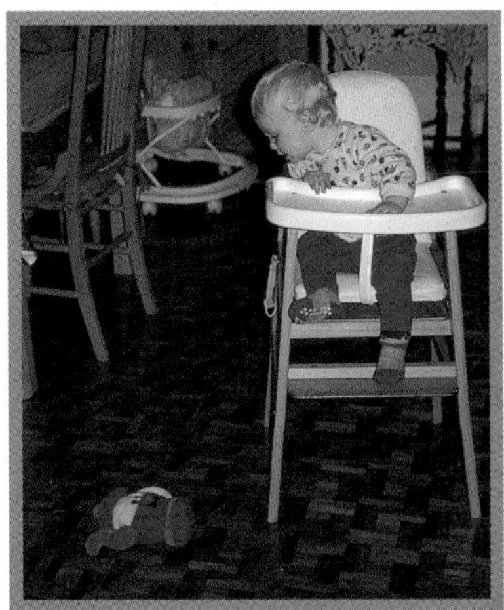

↑ 2.59

Figure 2.60 A ball is rolled toward an adult in reciprocal play.
Figure 2.61 Interest is shown in a book.

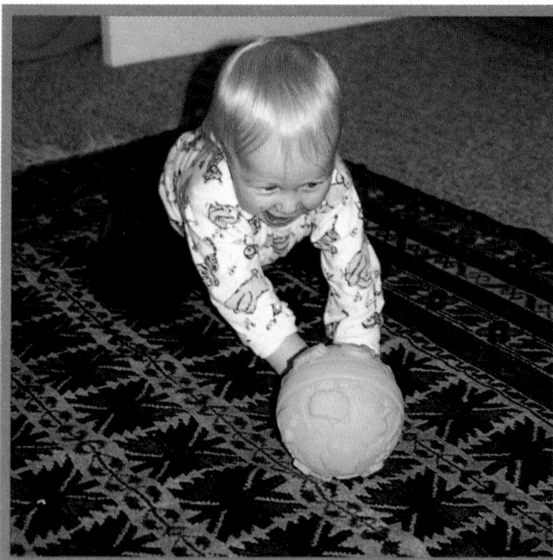

←2.60

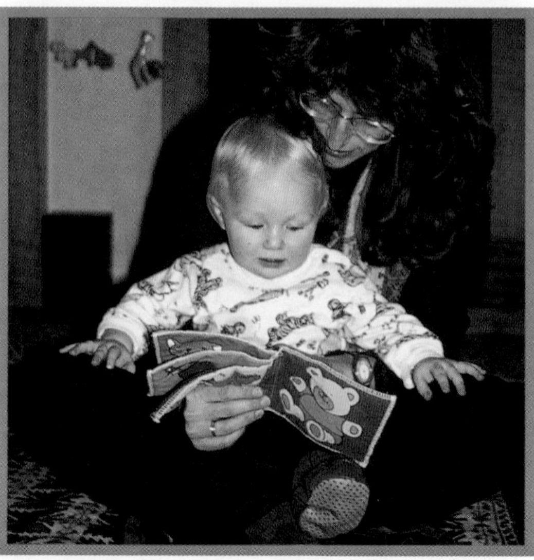

←2.61

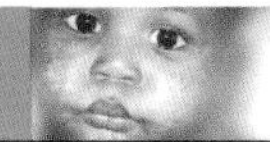

Hearing and Speech

Figures 2.62–2.64 show use of lifesized common objects. This indicates the beginning of comprehensive language.
Figure 2.65 No assistance is needed to drink from a cup.

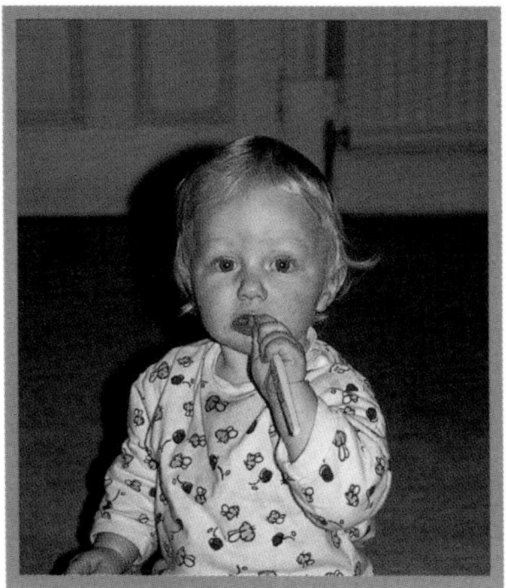

↑ **2.62**

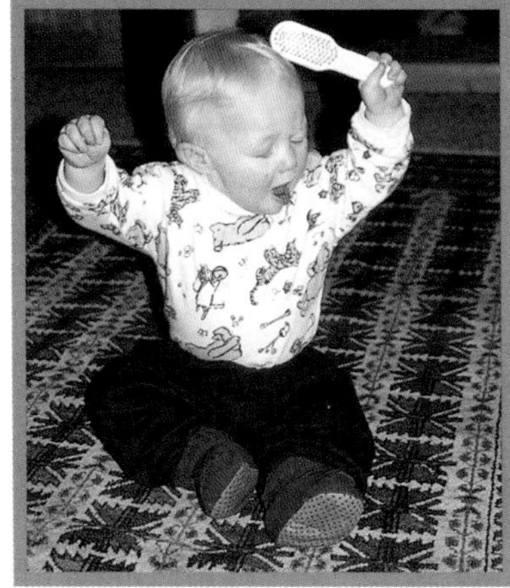

↑ **2.63**

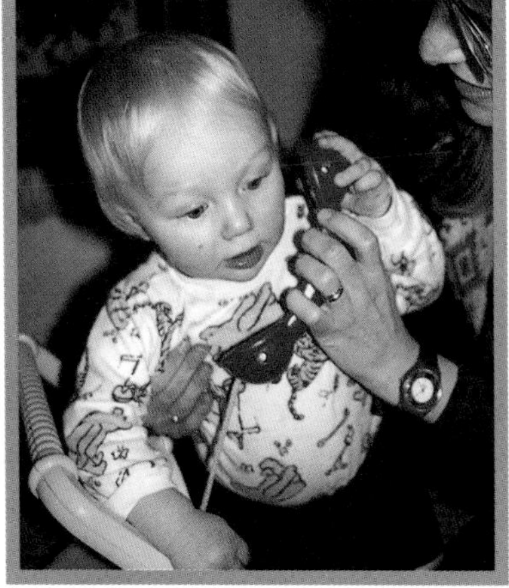

↑ **2.64**

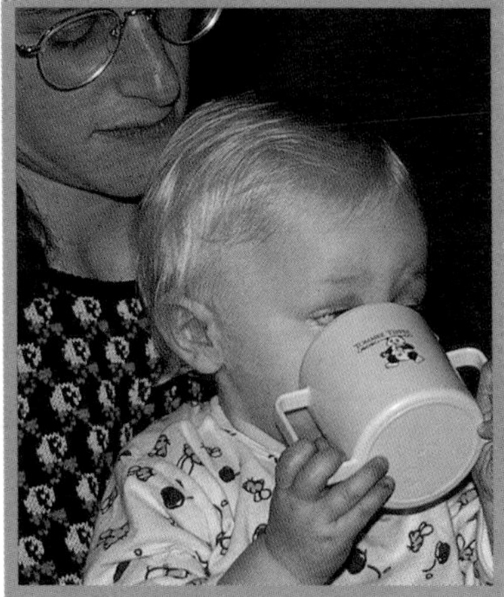

↑ **2.65**

Figure 2.66 The child waves 'bye-bye' on request.

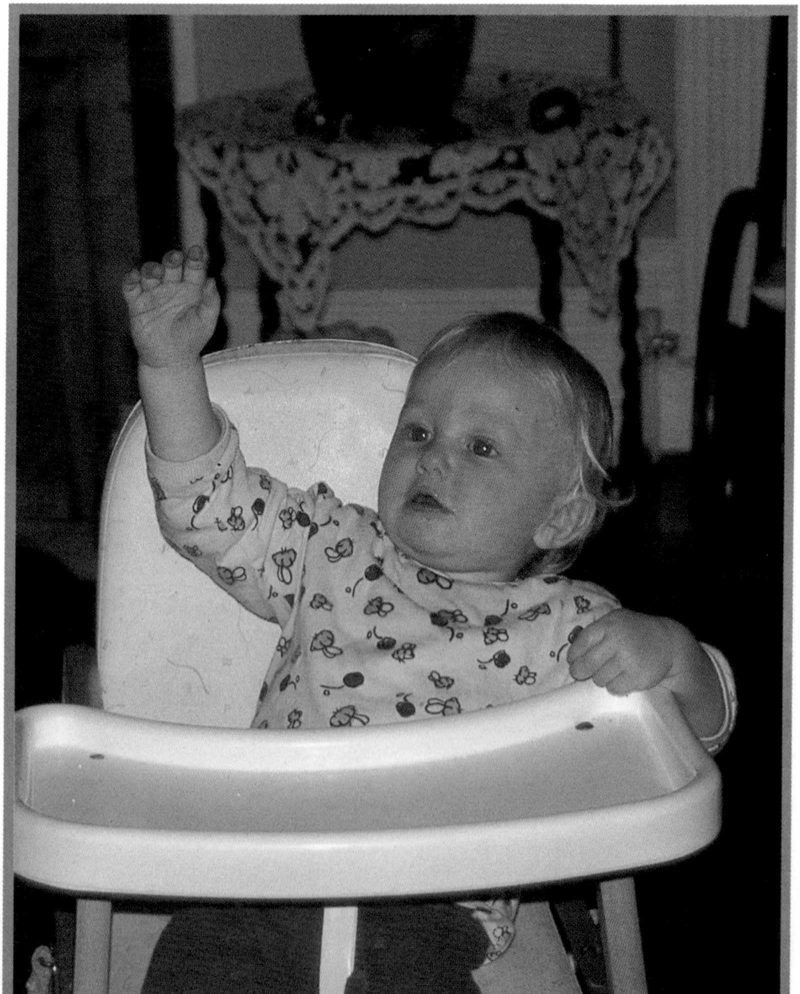

↑**2.66**

3 Cardiac disorders

Figure 3.1 Cyanosed Newborn. A newborn boy is shown with central cyanosis and no respiratory distress. On examination, no heart murmur could be heard but the second heart sound was single and accentuated. The hyperoxic test (the administration of > 90% oxygen for 10 minutes) was positive, *i.e.*, the partial pressure of arterial oxygen did not rise above 14 kPa. A chest X-ray showed the classic egg-on-side appearance with pulmonary plethora and a narrow vascular pedicle. Often, however, there are no chest X-ray changes. An echocardiogram revealed transposition of the great arteries with intact ventricular septum but without pulmonary stenosis.

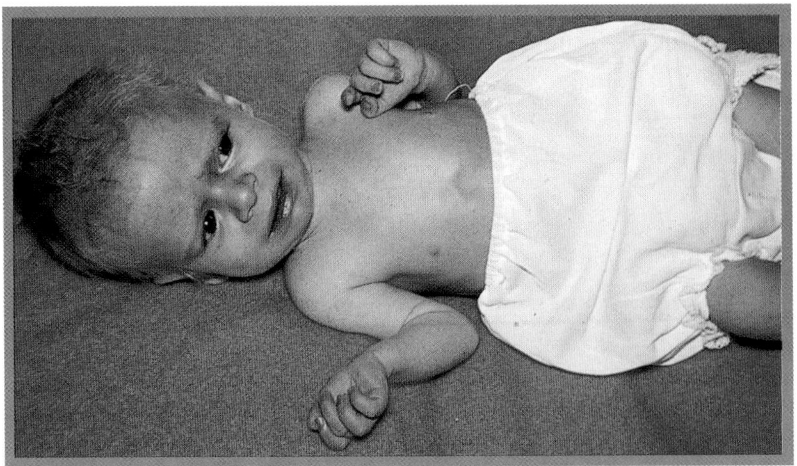

↑ 3.1

Following the diagnosis a Rashkind balloon septostomy was performed, enlarging the atrial–septal communication. The child underwent a switch operation of the great vessels to move them to their anatomically correct position in the first week of life. The differential diagnosis of cyanosis in the first week of life includes:

1. Transposition of the great vessels.
2. Severe tetralogyof Fallot. } these result in oligemic lung fields.
3. Pulmonary atresia. } these result in oligemic lung fields.
4. Tricuspid atresia. } these result in oligemic lung fields.
5. Ebstein anomaly.
6. Obstructive, total, anomalous pulmonary venous drainage, usually of the infracardiac variety.
7. Persistent pulmonary hypertension of the newborn.
8. Pulmonary pathology.
9. Neurological depression, *e.g.*, asphyxia.

Figures 3.2 and 3.3 Ebstein Anomaly. At 1 month of age, a child who was cyanosed from birth had shortness of breath and congestive heart failure, a grossly enlarged heart on chest X-ray with prominent right atrium and pulmonary oligemia.
The electrocardiogram (ECG) showed giant P-waves, prolonged PR interval and right bundle branch block. An echocardiogram confirmed the abnormal anatomy of the tricuspid valve. Differential diagnosis includes tricuspid valve dysplasia.

The respiratory difficulties are due to hypoplasia of the lung resulting from intrauterine compression. The cyanosis generally resolves as pulmonary vascular resistance falls during the first weeks of life. There are few causes of a large heart at birth, and these include a volume-overloaded heart, *e.g.*, common arterial trunk (truncus arteriosus), cerebral arteriovenous malformation, and disorders of the

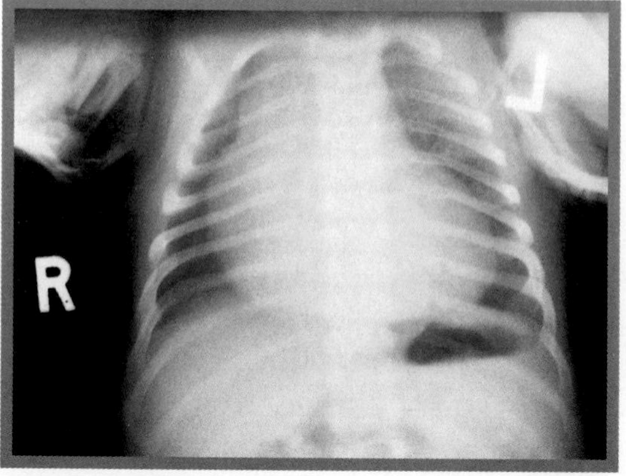

← 3.2

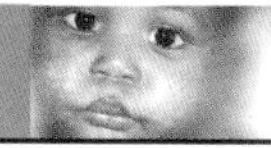

myocardium itself, *e.g.*, metabolic myopathy such as Pompé and dilated cardiomyopathy.

Figure 3.3 shows Ebstein anomaly in a 16-year-old. Note the enlarged heart with a specifically prominent right heart border due to right atrial enlargement. Additionally, there is abnormal convexity of the upper left heart border due to dilatation of the right ventricular outflow tract. There are normal pulmonary vascular markings present. In Ebstein anomaly, the greater portion of the valve is attached to the ventricular wall rather than the fibrous ring, resulting in atrialization of the inlet portion of the right ventricle. As shown above clinically, there is a wide spectrum of symptoms (depending on the degree of malattachment of the valve) from absence of symptoms through to death in early life. Rhythm disorders occur, so affected children are sometimes advised to avoid competitive sports.

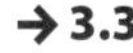
→3.3

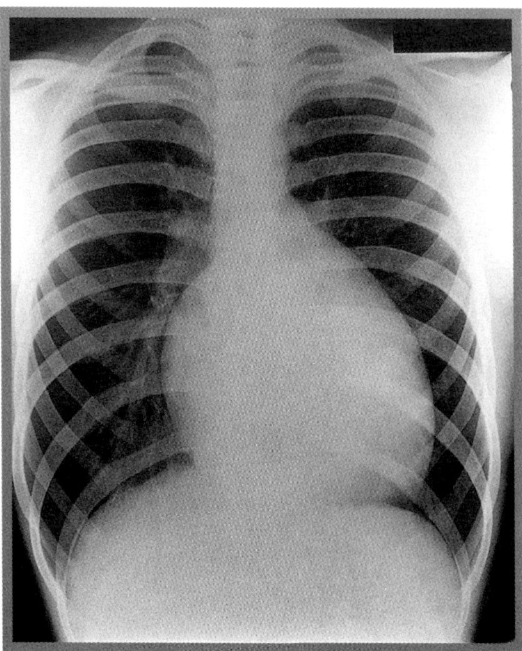

Figure 3.4 Central Cyanosis. The figure shows central cyanosis in a 12-year-old boy who presented with late-diagnosed tetralogy of Fallot. This child had increasing cyanosis, having been acyanotic at birth with hypercyanotic spells occurring from 6 years of age. The spells were precipitated by exercise and relieved by squatting. Note also the plethoric facies secondary to polycythemia. On examination, he had a pulmonary ejection systolic murmur with a single second heart sound.

Figures 3.5–3.8 Tetralogy of Fallot. Note the central cyanosis with a right thoracotomy scar from a Blalock–Taussig shunt (right subclavian to right pulmonary artery) that was inserted to increase pulmonary blood flow, by creating an artificial L to R shunt and increasing pulmonary blood flow.

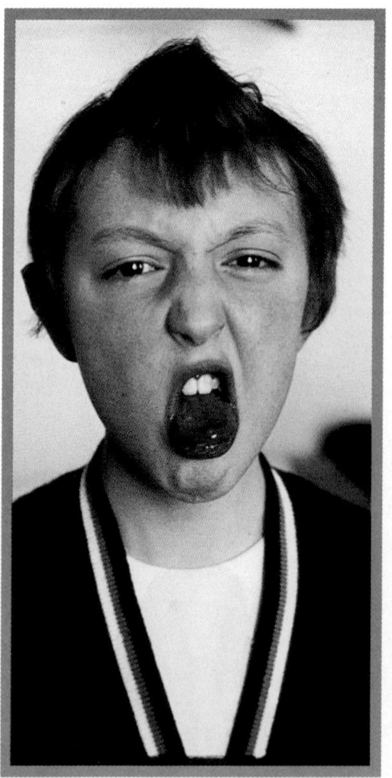

↑3.4

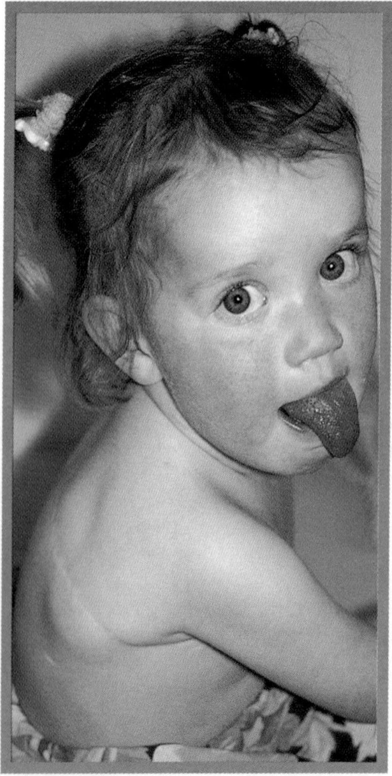

↑3.5

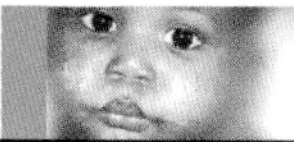

She also has clubbing of the fingers and toes (see **Figures 3.6** and **3.7**). Clubbing is seen in the feet first, starting with the great toe.

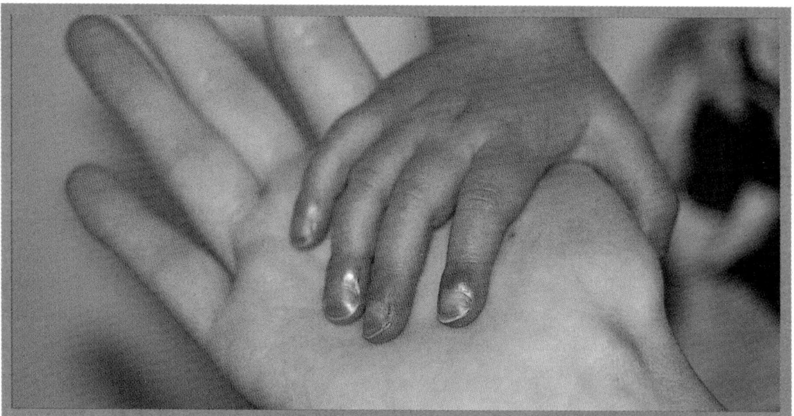

↑ 3.6

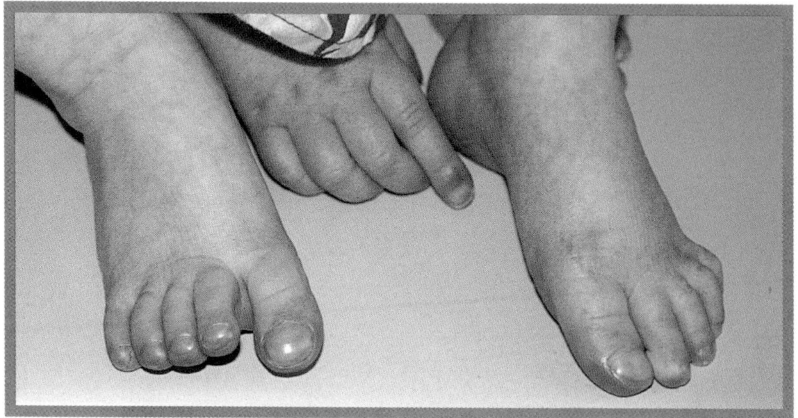

↑ 3.7

Figure 3.8 shows a chest X-ray of the same child prior to surgical intervention. Note the typical 'coeur en sabot' due to an upturned apex from the right ventricular enlargement. There is a right aortic arch, a pulmonary bay from hypoplasia of pulmonary outflow tract, and pulmonary oligemia. The electrocardiogram showed right axis deviation, right atrial enlargement and right ventricular hypertrophy.
Tetralogy of Fallot consists of:

1. Pulmonary outflow stenosis.
2. Ventricular septal defect.
3. Overriding aorta.
4. Right ventricular hypertrophy due to outflow tract obstruction.

Tetralogy of Fallot is the commonest of the cyanotic heart defects. Hypercyanotic spells (spelling) should be treated by putting the child in the knee–chest position (so increasing systemic vascular resistance),administrating oxygen, correcting acidosis and giving intravenous morphine and propanalol. Total repair of the defect is now usually performed within the first 2 years of life.

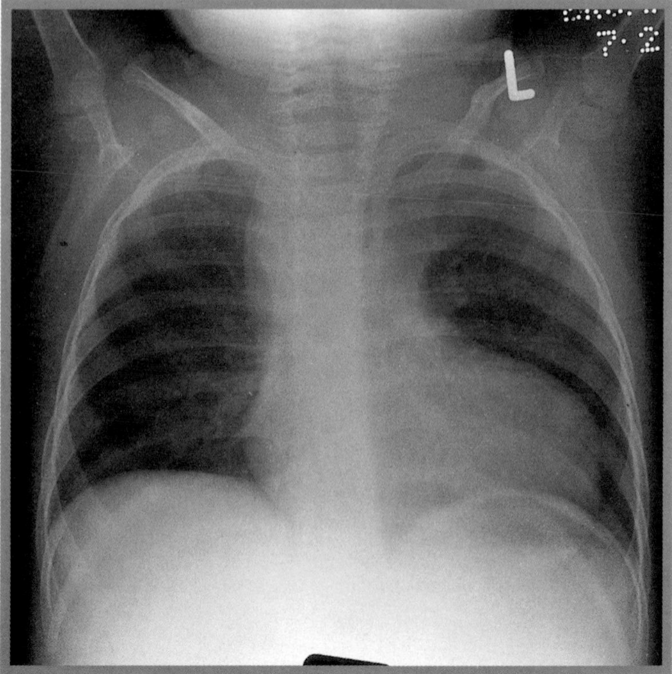

←3.8

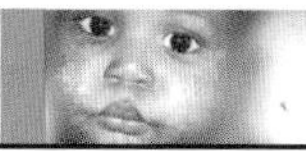

Figures 3.9–3.11 Ventricular Septal Defect. The 7-year-old boy shown in **Figure 3.9** has an untreated ventricular septal defect. He suffered from repeated chest infections. Note the chest deformity with precordial prominence and a bulging sternum due to cardiomegaly. Harrison sulci are present due to pulmonary edema, causing stiff lungs and increased breathing labour and subsequent failure to thrive. On examination, there was a right ventricular heave and left ventricular thrust. A thrill could be felt at the lower left sternal border associated with a pansystolic murmur. The second heart sound was normally split with a loud pulmonary component.

→3.9

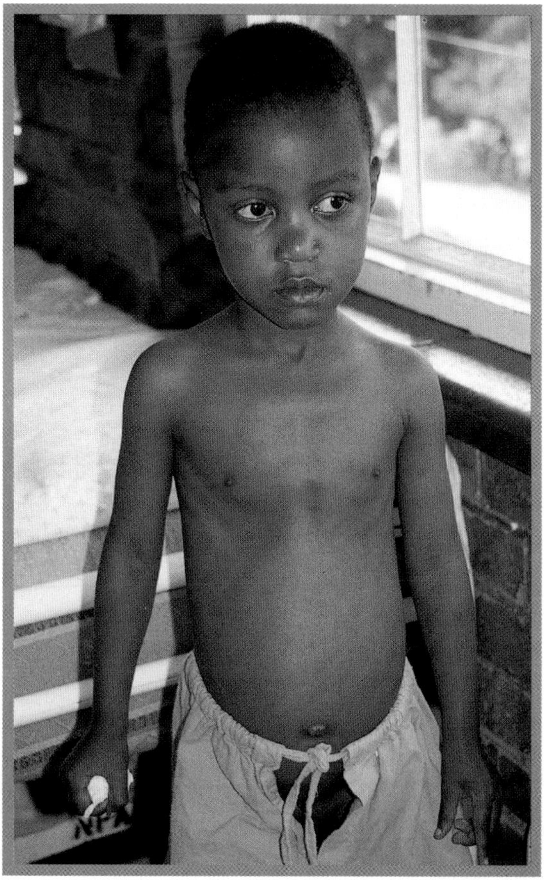

A chest X-ray of the same child shows pulmonary plethora associated with a prominent pulmonary artery (**Figure 3.10**). The heart size is normal. **Figure 3.11** shows the post-operative chest X-ray on another patient where despite surgical repair for ventricular septal defect, the patient went on to develop vascular disease. The chest X-ray reveals peripheral pulmonary vessel pruning and a large pulmonary artery typical of this condition.The echocardiogram showed equal systemic and pulmonary pressures.

A ventricular septal defect is the most common heart defect presenting with either a murmur or cardiac failure. The prognosis for ventricular septal defect is that 50% will close spontaneously. Of the remainder, and depending upon the degree of left-to-right shunt and subsequent development of pulmonary hypertension, operative closure may be necessary. If pulmonary hypertension is not reversible on administration of a high concentration of oxygen and vasodilators, *e.g.*, nitric oxide, then the condition is considered inoperable, and reversal of the shunt with cyanosis and later polycythaemia, with development of right-sided failure will occur, *i.e.,* Eisenmenger syndrome.

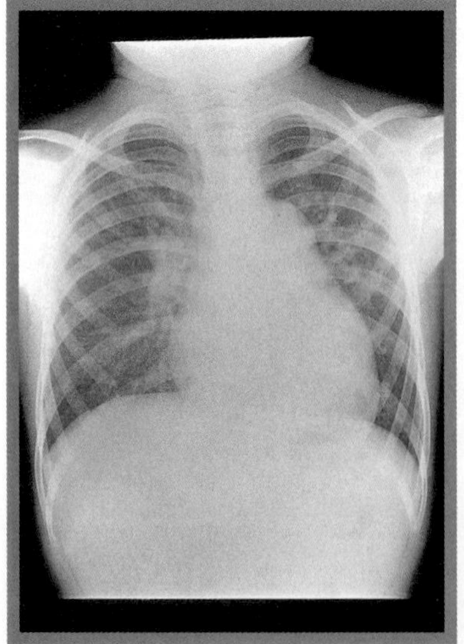

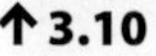

↑3.10

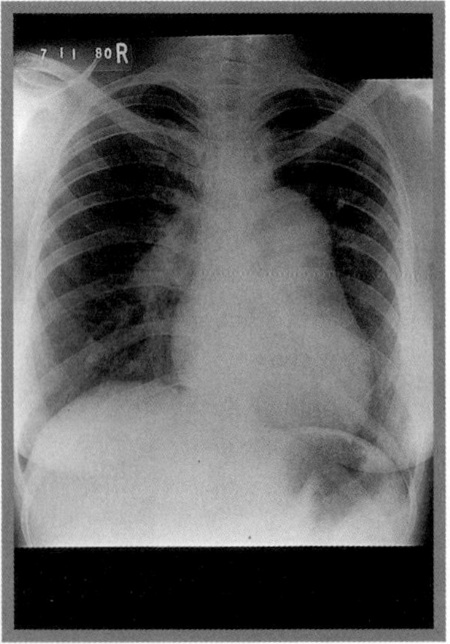

↑3.11

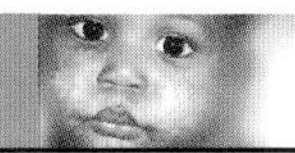

Figure 3.12 Transposition of the Great Arteries. The 10-year-old boy shown presented late with central cyanosis, clubbing, marked failure to thrive and polycythemia. He has a bulging precordium and central thoracotomy scar from a Rastelli operation – closure of the ventricular septal defect and insertion of a homograft between the right ventricle and pulmonary artery to restore a normalized circulation. This child had transposition of the great arteries, ventricular septal defect and pulmonary stenosis.

→3.12

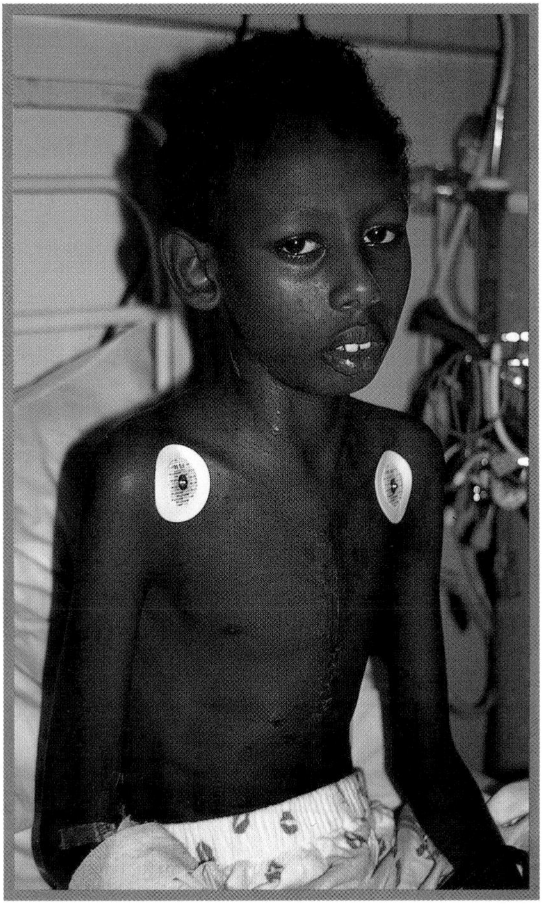

Figure 3.13 Right Lateral Thoracotomy Scar. The figure shows a 1-year-old child with pulmonary atresia who required a Blalock–Taussig shunt in the newborn period. Diagnosis had been made antenatally and the child had been treated initially with a prostaglandin infusion to maintain duct patency. Other conditions in which ductal patency needs to be maintained are: pulmonary atresia, critical pulmonary stenosis, aortic atresia, critical aortic stenosis, coarctation, and possibly transposition of the great arteries.
A left thoracotomy scar is seen after:
1. Blalock–Taussig shunt.
2. Patent arterial duct closure.
3. Coarctation repair.
4. Banding of pulmonary trunk .
5. Pulmonary surgery.

A right thoracotomy scar is seen after:
1. Blalock–Taussig shunt insertion.
2. Pulmonary surgery.

Figure 3.14 CHARGE Anomaly. A child with CHARGE anomaly is shown (see **Chapter 4, Respiratory Disorders** for a full description), with central thoracotomy scar following closure of an atrioventricular septal defect. A central thoracotomy scar generally indicates open heart surgery.

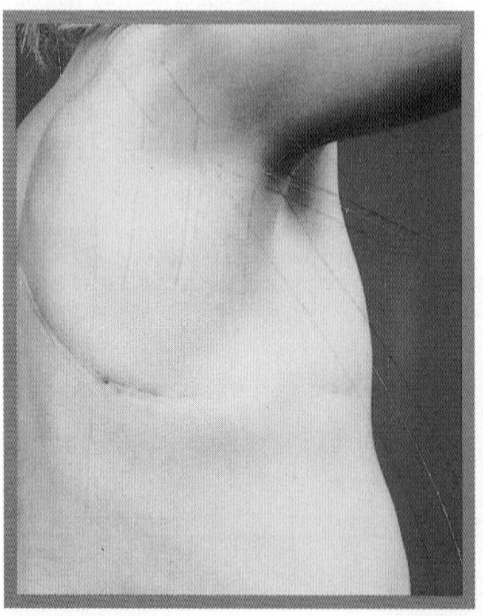

↑3.13

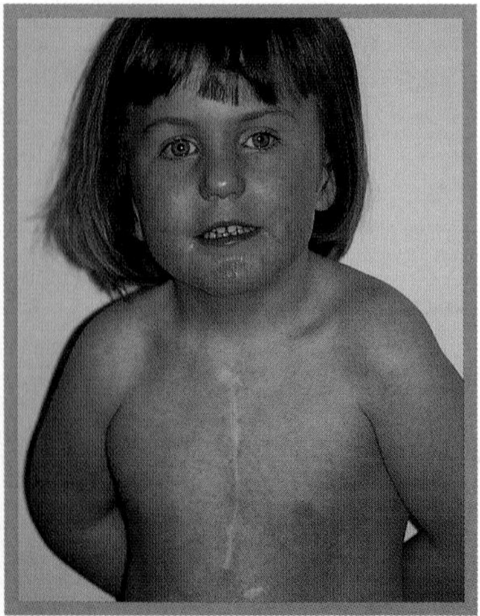

↑3.14

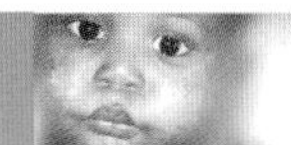

Congenital Heart Disease Associated with Syndromes

Figure 3.15 Down Syndrome. This is commonly associated with atrioventricular septal defect, ventricular septal defect, atrial septal defect, patent arterial duct and tetralogy of Fallot. For further details, see **figures 1.9–1.17**.

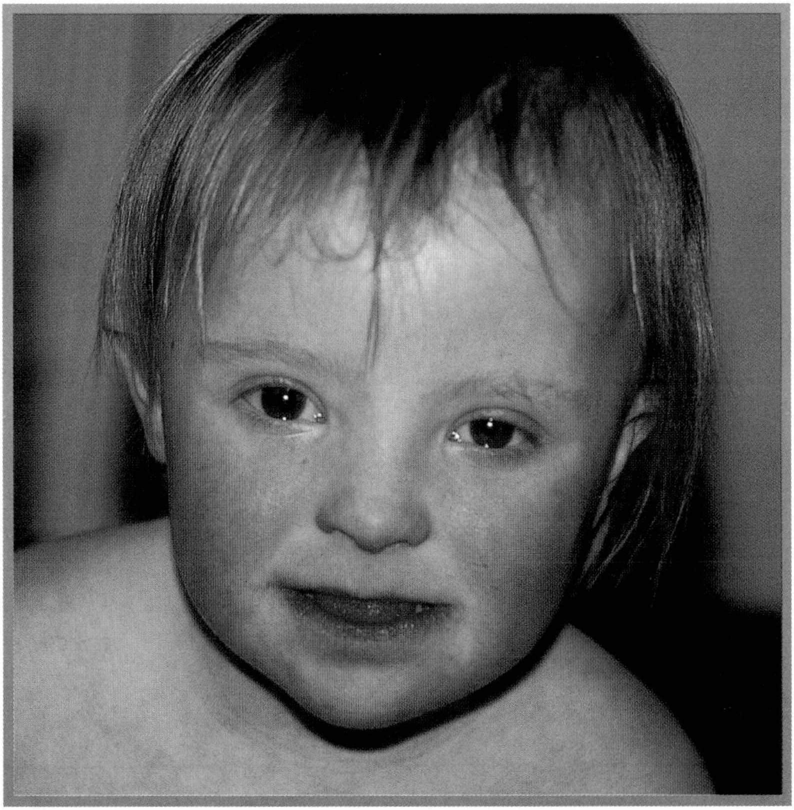

↑3.15

Figures 3.16 and 3.17 Williams Syndrome. Williams syndrome is shown here in a 1-year-old boy (left)and an 8-year-old girl (right). **Figure 3.16** shows the elfin facies, medial eyebrow flare, hypertelorism, the stellate pattern of the iris, periorbital fullness, drooping cheeks, long philtrum, fish lips, large open mouth, upturned nose and low-set ears. In **Figure 3.17**, this older girl had an inguinal hernia repair. She had been treated for a squint and had the typical cocktail party affect.

Both children had supravalvular aortic stenosis. Other heart diseases associated with this condition are peripheral pulmonary stenosis and coarctation of the aorta. Hypercalcemia was not detectable in either child at the time of diagnosis but is an important association during the neonatal period.

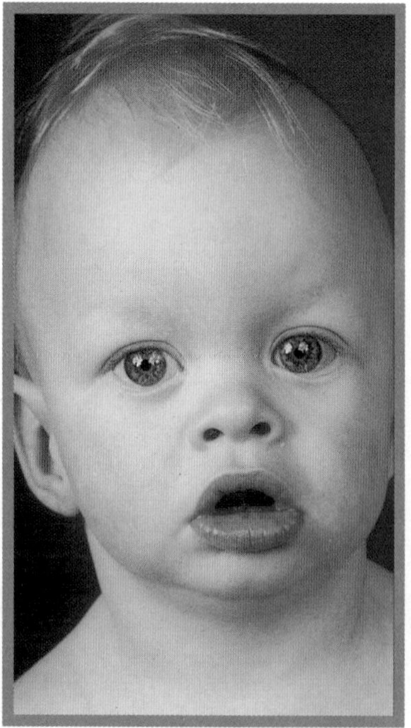

↑ **3.16**

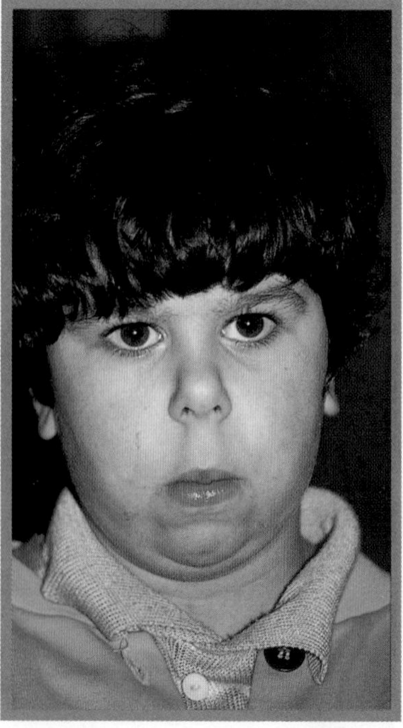

↑ **3.17**

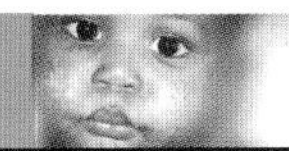

Figures 3.18 and 3.19 Noonan Syndrome. A 13-year-old boy (left) and a 7-year-old girl (right) are shown. Note the carrying angle, wide spaced nipples, neck webbing and short stature in **Figure 3.18**. **Figure 3.19** shows low-set, posteriorly rotated ears, ptosis and thick wavy hair. Additionally, the girl had pulmonary stenosis and the boy had hypertrophic cardiomyopathy. This condition should be differentiated from Turner Syndrome (see **Chapter 9, Endocrine and metabolic disorders**) which is phenotypically similar but associated with different cardiac lesions (coarctation of the aorta, aortic stenosis and atrial septal defect).

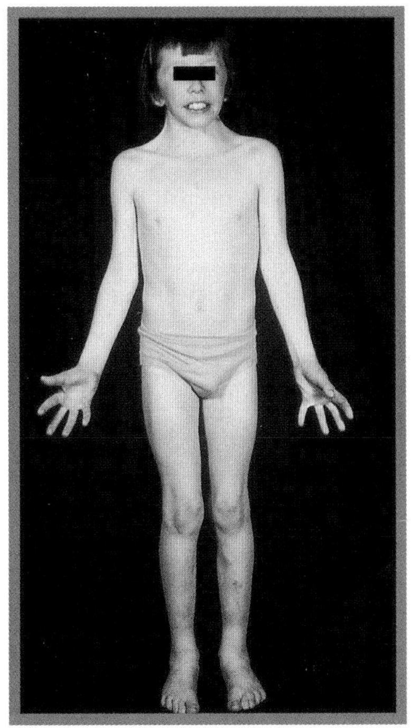

↑3.18

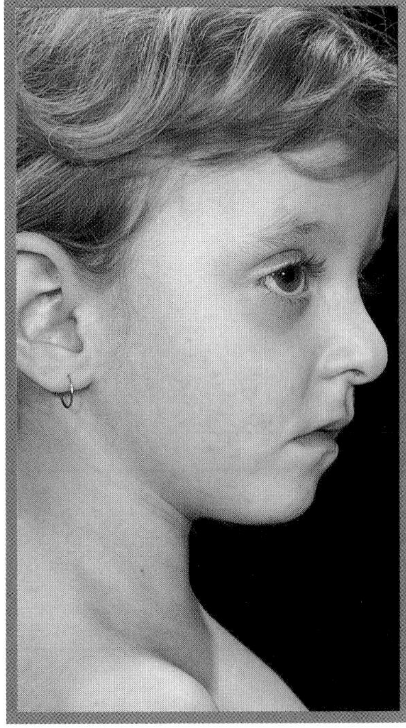

↑3.19

Figure 3.20 Di George Syndrome. This boy, aged 5, was diagnosed in the newborn period with DiGeorge syndrome. He shows low-set ears with mild hypertelorism, a small jaw, a short philtrum, and an upturned nose. He also had thymic hypoplasia and absent parathyroid glands. This syndrome is also associated with common artrerial trunk, Tetralogy of Fallot, a right-sided aortic arch and an interrupted aortic arch. Children with this syndrome often present with hypocalcemia in the first few days of life. Cytogenetic investigation may demonstrate chromosome 22q deletion by FISH (Fluorescent In-Situ Hybridization) techniques. The same phenotype is seen in Velo-Cardio-Facial (Shprintzen) syndrome.

Figures 3.21–3.23 Holt–Oram Syndrome. This boy, aged 5, presented with skeletal malformations: there was bilateral radial hypoplasia, which was more prominent on the left (**Figure 3.21**) an absent thumb on the left hand (**Figure 3.22**) and a hypoplastic thumb on the right (**Figure 3.23**), note the dressing covering the central thoracotomy scar that follows atrial septal defect repair. More rarely, children with this condition may have a ventricular septal defect or other lesions. This is an autosomal dominant condition with varied expression.

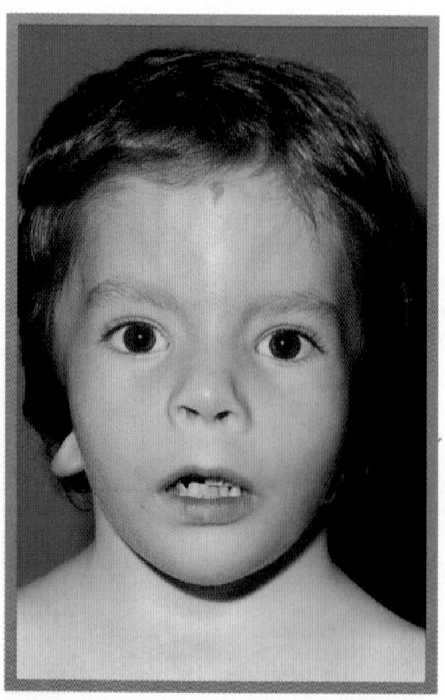

↑ 3.20

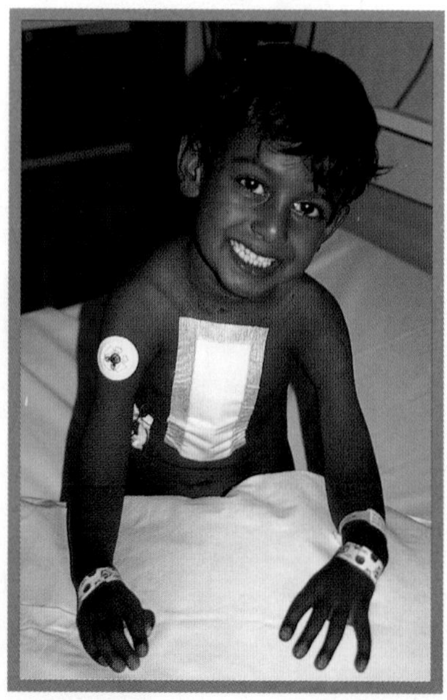

↑ 3.21

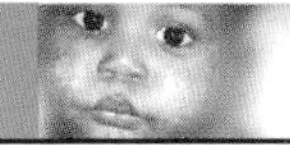

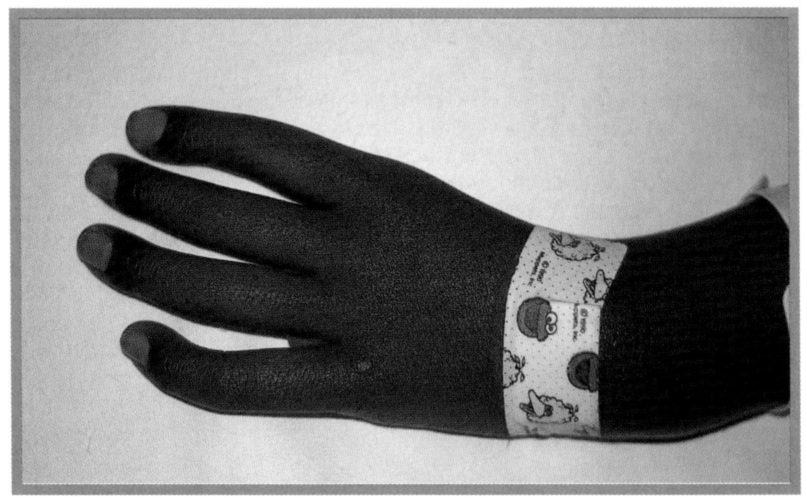

↑ 3.22

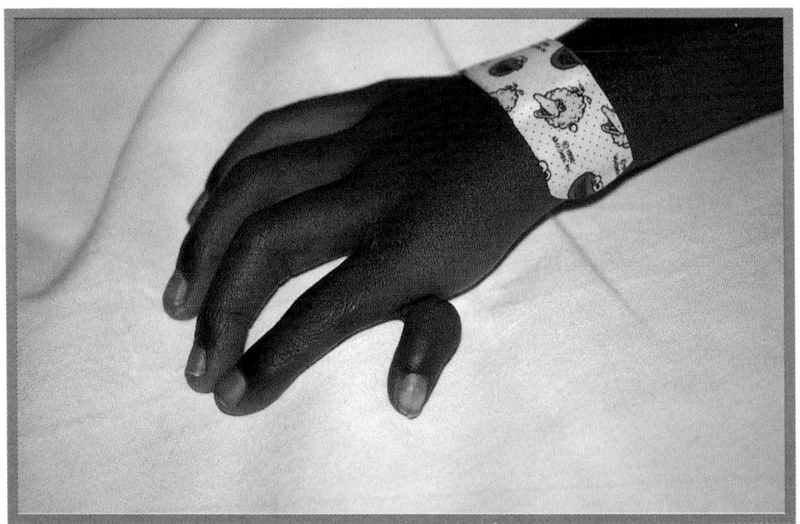

↑ 3.23

Figure 3.24 Obstructed Total Anomalous Pulmonary Venous Connection (Supracardiac). Shown is a chest X-ray of an 8-month-old child who presented cyanosed in the neonatal period. There is increased pulmonary vascular markings due to a combination of plethora and pulmonary edema. The heart size is normal, and there are dilated systemic veins in the supramediastinum. This demonstrates the classic 'cottage loaf' appearance. Treatment consists of correction of the anomalous venous return.

Figure 3.25 Pulmonary Embolism in Infectious Endocarditis. Note in this x-ray the clearly demarcated wedge-shaped opacity adjacent to the pleural edge in the right mid zone, and the prominence of the right heart border. This is a hazard of right-sided endocarditis in the presence of an additional right-to-left shunt. This patient may have presented with cerebral abscesses and systemic septic emboli.

Figure 3.26 Vascular Ring. This x-ray shows a barium swallow in an infant who presented with stridor in the newborn period. It demonstrates a (posteriorly) filling defect in the middle third of the esophagus due to double aortic-arch encircling the esophagus. Differential diagnosis of stridor in the newborn period includes:

1. Laryngomalacia.
2. Superior mediastinal mass compressing the trachea.
3. Gross gastroesophageal reflux with laryngospasm.
4. Anomalous vessels.

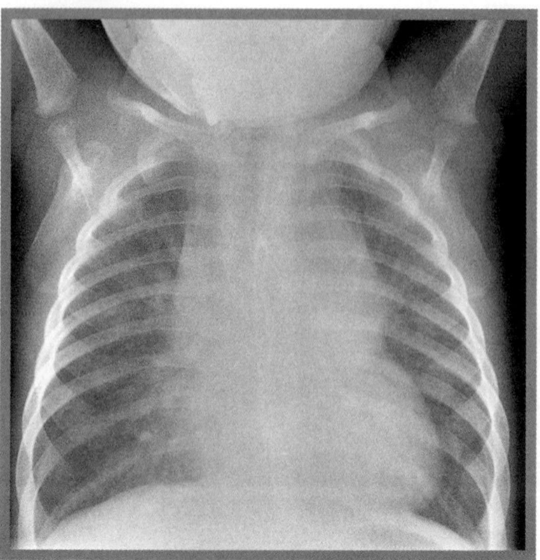

←3.24

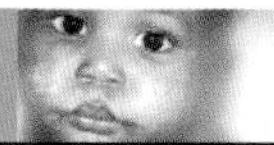

→3.25

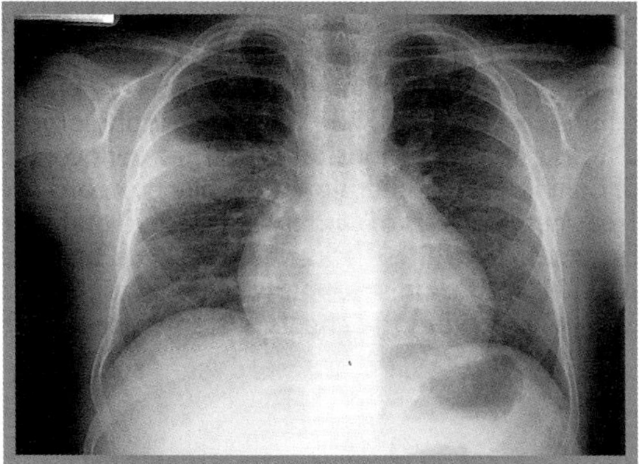

→3.26

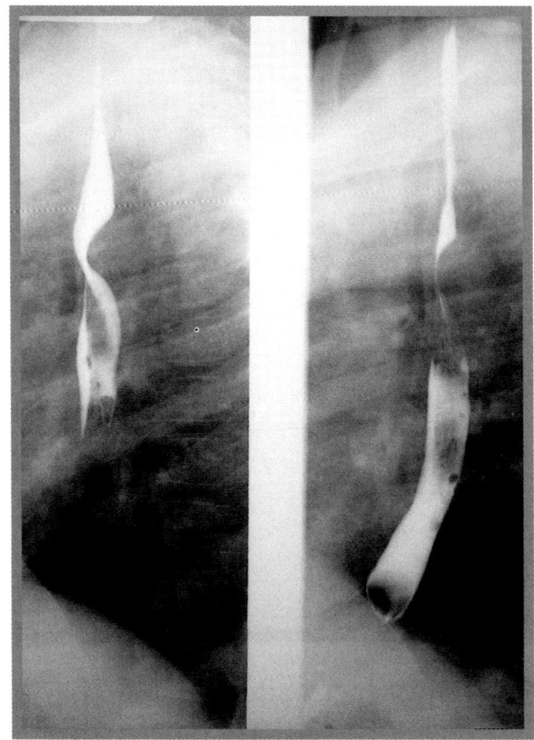

Figure 3.27 Arteriovenous Malformation in the Brain (Vein of Galen Malformation). This consists of massive cardiomegaly with congestive cardiac failure. The newborn infant discussed here presented with refractory heart failure and cyanosis. The heart is morphologically normal, but a cerebral ultrasound scan demonstrated a large arteriovenous malformation of the vein of Galen. A celebral bruit will usually be heard over the anterior fontanelle. Treatment consists of surgery or transcatheter embolization.

Figures 3.28 and 3.29 Pericardial Effusion. Chest X-rays of a child with massive pericardial effusion secondary to rheumatic heart disease are shown. **Figure 3.29** demonstrates the effects of steroids on the effusion.

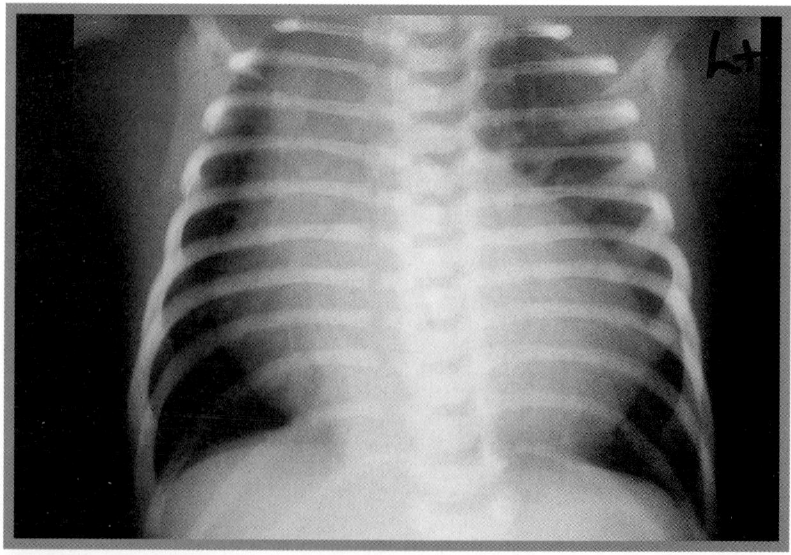

↑3.27

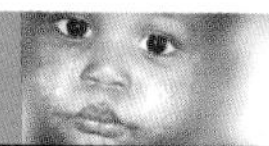

→ 3.28

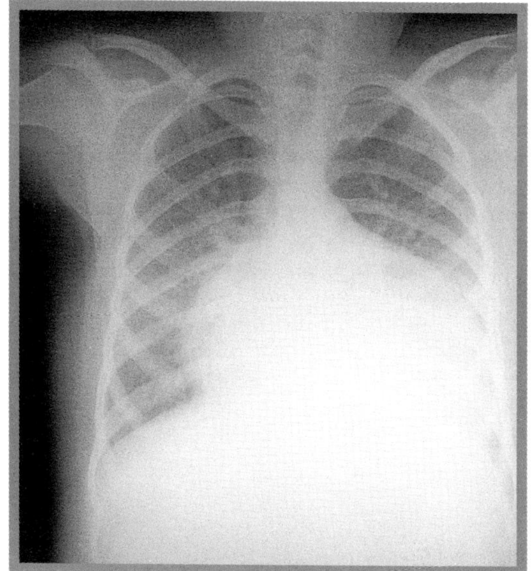

→ 3.29

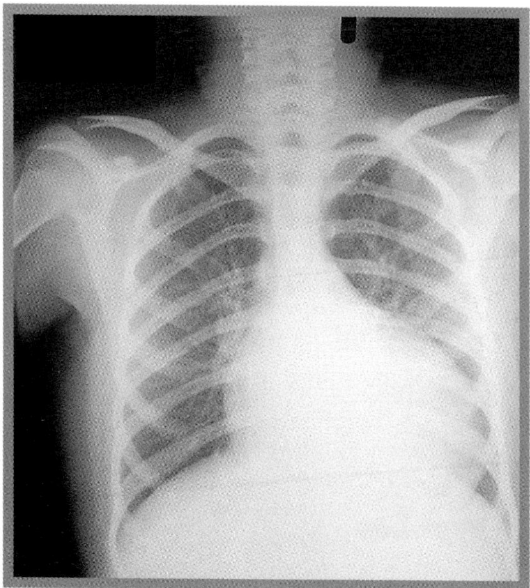

Figures 3.30 and 3.31 Pericardial Effusion. The pericardial effusion seen here was secondary to hemophilus pericarditis in an 8-month-old baby. The infant presented with septic shock. A chest X-ray revealed a large globular heart, and an echocardiogram revealed pericardial effusion. Percutaneous drainage (**Figure 3.31**) withdrew 200 ml of pus that grew *Hemophilus influenzae* type B. The child made a complete recovery.

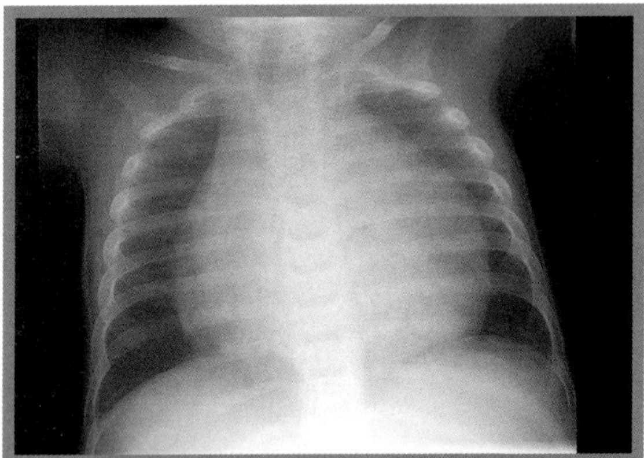

←3.30

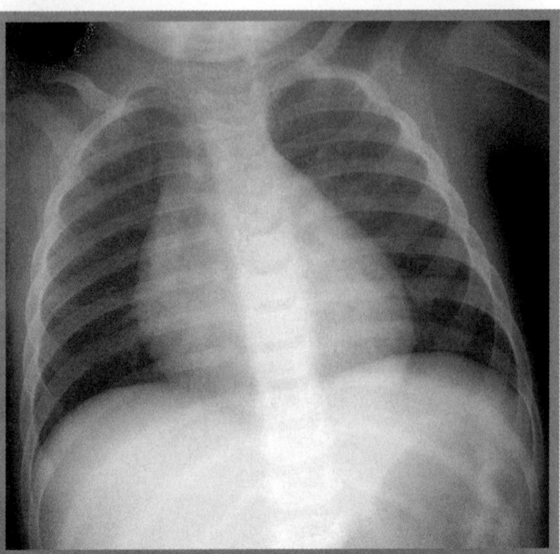

←3.31

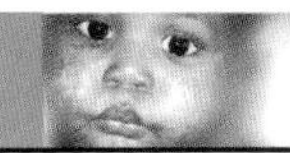

Figure 3.32 Large Patent Arterial Duct. This is a high, parasternal echocardiogram showing a left-to-right shunt (in red) through the arterial duct (D) connecting the aorta (AO) and pulmonary trunk (PT).

Figure 3.33 Echocardiogram of Rhabdomyoma. The 6-month-old baby discussed here presented with salaam attacks and was found to have tuberous sclerosis (see **Chapter 7**, **Neurology**). Echocardiography reveals a well-circumscribed, highly echogenic area in the region facing the left ventricular and septal aspect. This represents a rhabdomyoma. Interestingly, rhabdomyomas may resolve spontaneously before neurological diagnosis is made.

→3.32

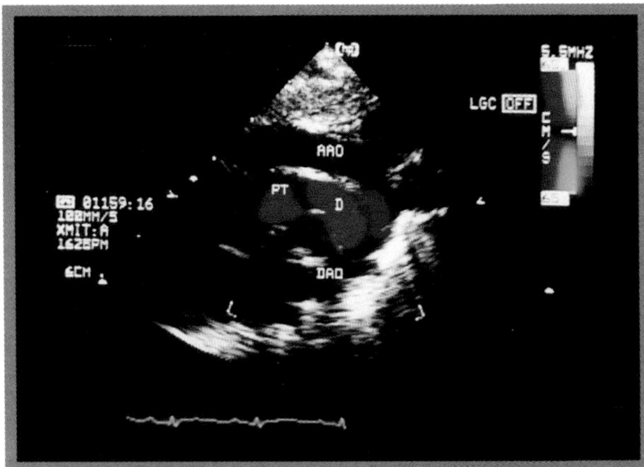

→3.33

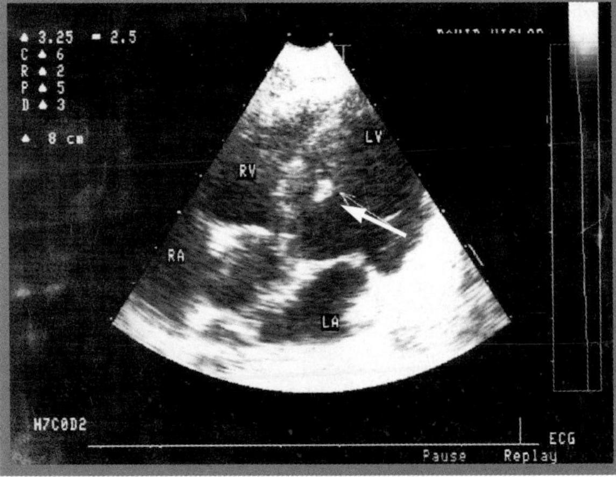

Figure 3.34 Ostium Primum Atrial Septal Defect. Echocardiogram of this partial atrioventricular septal defect. Note the obvious communication between the right and left atria above the atrioventricular valve in this (four-chamber view) echocardiogram.The atrio-ventricular valves take off at the same level (shown with arrow).

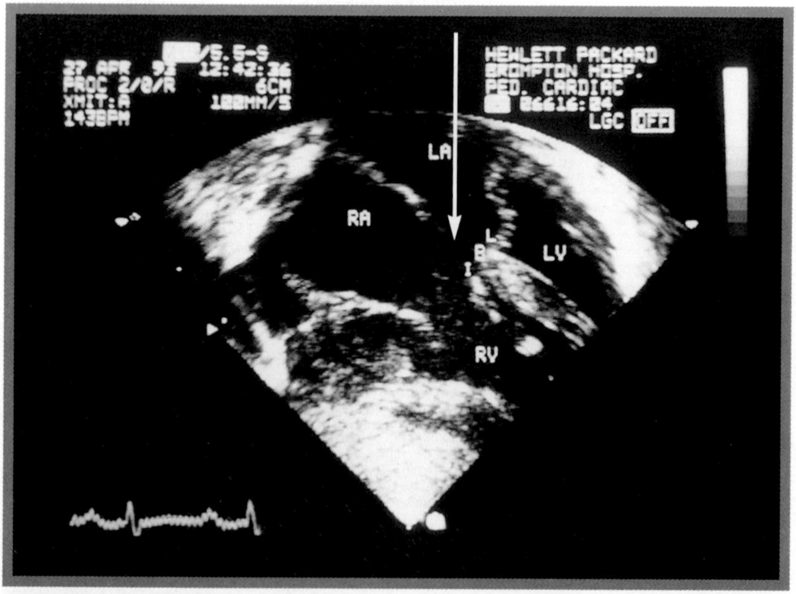

↑ 3.34

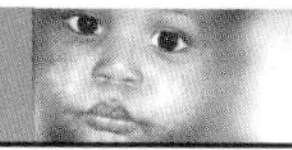

Figure 3.35 Large Muscular Ventricular Septal Defect. A large muscular defect can be seen in the septum (S) on both views, between the right ventricle (RV) and left ventricle (LV). **Figure 3.35a** shows a four-chamber view, and **Figure 3.35b** shows a short-axis view.

→ 3.35a

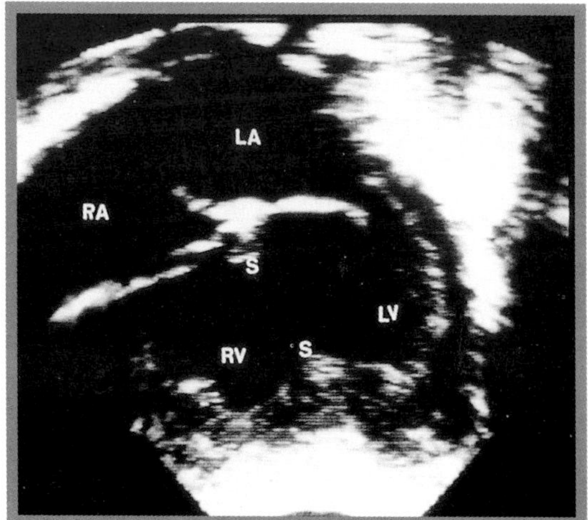

→ 3.35b

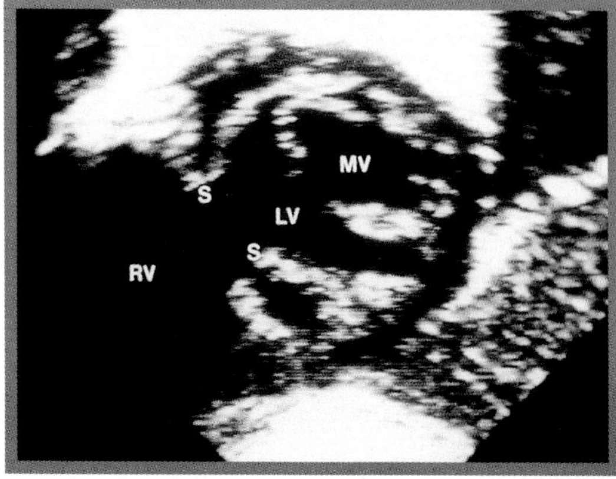

Figure 3.36 Kawasaki Disease. This echocardiogram shows a left coronary artery arising from the aorta (AO) in a child with Kawasaki disease. Note the saccular aneurysm at the proximal part of the left anterior descending artery (LAD).
Figure 3.37 Kawasaki Disease. This coronary arteriogram shows a massive aneurysm of the left anterior descending artery as well as diffuse involvement of the circumflex coronary artery. For more details of Kawasaki disease see **Chapter 12, Infection and immunity**.

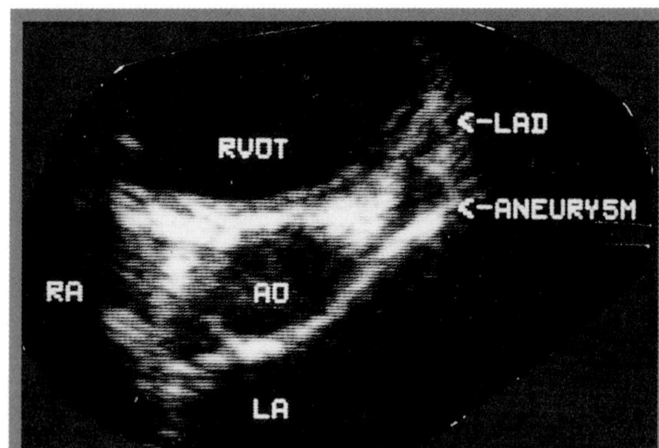

←3.36

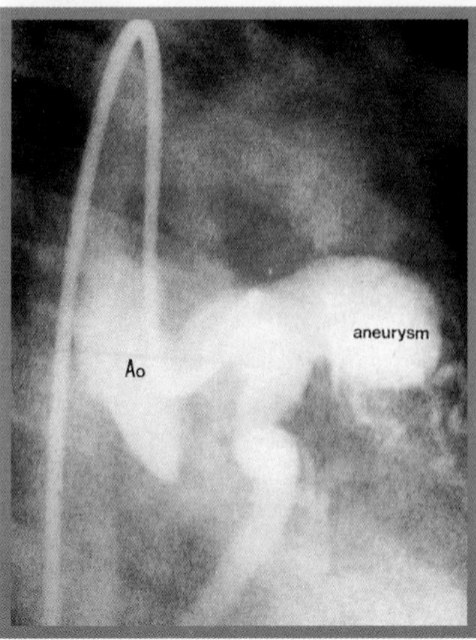

←3.37

4 Respiratory disorders

Cleft Lip and Palate. The following sequence of figures shows examples of cleft lip and palate in newborn infants. **Figure 4.1** shows a bilateral cleft lip which is often associated with a protrusion of the cleft premaxillary process as shown here. Unilateral cleft lips may vary from a small notch to a complete separation of the prolabium, usually unilateral on the left. **Figure 4.2** shows a combined cleft lip and palate. Cleft lip and palate occurs in approximately 1 in 1000 deliveries. A cleft palate alone is less common (about 1 in 2000 deliveries) but is more commonly associated with other congenital malformations. Generally, cleft lip and palate are diagnosed on antenatal scan screening.

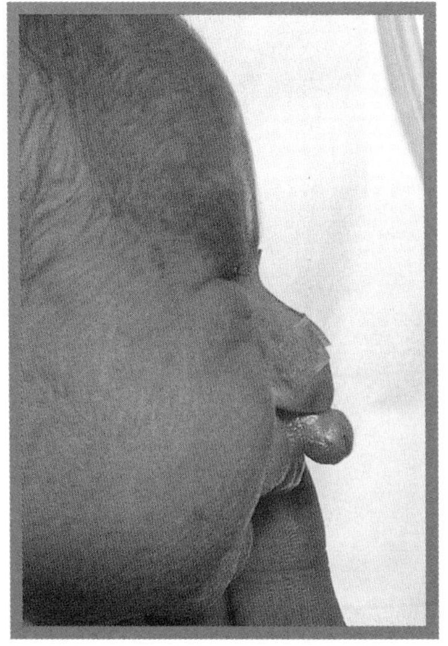

↑ 4.1

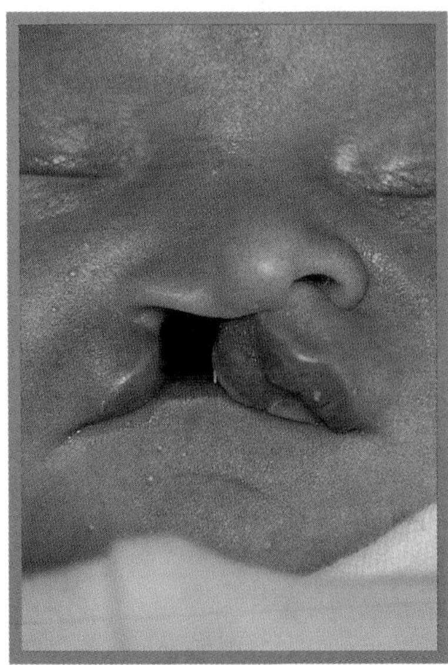

↑ 4.2

Figure 4.3 shows a feeding tube *in situ* with absence of the hard palate. Management of cleft lip and palate include full examination to exclude other significant congenital abnormalities and referral to a specialist unit. Management is based on a team approach with surgical (ENT, plastic and maxillofacial), dental and audiological assessment and speech therapy.

Complications include feeding problems (leading to failure to thrive), aspiration pneumonia, speech difficulties, abnormalities of dentition, hearing loss due to recurrent otitis media, and a cosmetic appearance that occasionally results in poor parental bonding. Long-term follow up is always required.

Clefts can either occur in isolation or as part of a more generalized syndrome. There are various associations:

- Environmental, *e.g.*, maternal anticonvulsant treatment, fetal alcohol syndrome, amniotic bands
- Chromosome abnormalities, *e.g.*, Trisomies 13 and 18 and deletions 4p (Wolf–Hirschhorn syndrome) and 5p (Cri du Chat syndrome).
- Single gene disorders, *e.g.*, Treacher–Collins syndrome and Stickler syndrome.

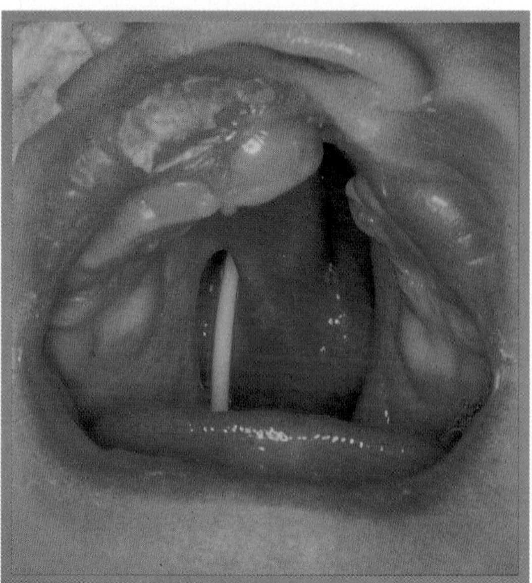

←4.3

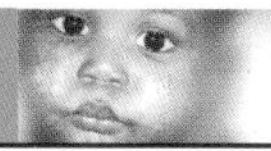

Figures 4.4 and 4.5 Pierre Robin Sequence. The Pierre Robin Sequence shown here in a newborn (**Figure 4.4**) and a 2-year-old child (**Figure 4.5**). The micrognathia seen here is associated with midline cleft palate or high arched palate, and upper airway obstruction due to glossoptosis and relative macroglossia. Babies with the Pierre Robin sequence often have severe upper airway obstruction. Feeding difficulties occur and tube feeding or gastrostomy feeding may be required. The child should be nursed prone. Growth of the mandible progresses, and by the age of 4–6 years the airway and lower jaw size are normal.

Less severe micrognathia occurs in other syndromes, *e.g.*, Treacher–Collins, Cri du Chat, Wolf–Hirschhorn, Bloom and Trisomy 18 .

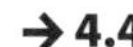

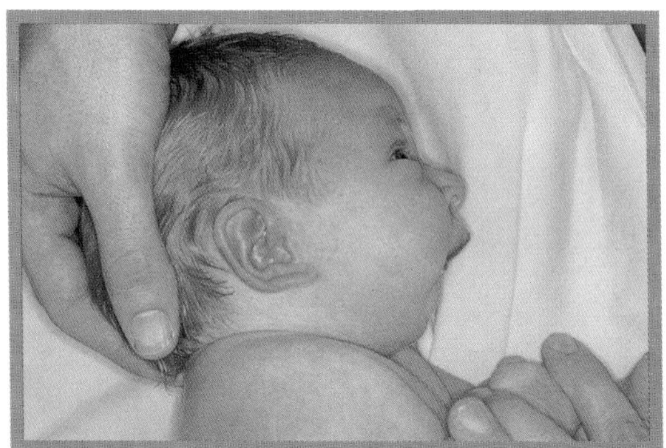

→4.5

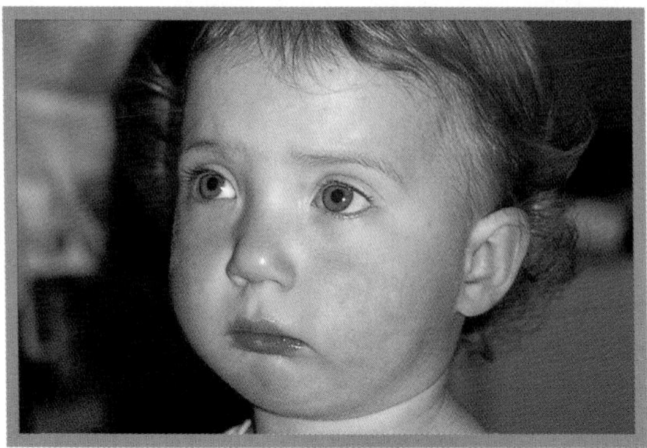

Figures 4.6 and 4.7 Abnormalities of Auricle. These are relatively common and vary from simple appendages to atresia of the auricle. In **Figure 4.6**, the accessory auricle was associated with cardiofacial syndrome. Associated abnormalities of the auditory meatus, middle and inner ear are more serious. Dermal pits may be found, and these occasionally become infected. Investigation may include detailed radiology of the inner ear, specialized audiological testing and clinical genetic assessment. ENT and plastic surgery referral for reconstructive and cosmetic surgery may be indicated.

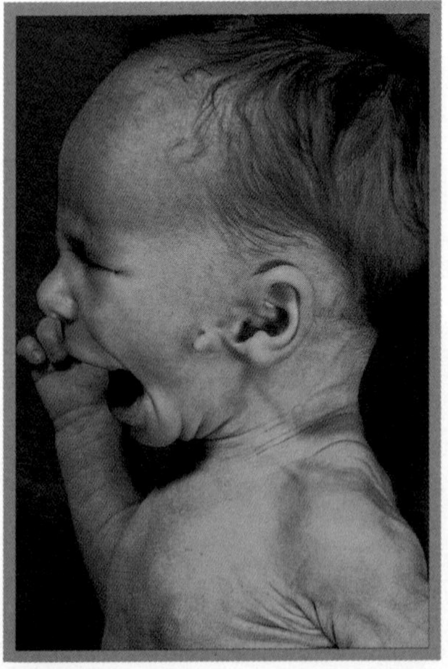

↑ **4.6**

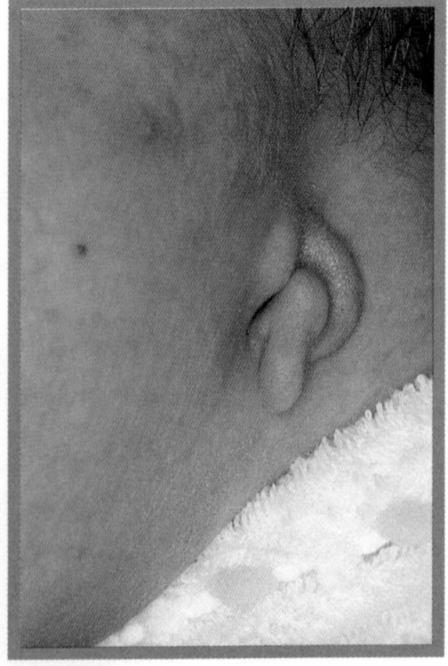

↑ **4.7**

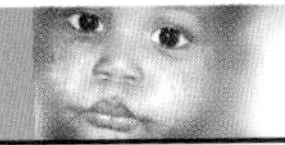

Figure 4.8 CHARGE Association Syndrome. This child had features of CHARGE association syndrome:

1. **C**oloboma of the retina.
2. **H**eart defects.
3. **A**tresia of the choanae.
4. **R**etardation of growth.
5. **G**enital anomalies (not seen in this child).
6. **E**ar anomalies: cup-shaped anteverted ears and sensory neural deafness requiring hearing aids.

Four of the above criteria need to be present to make a diagnosis.

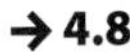

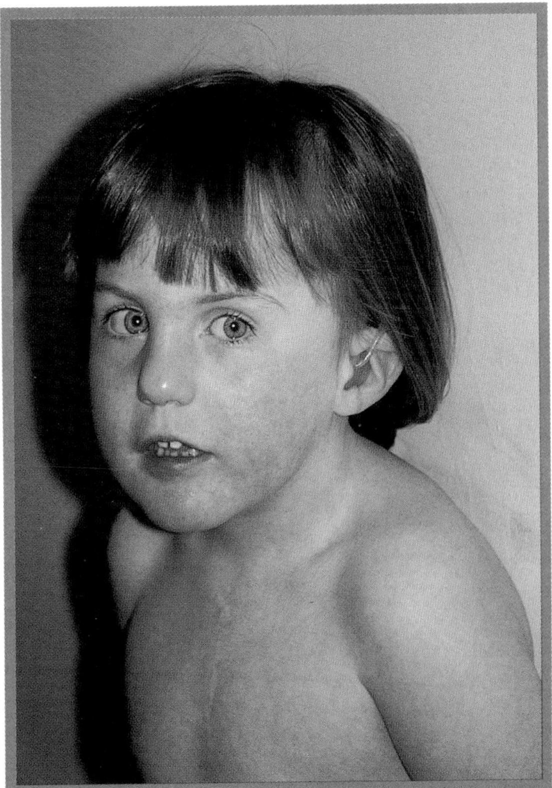

Figure 4.9 Retropharyngeal Abscess. Infection of the potential space between the posterior pharyngeal wall and the prevertebral fascia is seen. This is most common in children under the age of 4 years, as after this age the lymph nodes in the prevertebral fascia involute. It usually results from an abscess in the lymph glands that drains into the nasopharynx and posterior nasal passages. This commonly arises from group A hemolytic streptococcal or straphylococcal infection, and can result from penetrating trauma.

The child presents with a history of an upper respiratory tract infection followed by high fever, difficulty in swallowing, refusal of food, the neck being held in extension, and noisy respiration due to pooled secretions.

The clinical diagnosis is confirmed by careful digital examination or by lateral neck soft-tissue X-ray, showing the retropharyngeal space to be wider than the C4 vertebral body.

This is a surgical emergency because of the potential for airway obstruction and spread of infection.Treatment consists of incision and drainage performed by an ENT surgeon with care being taken to prevent aspiration of pus. Preoperative antibiotic treatment is indicated.

Differential diagnosis is peritonsillar (quinsy) or retrotonsillar abscess.

Figures 4.10 and 4.11 Epiglottitis. Figure 4.10 illustrates the 'cherry red' appearance on direct laryngoscopy of the inflamed epiglottis. **Figure 4.11** shows a comparison between the normal upper airway (left) and the obstructed airway of epiglottitis (right) on lateral X-ray of the neck. On the right, the soft tissue shadow of the epiglottis is grossly enlarged, extending anteriorly and obstructing the entrance to the larynx. Cervical lordosis is lost

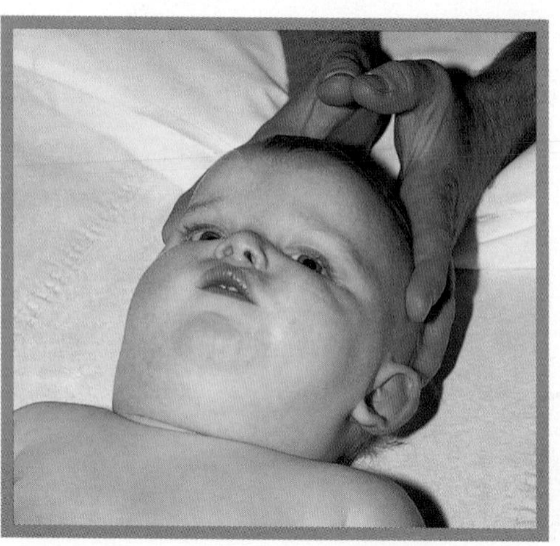

← 4.9

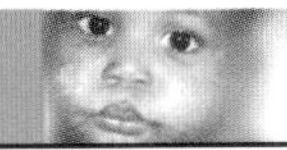

as the child is straining forward to overcome the obstruction, however hyperextension of the neck may also occur.

Epiglottitis is an acute infection of the epiglottis and associated soft-tissue structures. It is characterized by the acute onset of stridor, fever, dysphagia and drooling. The child adopts a 'tripod' position in order to minimize airway resistance. In the past, epiglottitis was usually caused by *Hemophilus influenzae* and is now much rarer because of Hib immunization. It can also be caused by group B β-hemolytic *Streptococcus.*

Differential diagnosis includes an aspirated foreign body, viral croup and severe bacterial tracheitis. Treatment consists in ensuring an adequate airway, preventing hypoxia and treating the infection. Intubation is usually essential and extubation is usually done within 48 hours. Ensure the absolute minimum of disturbance to the child before securing the airway. Life-threatening airway obstruction may occur rapidly. This is a medical emergency and **a lateral neck X-ray as shown is not indicated** as it may precipitate airway obstruction and delay securing of the airway.

→4.10

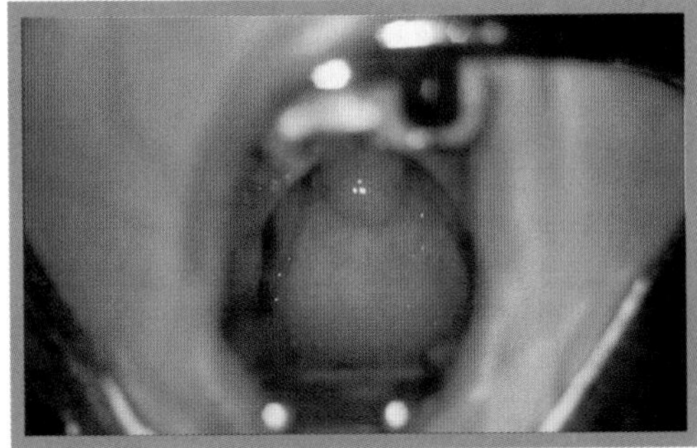

→4.11

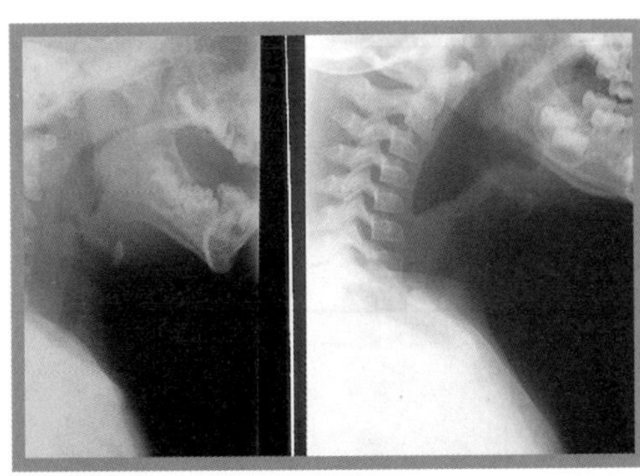

Figure 4.12 Tracheostomy. This figure shows a 1-year-old girl with a tracheostomy. The tracheostomy was required because of airway obstruction at the age of 4 months due to a hemangioma of the larynx. Follow-up laryngoscopy at 2 years of age demonstrated spontaneous resolution of the hemangioma. Granulation tissue at the site of tracheostomy delayed decannulation, which was successful at 28 months of age.

Figure 4.13 Ludwig Angina. This 1-year-old malnourished Asian infant presented with fever and tender swelling of the floor of the mouth. Upward displacement of the tongue caused drooling and dysphagia. This condition conistitutes a rapidly progressive spreading cellulitis of the submandibular space. The infection is usually precipitated by dental sepsis or occasionally trauma to the mouth, and is usually caused by Group A streptococci. Drainage of the infection is through the soft tissues of the mouth. Acute respiratory embarrassment and a toxic-shock-like picture may occur.

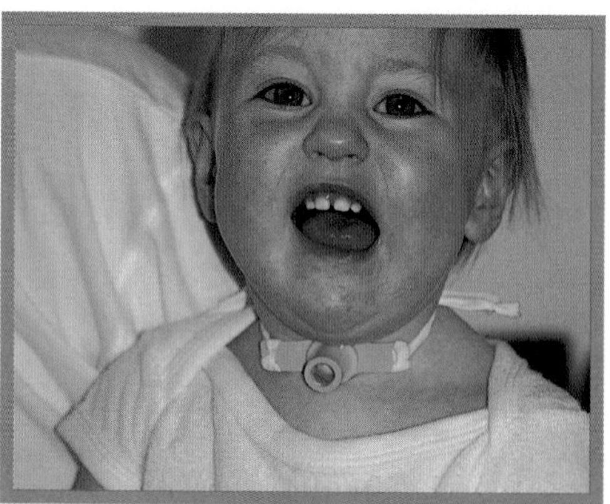

←4.12

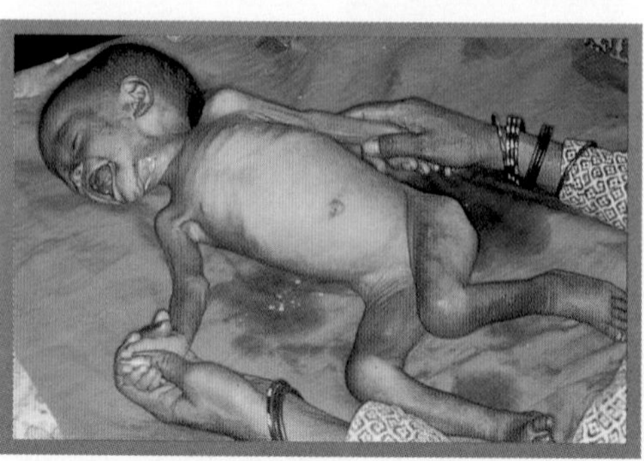

←4.13

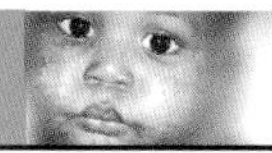

Treatment consists in diagnostic aspiration of the pus and administration of intravenous antibiotics. Intubation may be necessary.

Figures 4.14 and 4.15 Respiratory Distress in the Newborn. This is an 8-week-old male infant who had congenital lobar emphysema leading to respiratory distress. There is marked subcostal recession with recruitment of the accessory muscles of respiration.

Figure 4.15 demonstrates oxygen delivery via nasal catheters/prongs. In this case, surgical excision of the affected lobe was the treatment of choice.

Differential diagnosis of respiratory distress in a newborn infant includes surfactant deficiency, meconium aspiration, Group B streptococcal pneumonia, transient tachypnea of the newborn, pneumothorax, congenital heart disease, upper airway obstruction, pleural effusion, diaphragmatic hernia,primary ciliary dyskinesia and metabolic and neuromuscular diseases.

→4.14

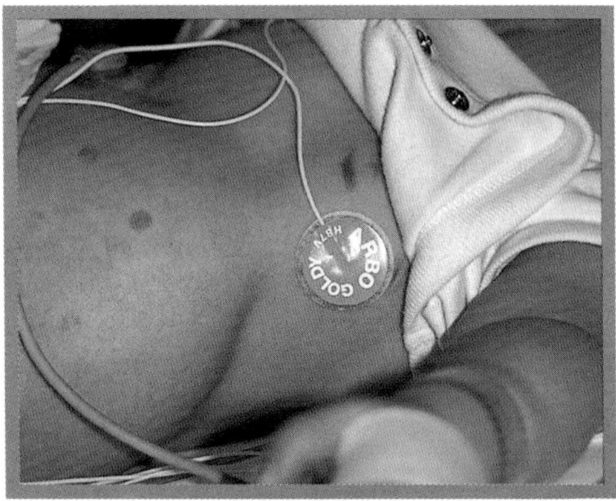

→4.15

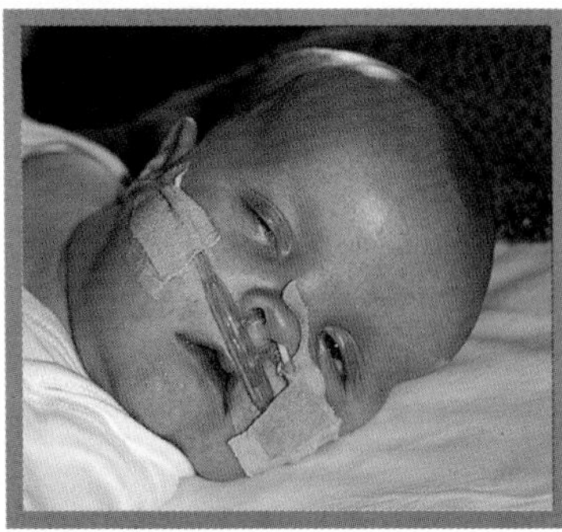

Figure 4.16 Congenital Lobar Emphysema – CT. Deviation of the mediastinum to the right with compression of the right lung is shown. The left lobe is over- expanded, with increased translucency. This, together with a clinical history such as that given above (see **Figure 4.14 and 4.15**), is consistent with the diagnosis of congenital lobar emphysema.

Figures 4.17–4.21 Chest Shape Variants. Figure 4.17 shows pigeon chest (pectus carinatum). This is a common chest-shape variant, and consists of a prominent anterior projection of the sternum. It is not usually associated with any underlying lung disease or functional impairment. Cosmetic improvement occurs as the child grows. Surgery may be indicated in severe cases.

Figure 4.18 Funnel Chest (Pectus Excavatum). Funnel chest consists of a marked depression of the sternum. It is often familial and appears to worsen in later childhood. Rarely, it is associated with functional impairment. Funnel chest can be found in Marfan syndrome, homocystinuria and Coffin–Lowery syndrome, and can be associated with thoracolumbar scoliosis. Some cases may be treated surgically for cosmetic benefit. Funnel chest may result from a midline sternotomy in infancy.

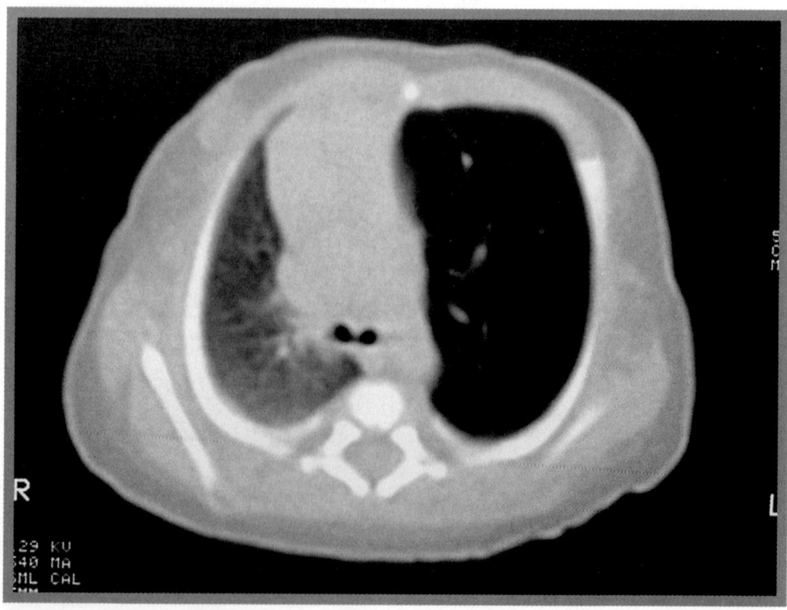

↑4.16

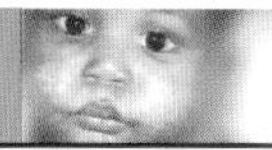

→ 4.17

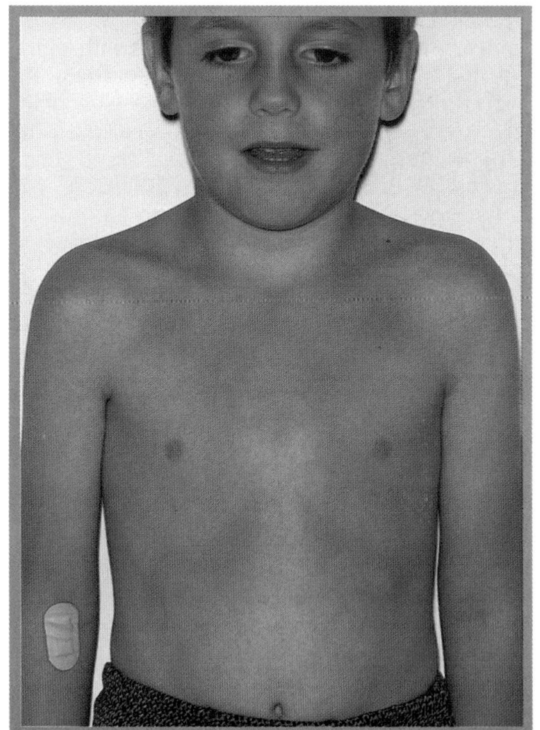

→ 4.18

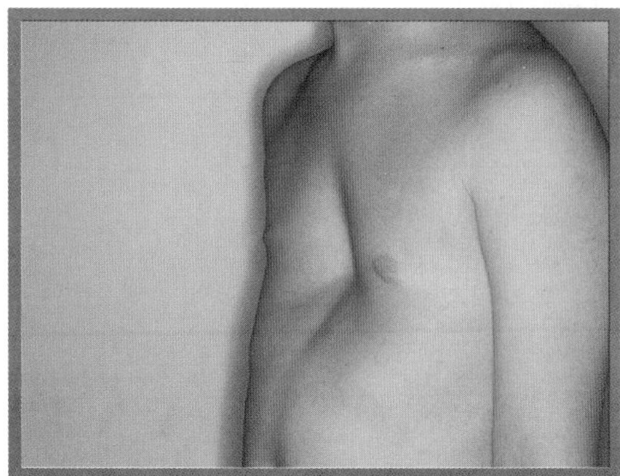

Figure 4.19 Barrel Chest. This figure shows an increased anterior–posterior diameter, and a barrel chest, associated with air trapping in chronic asthma.
Figure 4.20 Harrison Sulcus and Intercostal Recession. This prominent sulcus running parallel to the ribs at the level of the diaphragmatic insertion is referred to as Harrison sulcus. The 4-year-old asthmatic boy shown here also demonstrates intercostal recession.
Figure 4.21 Prominent Harrison Sulcus. A prominent Harrison sulcus is shown here in a 7-year-old girl with chronic asthma. With severe chest deformity of this nature one should consider cystic fibrosis as an alternative diagnosis.
Figure 4.22 Asthma. This child is receiving nebulized drugs (through a mask) for an acute exacerbation of asthma. Home and hospital care of asthma involves the appropriate use of delivery systems, including nebulizers, in order to treat the symptoms effectively.
Asthma is a disorder associated with wheezing and coughing and occurs in up to 20% of the child population. It is a chronic disease resulting in reversible obstruction of the airways, and is precipitated by multiple factors, including

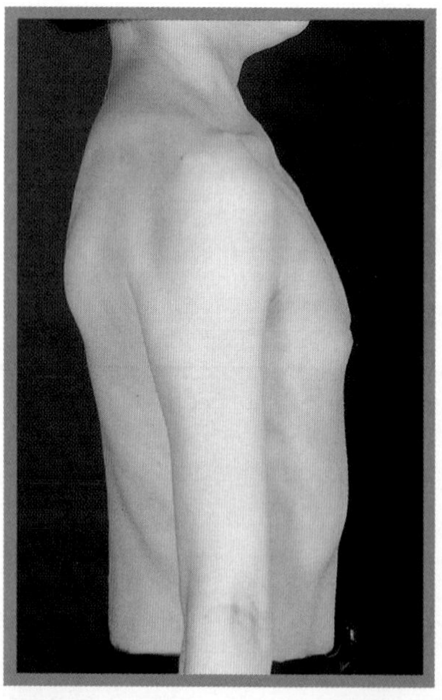

↑4.19

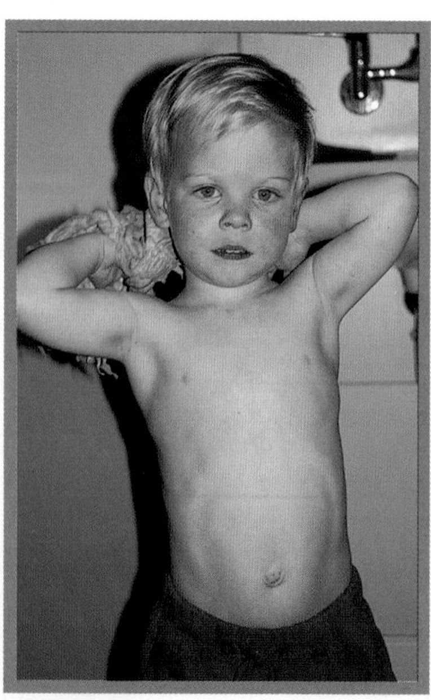

↑4.20

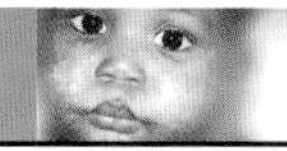

infection, gastroesophageal reflux, cigarette smoke, atmospheric pollution, exercise and aeroallergens. There is frequently a family history of atopy, and symptoms may be more persistent in atopic individuals.

Treatment may involve the use of inhaled bronchodilators and prophylactic therapy. A clear history and examination are essential to the successful management of this common disorder.

→4.21

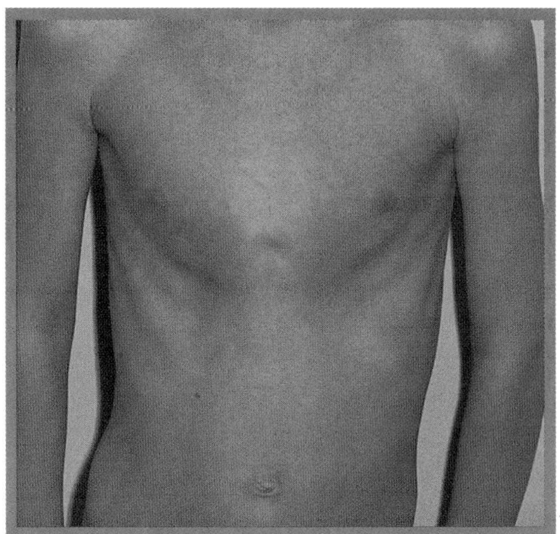

→4.22

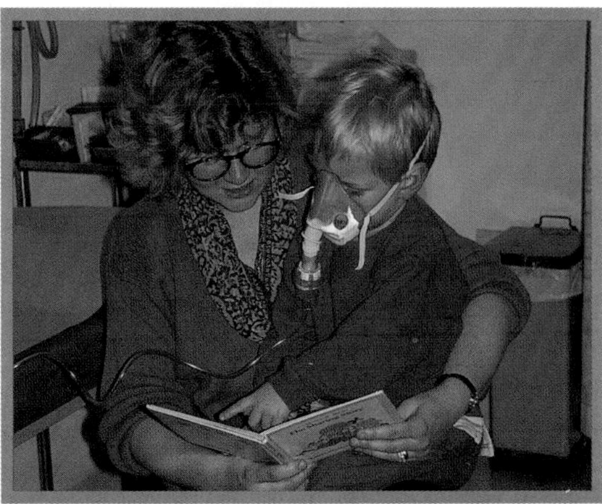

Figures 4.23–4.30 Cystic Fibrosis. This common, autosomal recessive condition is due to a defect in the transmembrane chloride transport mechanism (the cystic fibrosis transmembrane regulator protein–CFTR). Over 600 different gene defects have been identified on the CFTR locus of chromosome 7 to account for this. The most common is the Δf 508 deletion. Thick secretions block the airway, resulting in local destruction of lung tissue and associated chronic infection.

Diagnosis may be made based on the concentration of sweat sodium or chloride ions (a sweat test) or on the identification of the abnormal gene. Treatment is aimed at clearing respiratory secretions, treating infection and ensuring adequate nutrition.

Figure 4.23 shows twins displaying the effects of chronic infection in cystic fibrosis on growth, with the affected twin being on the right. There is associated hyperinflation and pallor in the affected child.

Figures 4.24 and 4.25 show a 6-year-old boy with cystic fibrosis. He has hyperinflation, marked intercostal recession and a Harrison sulcus. There is an implanted, subcutaneous, venous access device located at the left clavicle and a percutaneous gastrostomy for additional calories. Note the generalized malnourished appearance.

Figure 4.26 Polyp. This figure shows a polyp in left nostril of a child with cystic fibrosis.

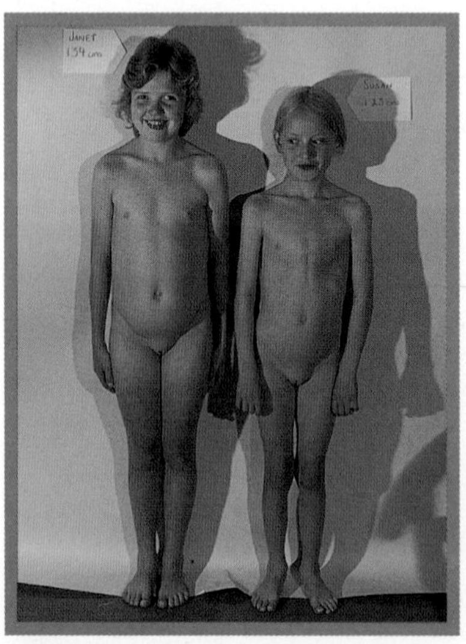

↑ **4.23**

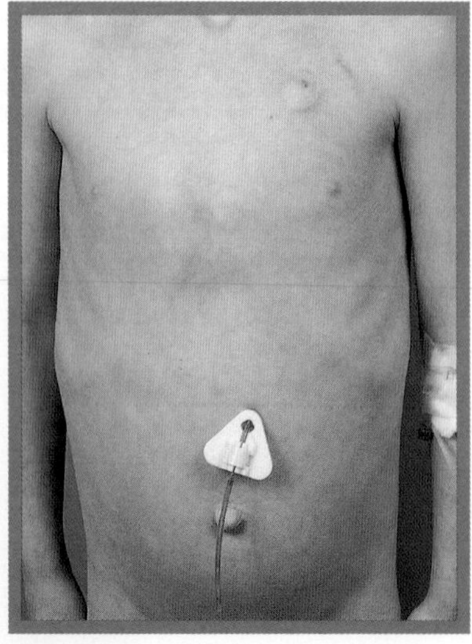

↑ **4.24**

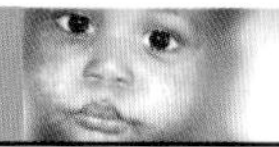

→ 4.25

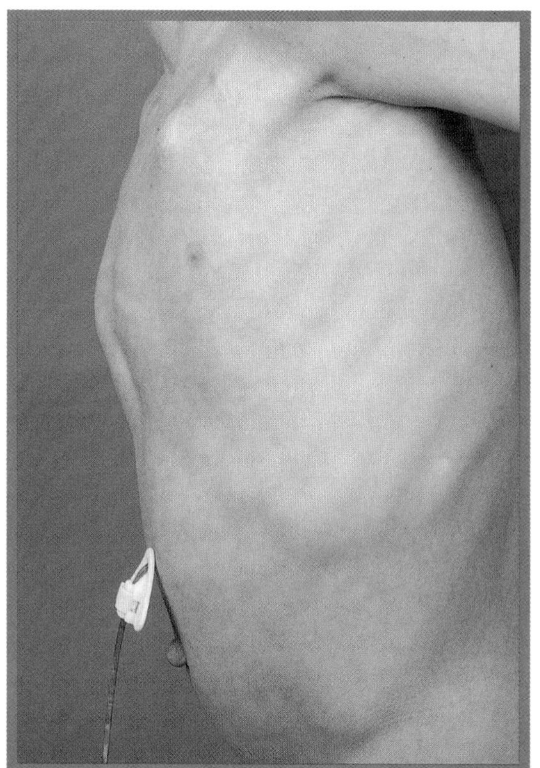

→ 4.26

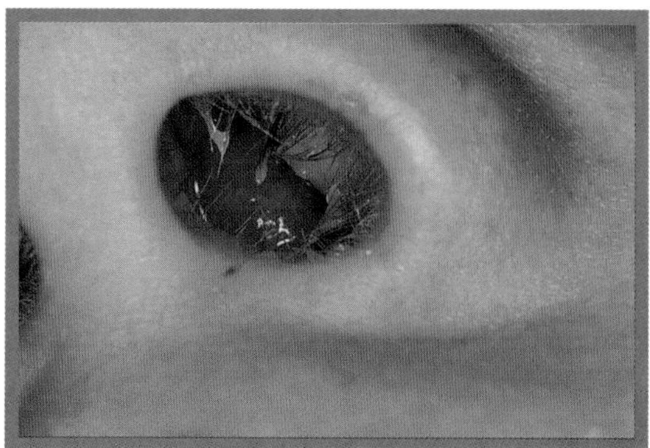

Figures 4.27 and 4.28 Clubbing. These figures show clubbing in cystic fibrosis associated with either pulmonary or hepatic involvement. There is loss of the soft tissue at the angle of the nail bed.

Note the loss of the 'diamond' usually found at the angle of the opposed nail beds of the second fingers.

Figure 4.29 Chest X-ray of Child with Cystic Fibrosis. This figure shows hyperinflation, increased lower-zone bronchial wall thickening and cyst formation. There is increased perihilar shadowing due to infection and hilar lymphadenopathy.

Figure 4.30 CT of Chest in Cystic Fibrosis with Allergic Bronchopulmonary Aspergillosis (ABPA). Ectasia of the bronchial branches with distal obstruction has produced segmental collapse. This is seen here asymmetrically and bilaterally. ABPA leads to further lung damage in children with CF, so early diagnosis and treatment with high-dose oral steroids is important. The features

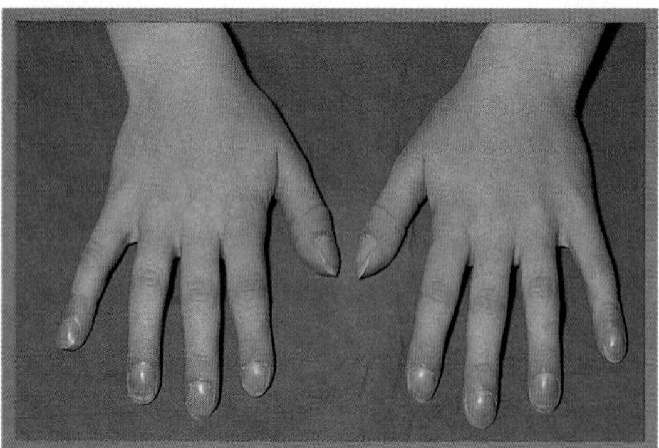

←4.27

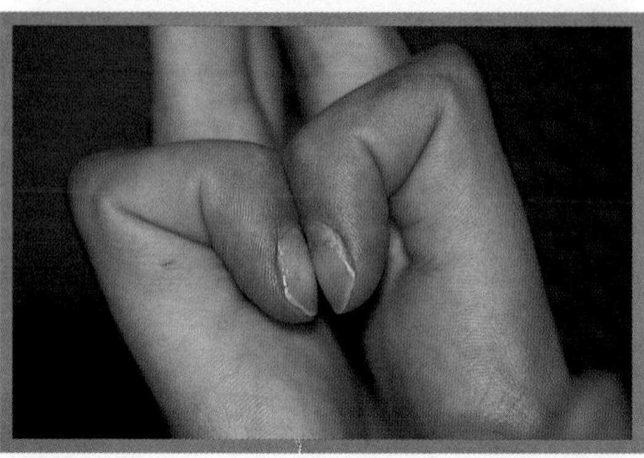

←4.28

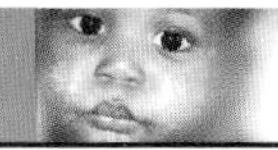

may be similar to an exacerbation of respiratory infection. There is a pyrexia and cough, but no improvement on antibiotic therapy. Investigations supporting a diagnosis are the presence of aspergillosis precipitans, an elevation in total IgE, positive RAST tests, and a chest X-ray showing segmental collapse.

→4.29

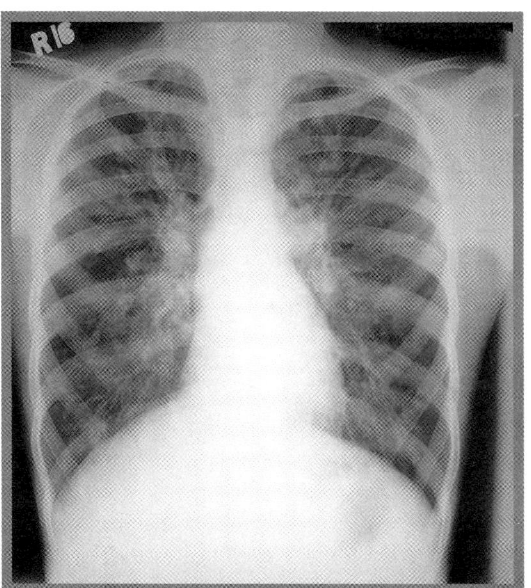

→4.30

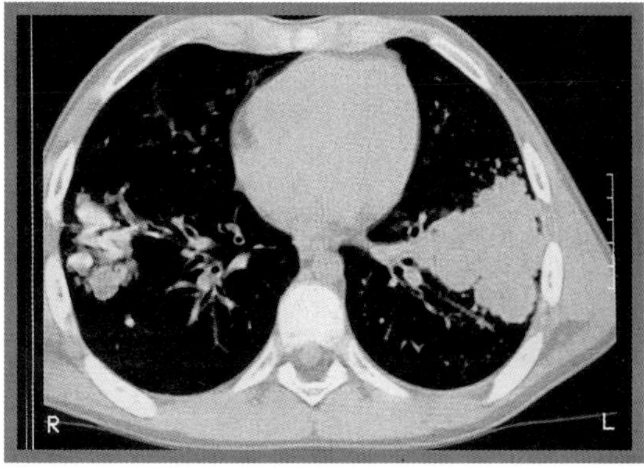

Figures 4.31–4.40 Tuberculosis (TB). Figures 4.31 and 4.32 show tuberculous lymphadenitis on the left side in both cases. This may be a primary lesion or, more commonly in the tropics, a secondary lesion. In the Western world, however, tuberculosis may be due to atypical mycobacterium. The skin has an irregular surface, is often discolored, and draining sinuses may form.

Diagnosis is usually based on excision biopsy, which is the treatment of choice, in atypical mycobacterial infection. However, tuberculous lymphadenitis requires chemotherapy.

Differential diagnosis includes simple reactive lymphadenopathy, lymphoproliferative disorders, disseminated malignancy, connective tissue diseases, and bacterial, fungal and protozoal infections, including cat-scratch disease and toxoplasmosis.

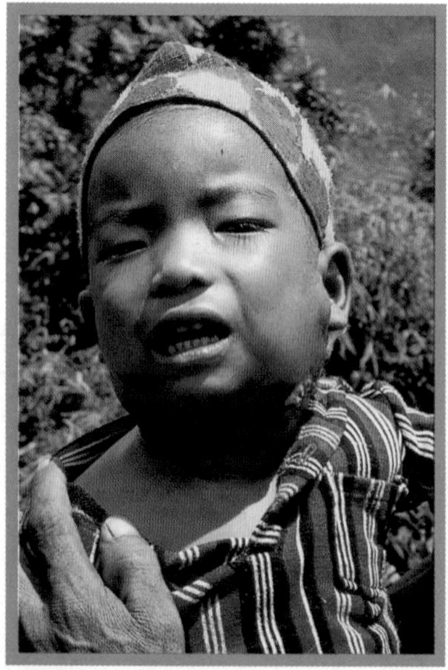

↑ 4.31

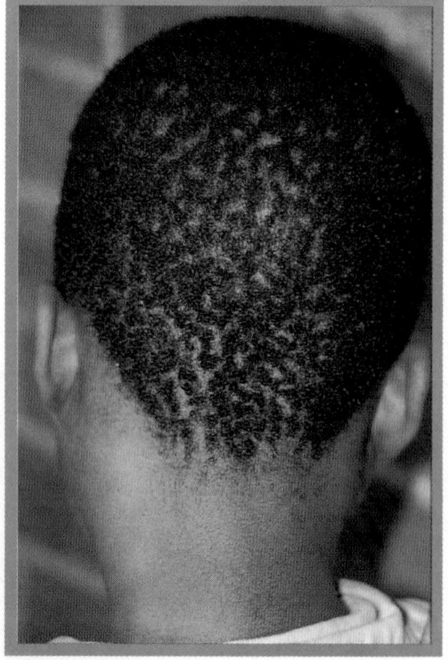

↑ 4.32

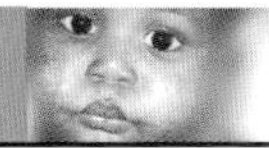

Figure 4.33 Disseminated TB Associated with Gross Malnutrition. In the developing world this is still a common problem and has high mortality and morbidity rates.

Figure 4.34 Jaundice in a 2-year-old Treated for TB with Triple Therapy. Liver dysfunction due to isoniazid therapy is shown presenting as hepatitis. This is rare in children, and liver function tests should be considered in children receiving antituberculous therapy.

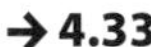

→4.33

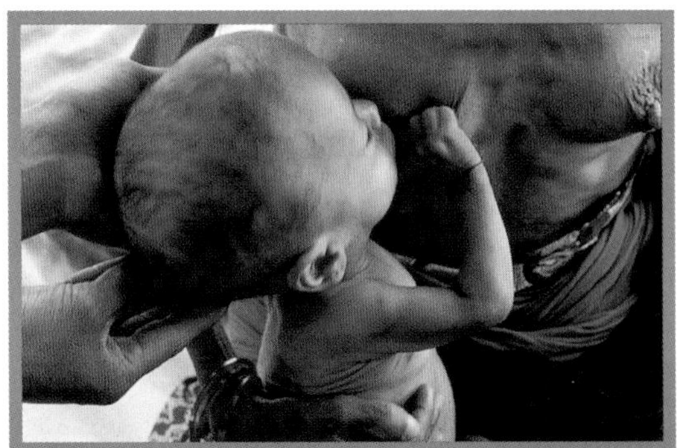

→4.34

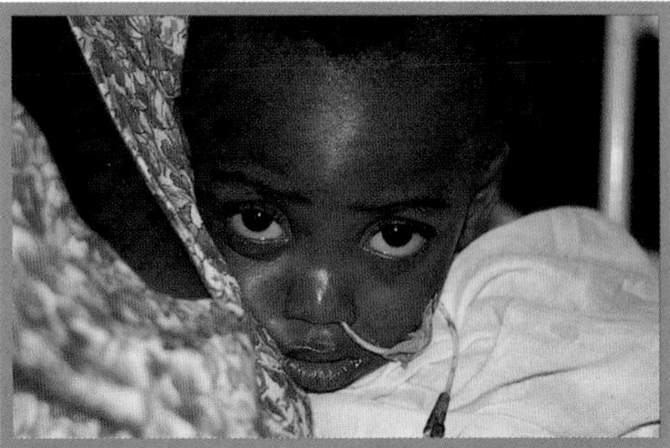

Figures 4.35 and 4.36 Positive Intradermal (Mantoux or Jet Injector-Heaf) Skin test. A 20 mm ring of induration is shown in **Figure 4.35**, and a ring associated with superficial ulceration is shown in **Figure 4.36**.

A reaction of 10 mm or more is regarded as positive (when using 5 tuberculin units), 5–9 mm is doubtful and 0–4 mm is negative. False negative results may occur in immunocompromized patients, in disseminated TB, and in patients on steroid therapy. Doubtful tests should be repeated and the result should be treated as positive if the patient has an indicative clinical history, close-contact history, or a positive chest X-ray.

Intradermal tests for atypical mycobacteria are available, but diagnosis is usually based on excision biopsy specimens showing acid-fast bacilli with negative intradermal tests to human TB.

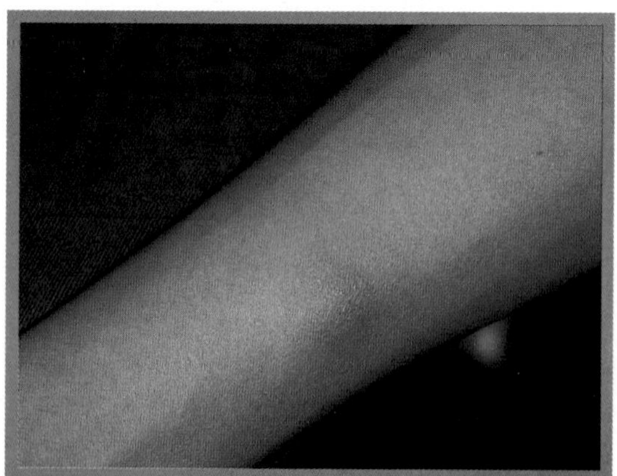

←4.35

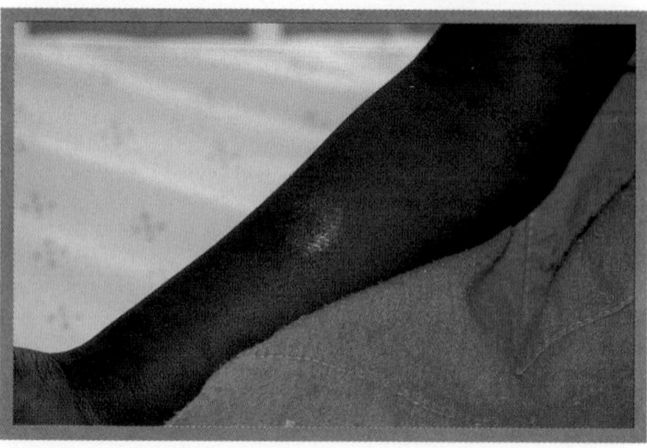

←4.36

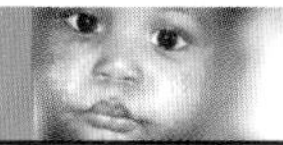

Figures 4.37–4.40 Pulmonary TB. Figure 4.37 shows bronchogenic spread from rupture of a tuberculous gland into a bronchus. Infected pus spreads distally as in this case, to the left lower lobe and lingula of the lung. The child is usually very sick, with associated cough and fever. Chest X-ray shows dense consolidation of the left middle and lower zones with complete effacement of the left heart border and the left hemidiaphragm.

Figure 4.38 shows the development of tuberculous pneumonia with the formation of pneumatoceles. There is a relative lack of hilar lymphadenopathy because this patient was receiving chemotherapy for leukemia. Pneumatoceles result from the breakdown of tuberculous abscesses. This later and more penetrated film shows the formation of irregular cavities within pneumonic consolidation.

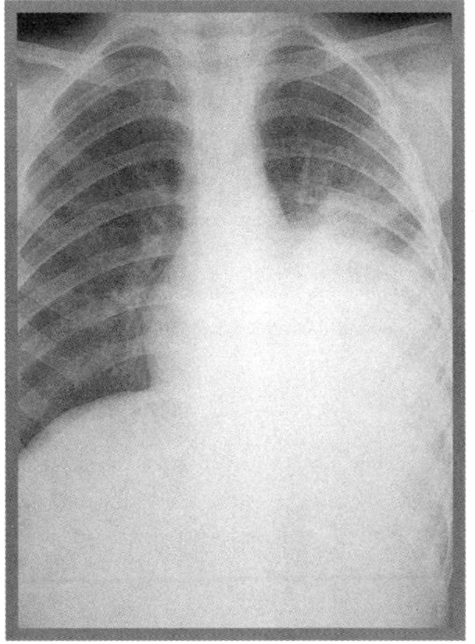

↑4.37

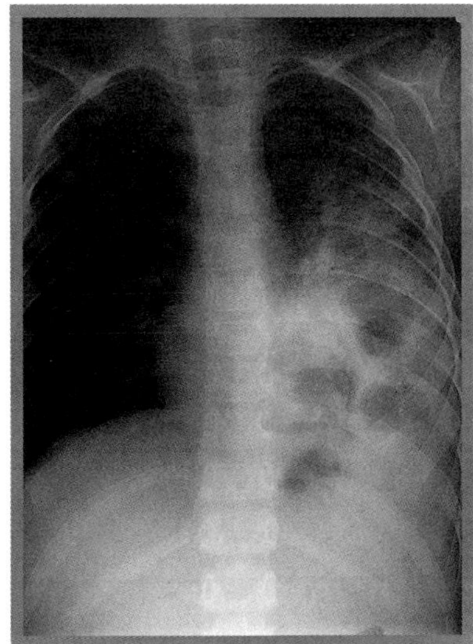

↑4.38

Figure 4.39 shows miliary spread from rupture of an infected gland into a bronchial blood vessel. This is more common in younger infants and can result in widespread lesions throughout the body. The X-ray appearance of miliary (micronodular) shadowing in the lung appears relatively late in the course of the disease, and late diagnosis has a high mortality rate.

Figure 4.40 shows acid-fast bacilli in a bone marrow specimen. This specimen is from a neonate born with congenital TB to a mother with disseminated TB. Pink-stained bacilli are seen surrounded by a giant cell reaction (granuloma). In the absence of acid-fast bacilli, an alternative diagnosis would be sarcoidosis.

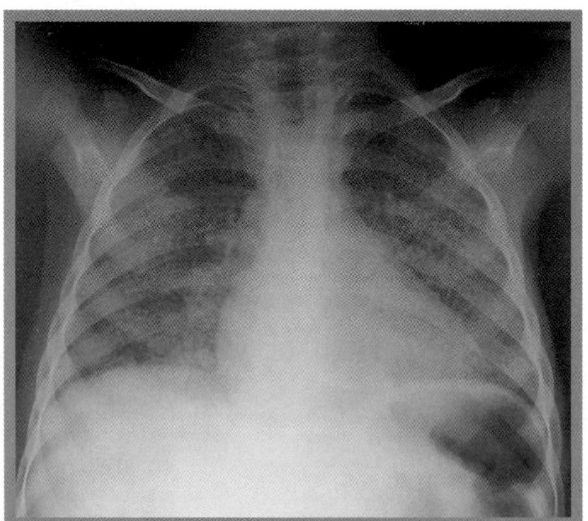

← 4.39

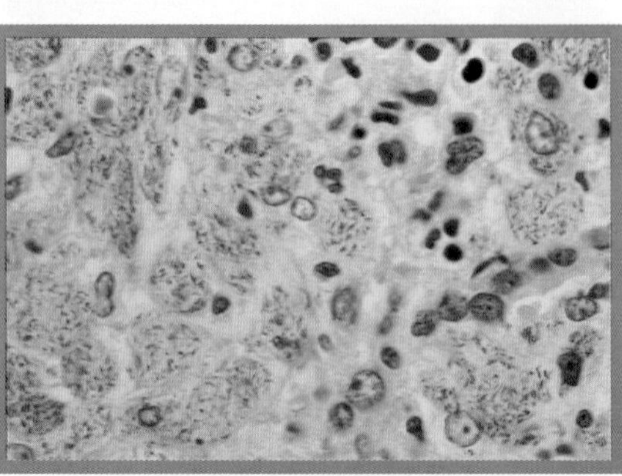

← 4.40

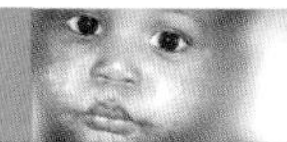

Figures 4.41–43 Chest Infection in HIV Positive Children. Figure 4.41 shows a chest X-ray of lymphocytic interstitial pneumonia (LIP).

Not uncommonly, the first presentation of vertical transmission HIV is indolent LIP. Note the bilateral, symmetrical, reticular, nodular shadowing with hilar lymphadonopathy. This appearance can also be seen in miliary TB but is becoming increasingly common with HIV. LIP maybe associated with clubbing and may run an indolent course often requiring no treatment.

Figure 4.42 Interstitial pneumonia which was shown on immunofluorescence of broncho-alveolar lavage to be due to *Pneumocystis carinii*. The figure shows bilateral midzone shadowing of a predominantly interstitial nature, and a treated pneumothorax. The X-ray also shows a radio-opaque cannula in the pulmonary artery to measure pulmonary pressures.

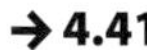

→4.41

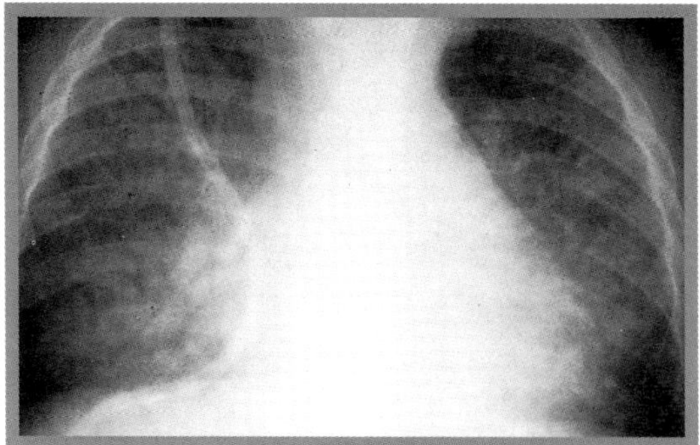

→4.42

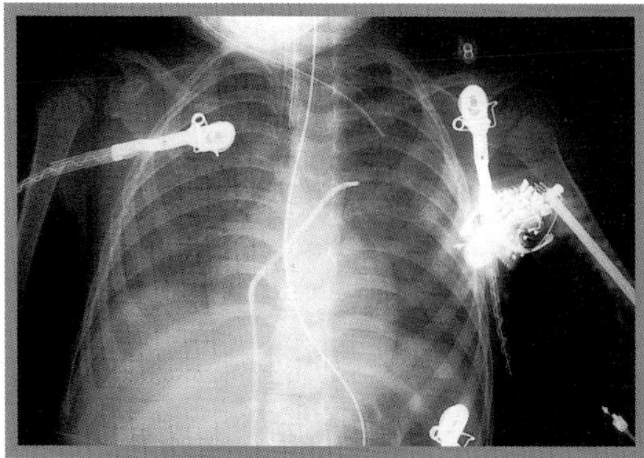

Figure 4.43 Positive immunofluorescence. Treatment is with intravenous high-dose septrin (trimethoprim/sulfamethoxazole) or pentamidine and steroids. There is a high mortality related to the underlying immunocompromized status, associated infection, and nutritional status.

Figure 4.44 MRI of a Bronchogenic Cyst. This T_1-weighted coronal MRI scan shows a well-demarcated ovoid lesion of uniform signal intensity. This is consistent with fluid in a post-mediastinal, extrapleural, left paraspinal position. Differential diagnosis include tumor of neurofibromatosis.

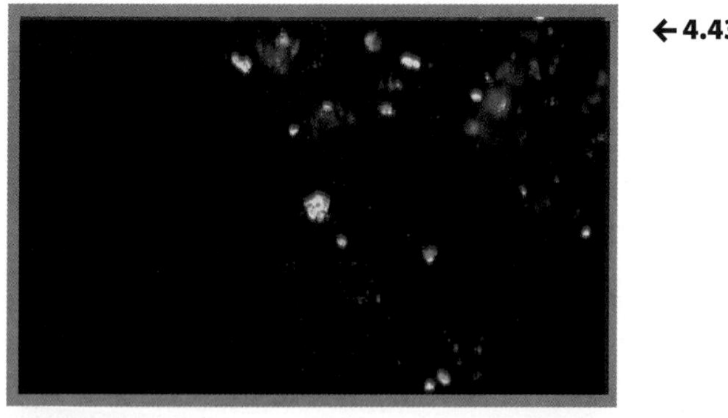

←4.43

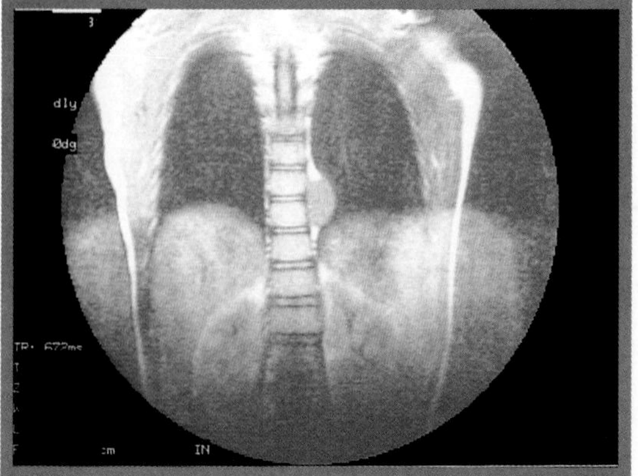

←4.44

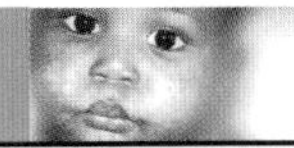

Figures 4.45 and 46 Bronchiectasis. Lobar bronchiectasis is shown here on an AP (left) and lateral (right) bronchogram. Note the ectasia of the lower left lobe bronchi with peripheral bronchial pruning. Consequent loss of acini results in crowding of bronchi in the affected lobe. Currently bronchograms are rarely done and modern imaging would include CT scans of the affected lung. Symptoms include a productive cough and clinical findings of clubbing and persistent crackles, suggesting suppurative lung disease. A sweat test, ciliary function test, α1-antitrypsin activity assessment and immunological investigations are essential. Treatment can be surgical if a single lobe is affected. Prophylactic antibiotics may be given and all children require physiotherapy.

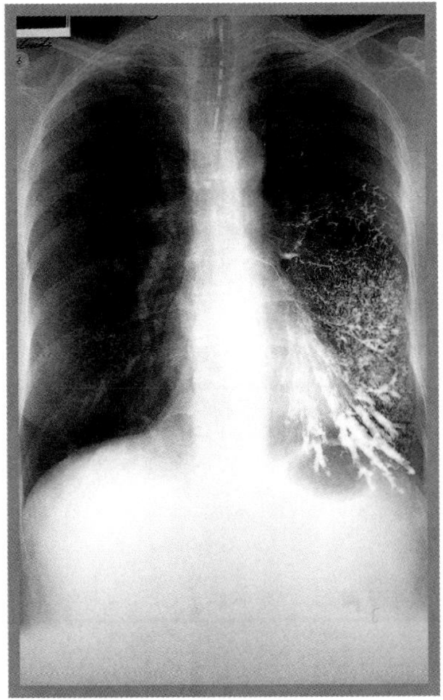

↑ **4.45**

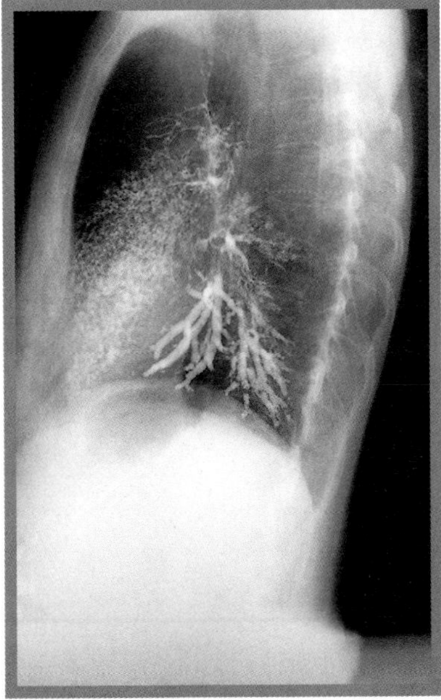

↑ **4.46**

Figures 4.47–4.49 Primary Ciliary Dyskinesia. The 11-year-old boy shown presented with recurrent chest infections, sinusitis, otitis media and later failure to thrive secondary to severe lung disease. This indicates Kartagener syndrome. Cor pulmonale developed with respiratory failure. Appropriate treatment consists of lung transplantation. **Figure 4.48** shows marked clubbing of the toes due to underlying suppuration

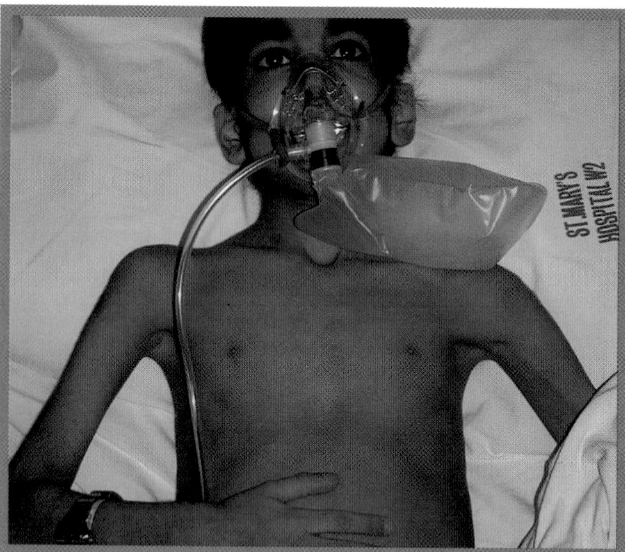

←4.47

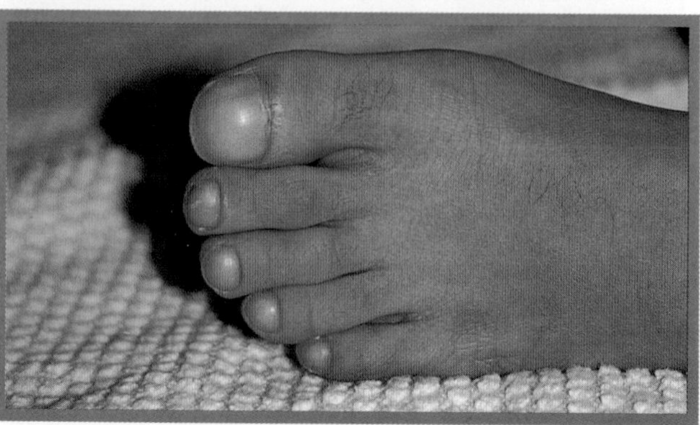

←4.48

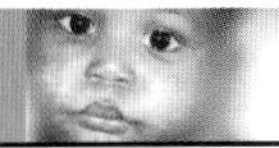

Figure 4.49 A CT in another child with primary ciliary dyskinesia shows that the heart was situated to the right (dextrocardia) and that there is bronchiectasis in the middle lobe situated on the left.

Figure 4.50a Complete Collapse of the Right Lung. This asthmatic patient's lung was reinflated (see **Figure 4.50b**) within 24 hours using only physiotherapy and bronchodilators .

→ **4.49**

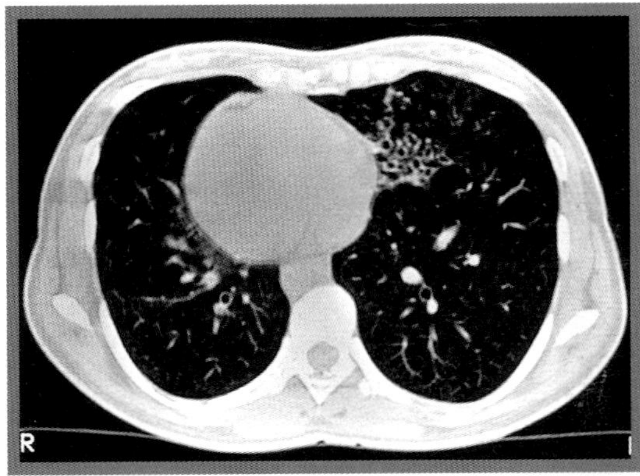

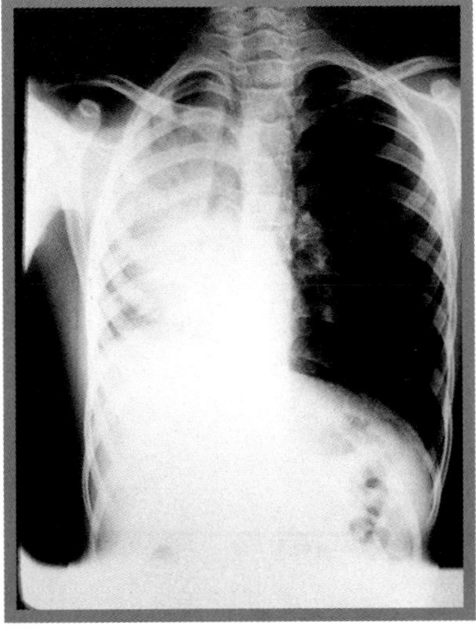

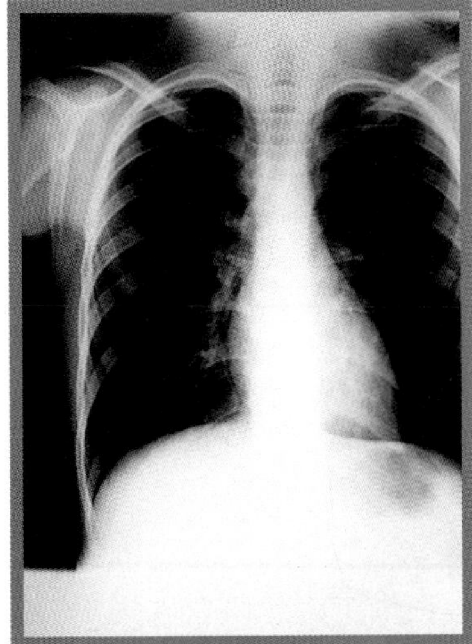

↑ **4.50a**

↑ **4.50b**

Figure 4.51 Right Upper Lobe Lung Consolidation. The X-ray shows pneumococcal pneumonia infection, but similar findings would be expected in *Hemophilus pneumoniae*, *Mycoplasma* and *Legionella* infections. Intravenous antibiotic therapy is preferred for the first 48 hours, followed by oral therapy.

Figure 4.52 Right Middle Lobe Lung Collapse. Note the loss of clarity of the right heart border and the patchy shadowing in a triangular configuration extending into the midzone (**Figure 4.52a**). The lateral view (**Figure 4.52b**) shows the complete and isolated collapse of the lung lobe. In this case, an enlarged right hilar lymph node obstructed the middle lobe bronchus. Pneumonia, mucus plugging, aspiration and inhalation of a foreign body are

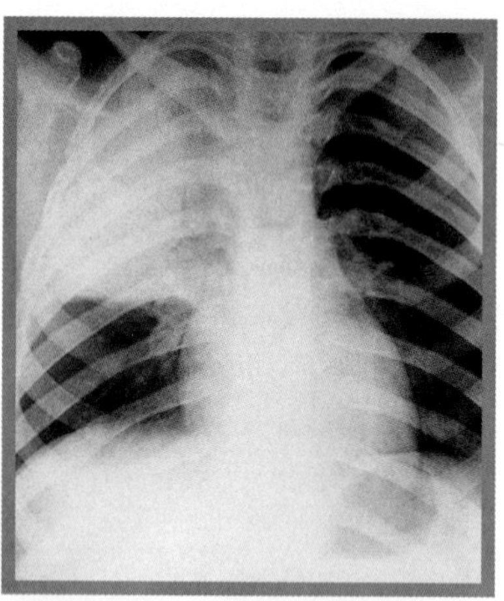

←4.51

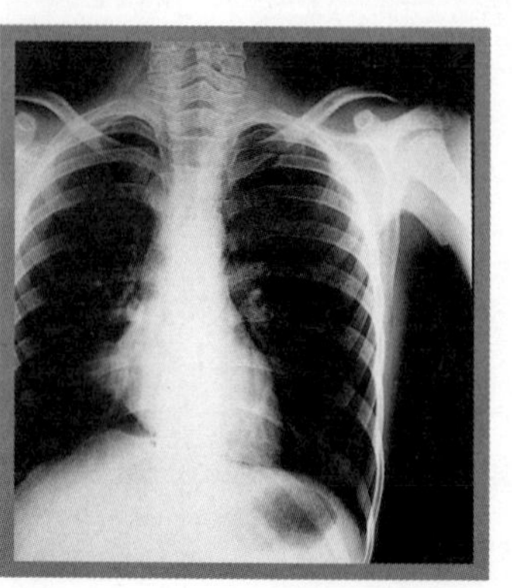

←4.52a

→4.52b

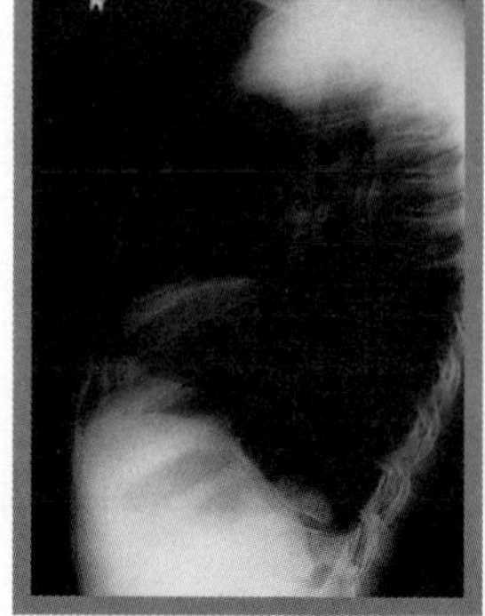

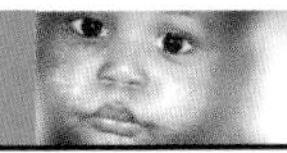

causes. Investigation is usually by X-ray only, but bronchoscopy may be valuable in cases that fail to respond well to antibiotics or bronchodilators. Removal with a rigid bronchoscope is essential in obstruction due to foreign bodies.

Figure 4.53 Left Lower Lobe Lung Collapse. This is the classic appearance of left lower lobe collapse. There is loss of the left hemidiaphragm with an increased density, and a clear margin behind the heart.

Figure 4.54a Complete Collapse of the Left Lung. This case was due to mucus plugging in an asthmatic. Bronchoscopy revealed a thick mucous plug in the left mainstem bronchus. The case was relieved by aspiration of the mucous plug at bronchoscopy **(Figure 4.54b)**. Vigorous physiotherapy and exercise will sometimes have a similar effect. Differential diagnosis include an inhaled foreign body or pneumonia.

→4.53

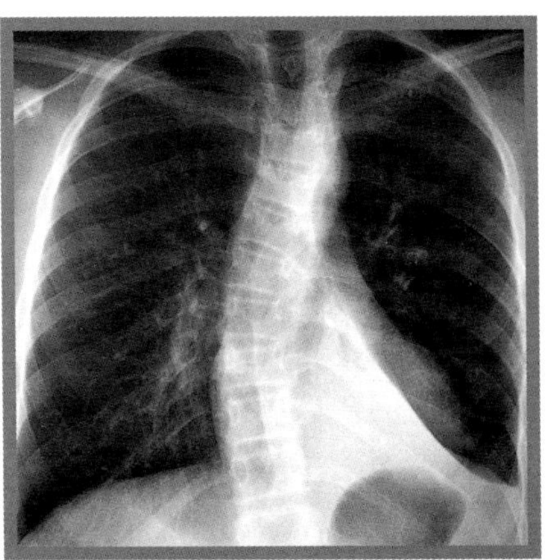

←4.54a

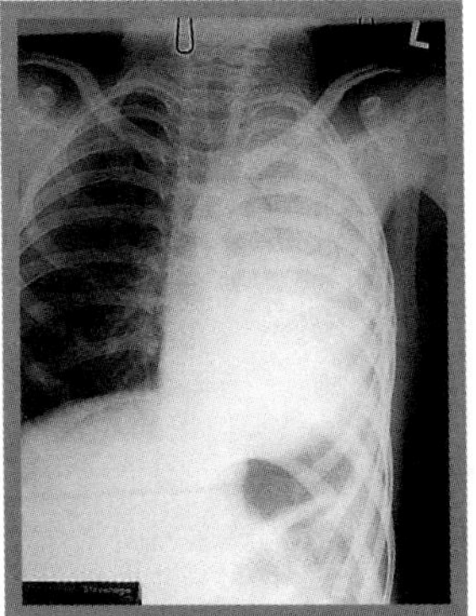

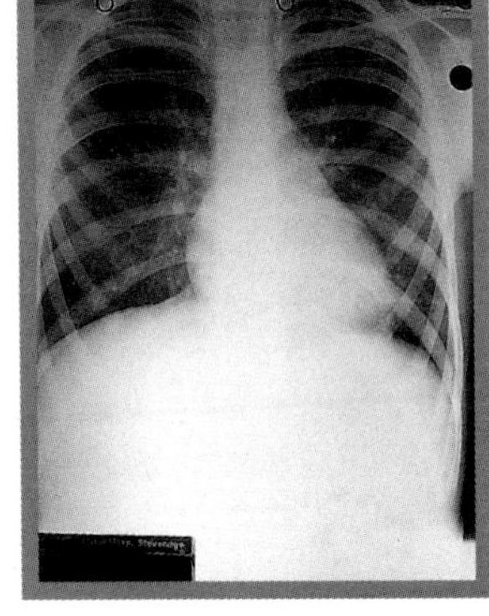

→4.54b

Figure 4.55 X-ray of Aspirated Coin in Upper Airway. Foreign bodies in the upper airway are an important cause of mortality and morbidity in children. Urgent management of the obstructed airway is essential if the child is to survive. The coin shown was removed endoscopically.

Figures 4.56 and 4.57 Right-sided Foreign Body – Tic-tac Top. Figure 4.56 shows a first chest X-ray. It was taken on inspiration and seems normal. On expiration however, the left lung collapses appropriately but the right lung is held in full inspiration by the obstructing 'valve' effect of the foreign body.

Figure 4.58 Foreign Body in Right Main Bronchus. The X-ray shows a screw in the right main bronchus.

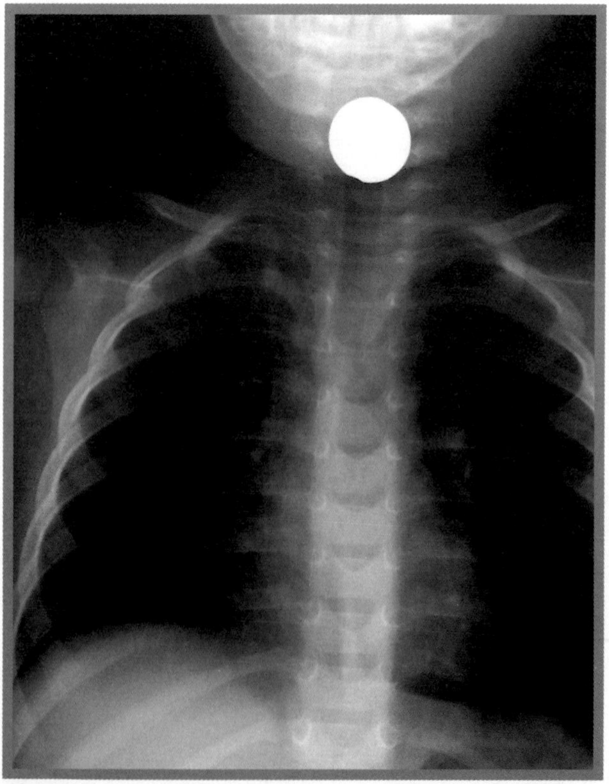

↑4.55

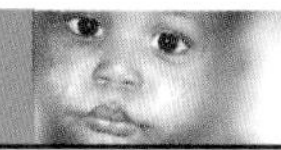

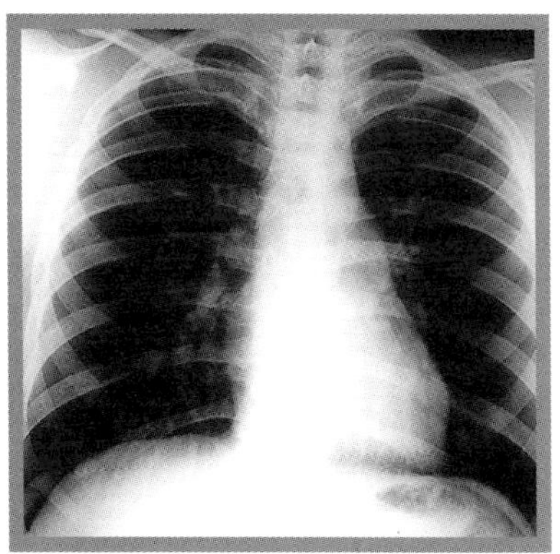

↑ 4.56

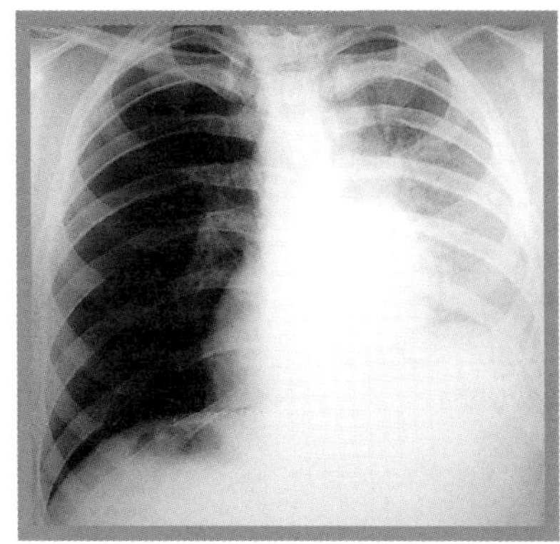

↑ 4.57

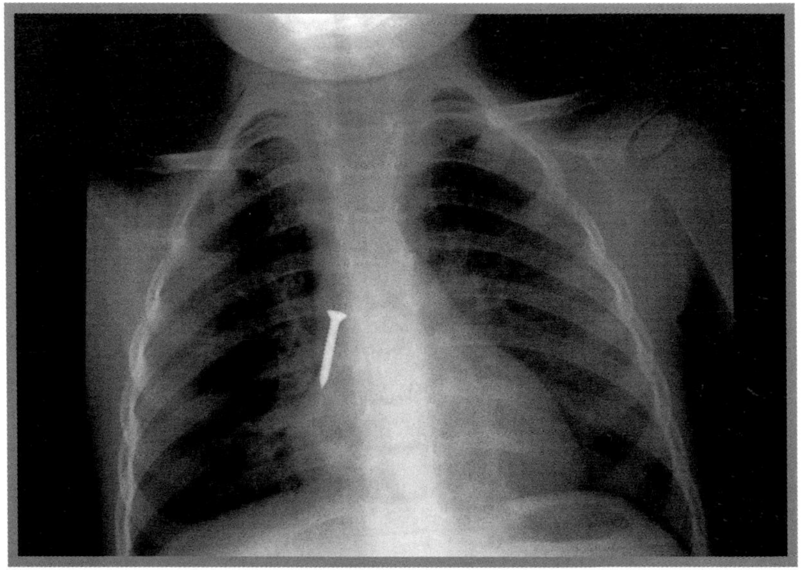

↑ 4.58

Figure 4.59 Aspiration Pneumonia from Gastroesophageal Reflux. The x-ray shows patchy shadowing bilaterally in a non-specific distribution resulting from aspiration. In this case this was due to gastroesophageal reflux.
Figures 4.60 Empyema. (Infected Parapneumonic Effusion). The 11-year-old boy discussed here presented with typical signs of lobar pneumonia: fever, tachypnea and a cough. There was also chest pain and reduced breath sounds on the infected side. In this case, the infecting organism was *Pneumococcus.*

The presence of effusion was confirmed by ultrasound, and loculation had occurred. The child required thoracotomy and decortication. Commonly, the severe cases are associated with Group A streptococcus and *Hemophilus*

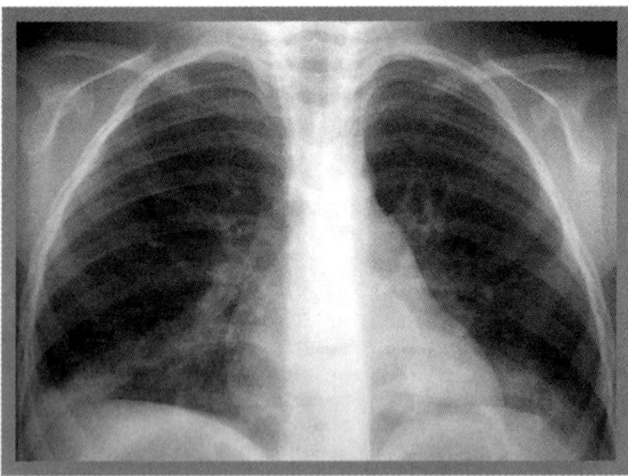

←4.59

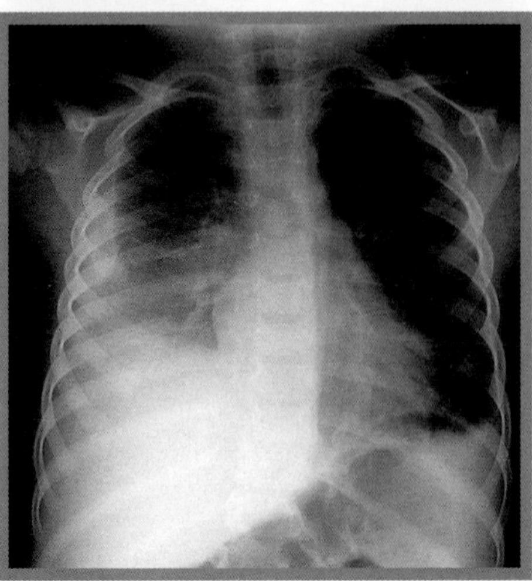

←4.60

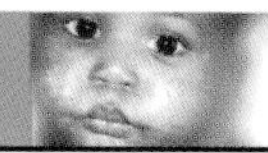

infection and rarely Gram-negative or anaerobic organisms.

The chest X-ray shown here reveals a large pleural effusion on the right lung base that tracks towards the apex and irregular pleural line suggesting loculation.

Figure 4.61 CT scan of right empyema in another child is shown. There is a pleural basal opacity, consisting of fluid surrounded by a thick pleural peel.

Figure 4.62 Cuirass Ventilation in a Child with Upper Airway Obstruction and Central Hypoventilation complicating Hurler Syndrome. Note the nasotracheal tube *in situ* to overcome upper airway obstruction. Increasingly, children with complex disorders are surviving longer, and the management of respiratory failure for many different causes results in the need for long-term continuous or intermittent ventilation, particularly at night. Shown below is an example of ventilation that may be encountered in a home-care setting.

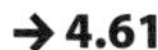

→4.61

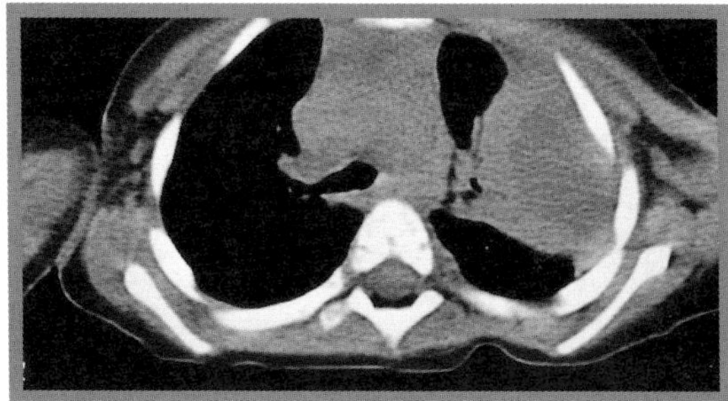

→4.62

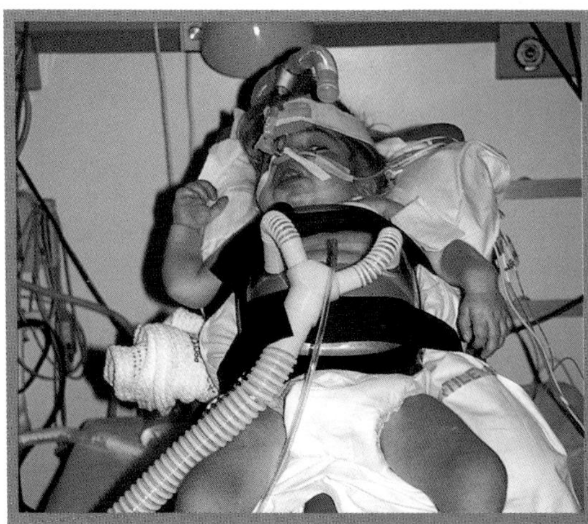

Figures 4.63–4.65 Treacher–Collins Syndrome. Figures 4.63 and **4.64** show a 4-year-old girl who presented with obstructive sleep apnea due to maxillary hypoplasia and micrognathia. The child had failed to thrive, and other anomalies were ear abnormalities (see **Figure 4.64**) and conductive hearing loss. The differential diagnosis includes Goldenhaar syndrome. Treacher–Collins syndrome is autosomal dominant.

Figure 4.65 Treacher–Collins syndrome in a newborn child. The facial features shown are an antimongolian slant, notching of the lateral part of the lower eyelids (coloboma), deficient eyelashes, hypoplasia of the zygomatic bones and micrognathia.

Figure 4.66 Goldenhaar Syndrome. This figure shows malformed ears with preauricular ear tags distributed along the line between the angle of the mouth and ear, and a small jaw. The face was also asymmetric. This condition usually occurs sporadically.

Figure 4.67 Obstructive Sleep Apnea. This X-ray of the postnasal space shows enlarged adenoids. Note the soft-tissue swelling on the roof of the nasopharynx. To investigate the extent of obstructive sleep apnea a sleep study needs to be done.

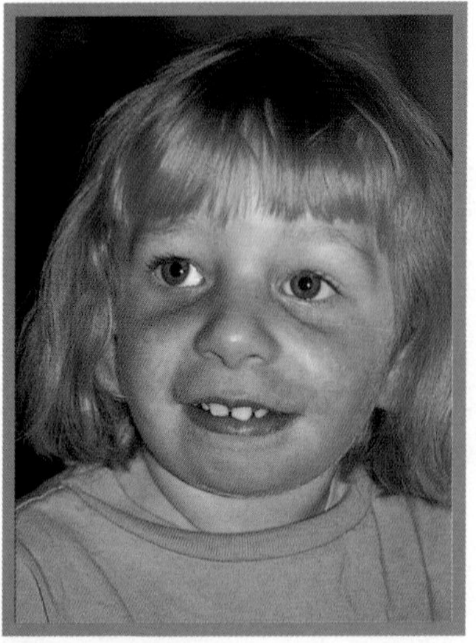

↑ 4.63

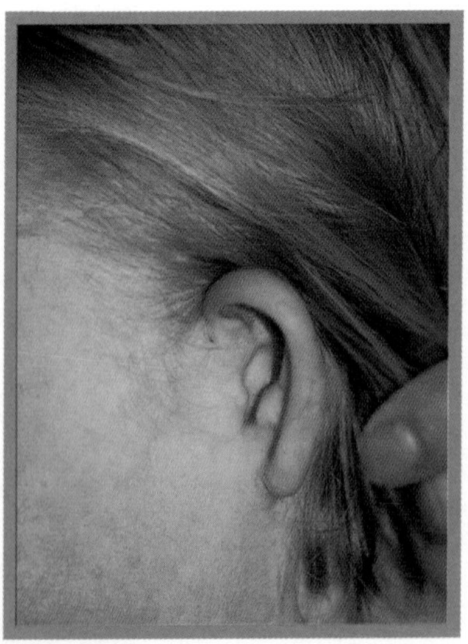

↑ 4.64

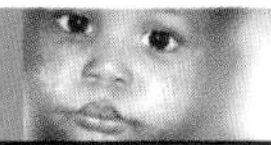

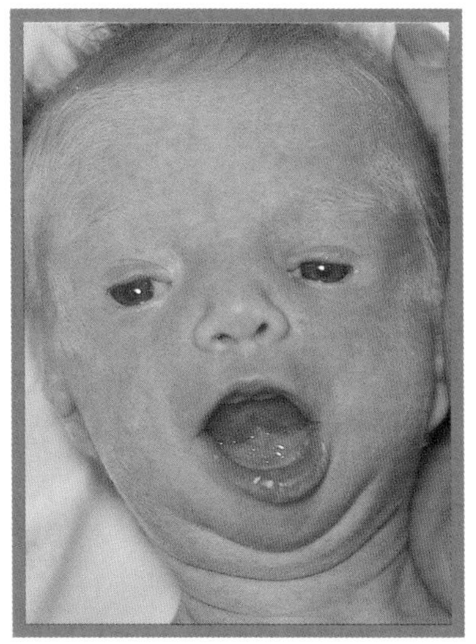

↑ 4.65

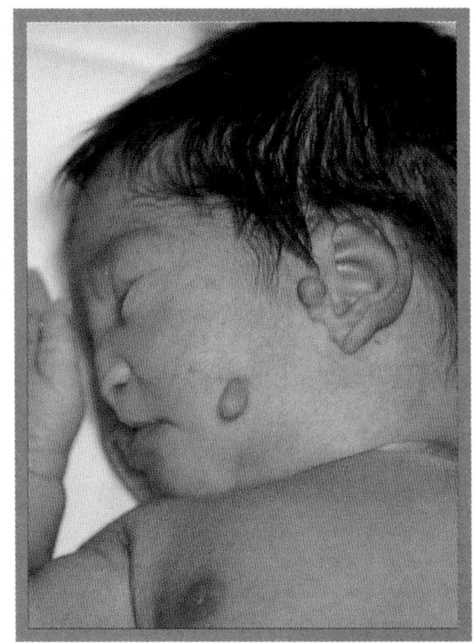

↑ 4.66

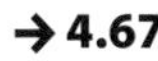

→ 4.67

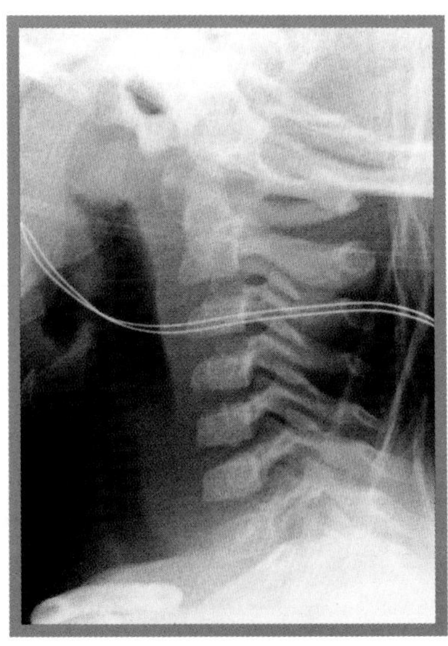

Figures 4.68 and 4.69 Alveolar Proteinosis. The chest X-ray shows ground glass shadowing.The CT demonstrates outlines of secondary pulmonary lobules with micronodular shadowing. This case was due to alveolar proteinosis.

Figure 4.70 Artifact on Chest X-ray. The elongated shadow over the left lung apex can be traced beyond the border of the thoracic cavity and is therefore artifactual. In this case it was due to a hair braid.

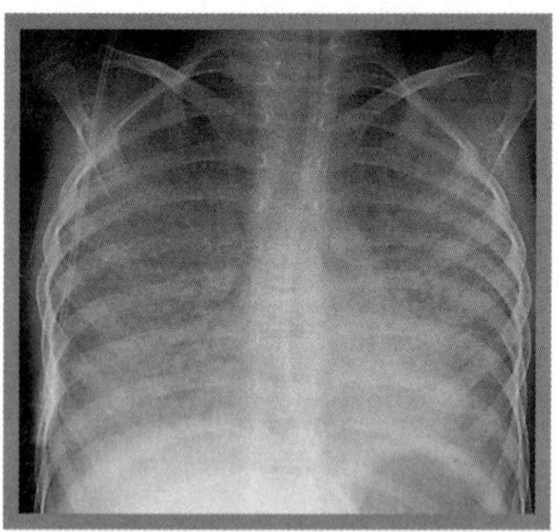

↑4.68

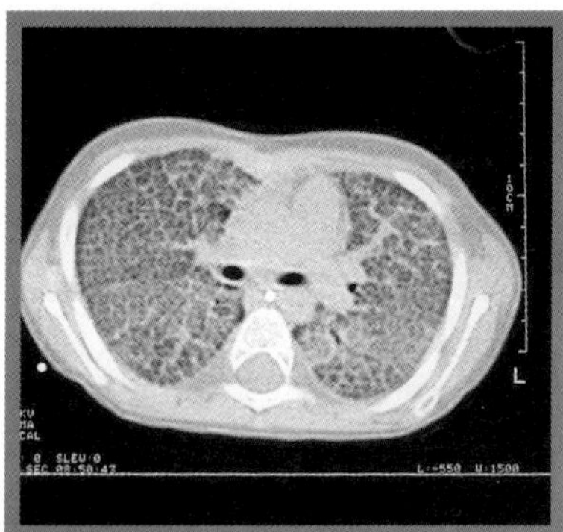

↑4.69

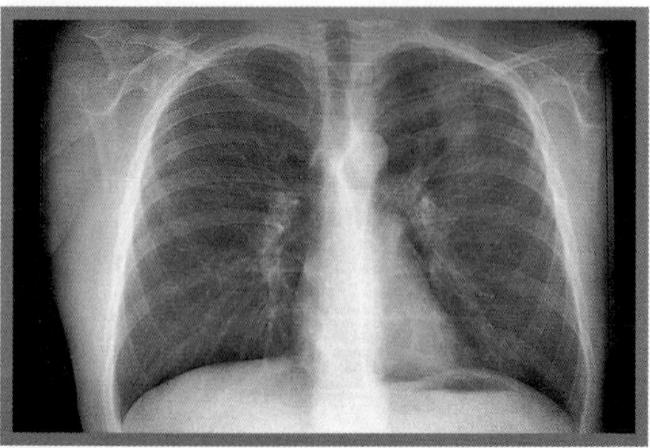

←4.70

5 Gastroenterology

Figures 5.1–5.3 Gastroenteritis with 12–15% Dehydration. The 11-month-old boy shown here presented with 12–15% dehydration resulting from a 3-day history of watery diarrhea, vomiting, pyrexia and loss of weight. At presentation, his weight of 6.2 kg was below the third centile, having previously been on the 50th centile. A clinical assessment of 15% dehydration was made, as indicated by a reduced level of consciousness, sunken eyes, dry oral mucosa, reduced skin turgor (**Figures 5.2 and 5.3**) with a doughy feeling, and shock. Investigations revealed raised plasma sodium (185 mmol/l), potassium and urea, with a metabolic acidosis.

Treatment of shock and intravenous rehydration are indicated, following which oral/nasogastric rehydration should be tried.

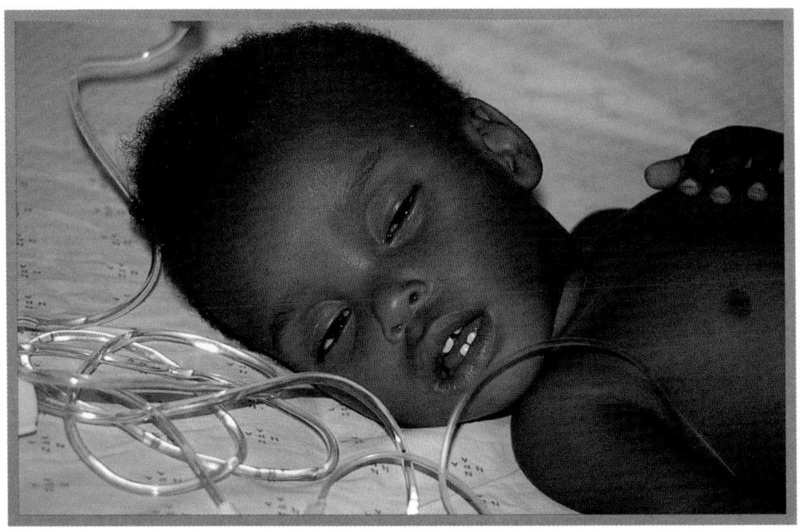

↑ 5.1

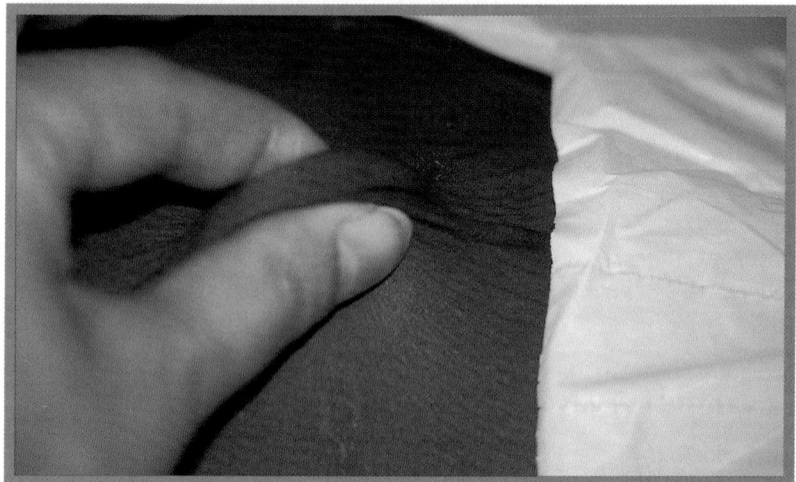

↑ 5.2

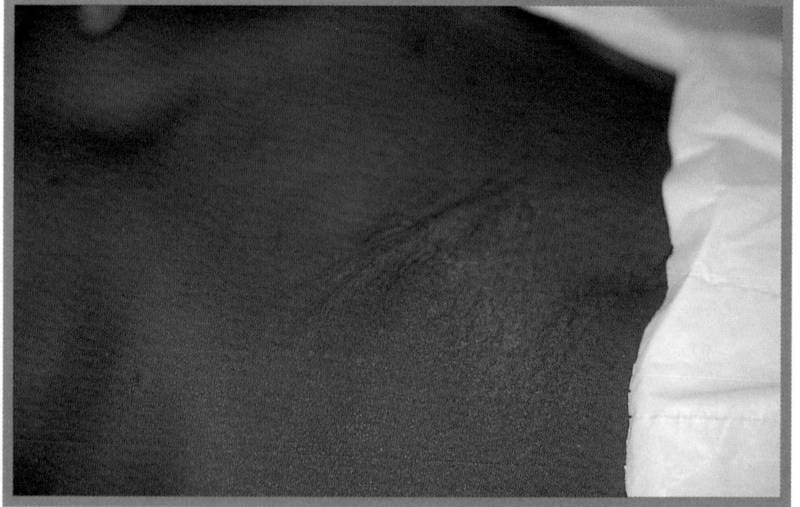

↑ 5.3

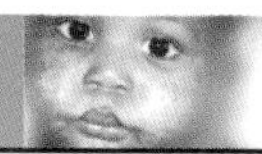

Figures 5.4–5.9 Enteropathies.

Protein Energy Malnutrition (Wellcome Classification)

	60–80% Expected weight	<60% Expected weight
No edema	Underweight	Marasmus
Edema	Kwashiorkor	Marasmic kwashiorkor

Figures 5.4 and 5.5 Kwashiorkor. Kwashiorkor occurs when the diet has a low protein-to-energy ratio, and is an edematous form of protein–energy malnutrition. Low albumin levels lead to edema. A reduced synthesis of alipoprotein predisposes to a fatty liver. Recurrent infection further diverts amino acids for the synthesis of acute phase proteins, which further reduces the hepatic synthesis of albumin.

The clinical features are shown in this 8-month-old child, whose weight of 7.7 Kg was 70% of the expected weight. There was a history of fever, oral ulceration, body swelling and absence of breast feeding. Clinically, the child demonstrates edema and areas of skin hypo- and hyperpigmentation, desquamation and ulceration. Sparse hair growth, with a classic ginger discoloration, is also seen.

The hair could be pulled out easily. Small hemorrhages are often seen around the hair follicles. An apathetic appearance is a feature.

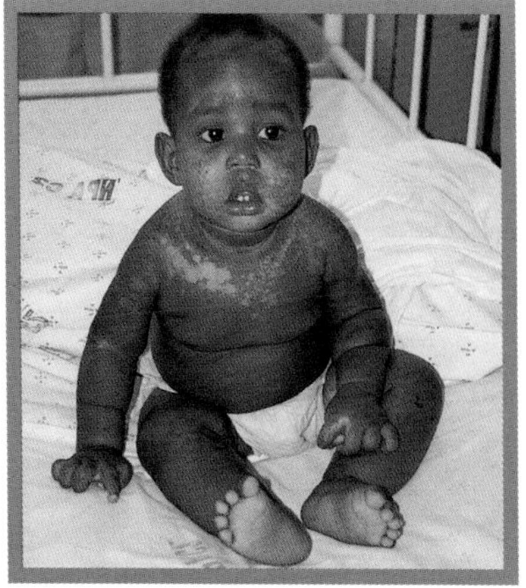

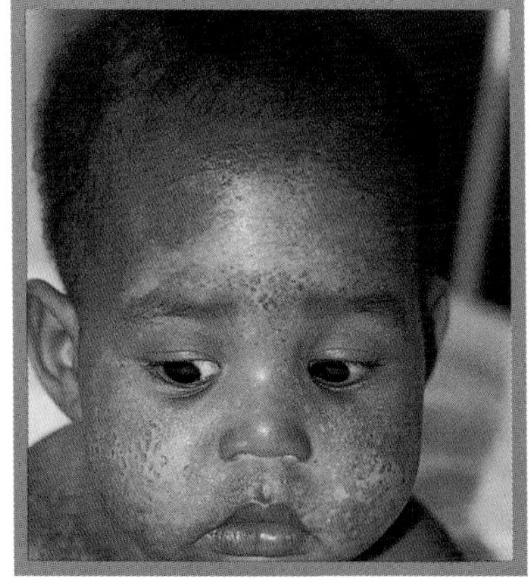

↑ 5.4

↑ 5.5

Figure 5.6 Marasmus. The 18-month-old Indian child shown here has severe malnutrition. Her weight of 6 kg is less than 60% of the expected weight for her age. Note loss of subcutaneous fat and muscle wasting. This child had candidal stomatitis, developmental delay and tuberculosis. Marasmus results from inadequate food intake, usually complicated by chronic infection.

Absence of edema in the presence of severe muscle wasting is characteristic of marasmus.

Figures 5.7–5.9 Marasmic Kwashiorkor. Marasmic kwashiorkor covers intermediate forms of protein–energy malnutrition wasting with a variety of clinical dermatoses and/or the edema characteristic of kwashiorkor. The children shown here are typically thin, with a weight of less than 60% of that expected.

Figures 5.7 and 5.8 show a 2-year-old girl with hypo- and hyperkeratosis, dry skin that is ulcerating in parts, facial edema, sparse hair growth, a reduction in linear growth, irritability, apathy.and marked muscular weakness resulting in immobility.

Figure 5.9 shows a girl with severe protein–energy malnutrition. She died shortly after the slide was taken. She has typical features, including hair discoloration, hypo- and hyperpigmentation of the skin, angular stomatitis, periorbital edema, and hepatomegaly due to fatty change in the liver. Her INR (clotting ratio) of 2.2 gives an indication of the disease severity, and Hb was 9 gm, with a microcytic, hypochromic picture. She died of overwhelming sepsis.

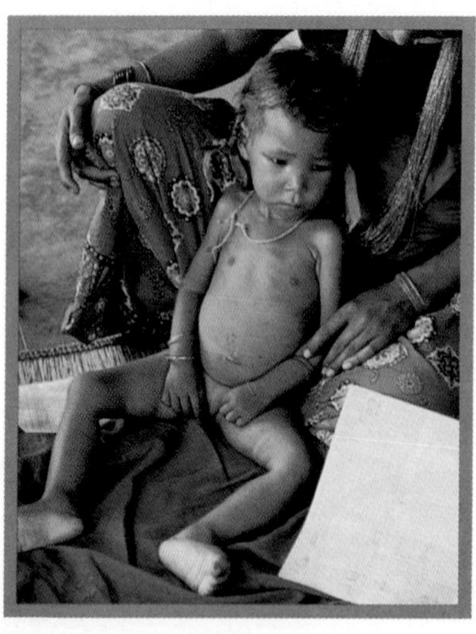

↑5.6

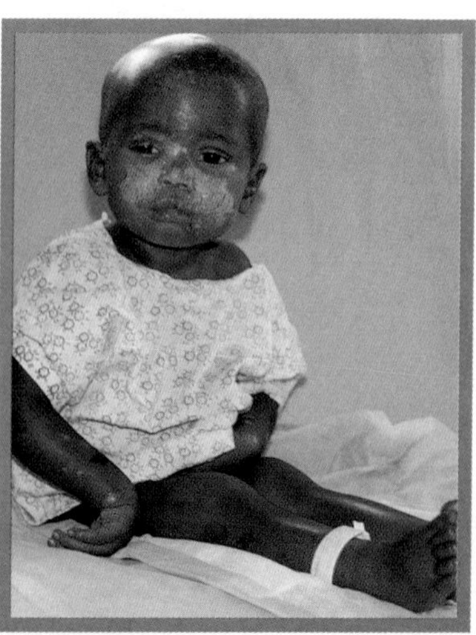

↑5.7

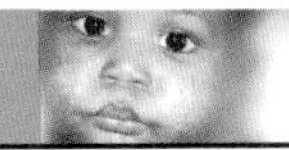

→ 5.8

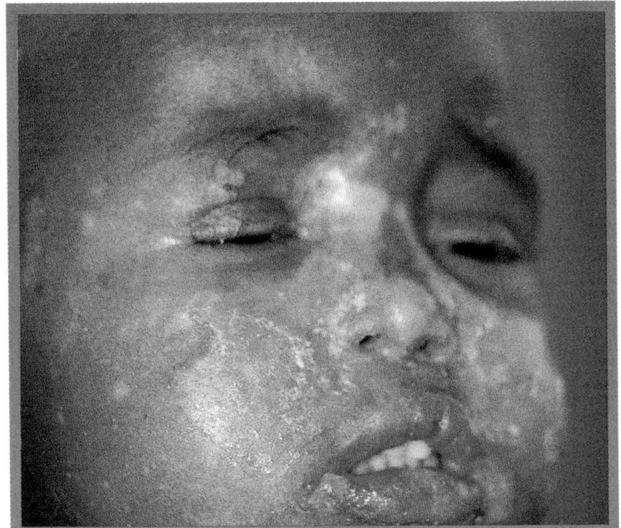

→ 5.9

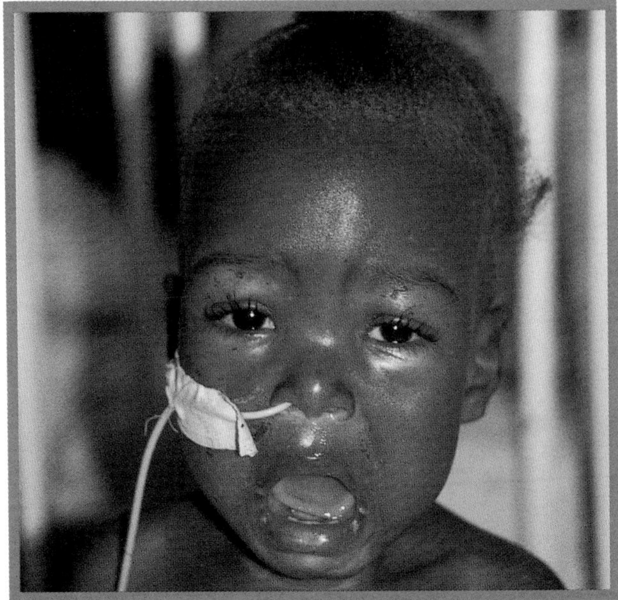

Figures 5.10 and 5.11 Perforated Ileum Secondary to Typhoid Enteritis. The 14-year-old boy from Nigeria shown here had a history of 1 week of a flu-like illness. In the second week he developed a headache, drowsiness, anorexia and vomiting, abdominal pain, diarrhea and a swinging temperature. In the beginning of the third week of the illness the child deteriorated suddenly, with tachycardia, hypotension and a rigid abdomen. An erect abdominal X-ray (**Figure 5.11**) showed free air under the left hemidiaphragm, and at laparotomy a perforated terminal ileum was noted. This is the most common complication of typhoid in this age group.

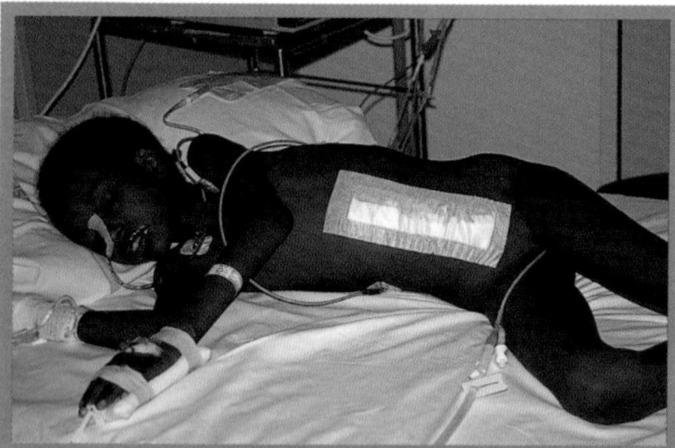

←5.10

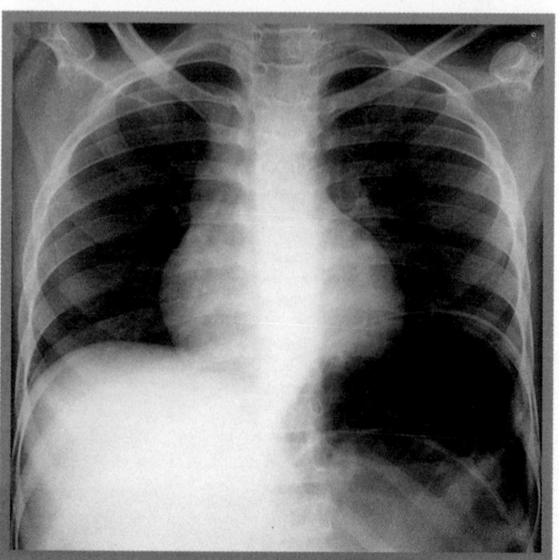

←5.11

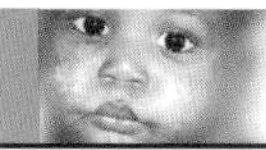

Figures 5.12 and 5.13 Hepatitis. The 5-year-old girl shown here has hepatitis B resulting from infected instruments used either in the piercing of her ear or the traditional facial scarification. Her mother was seronegative for hepatitis B. Clinical features in this case were those of acute severe hepatitis, with ascites, everted umbilicus, distended veins across the abdomen due to portal hypertension, fever, lassitude and jaundice. Note the flank bruising due to clotting abnormalities. Treatment is supportive and consists of dietary manipulation, management of ascites, vitamin K administration and, rarely, liver transplant in acute severe fulminant hepatitis.

→5.12

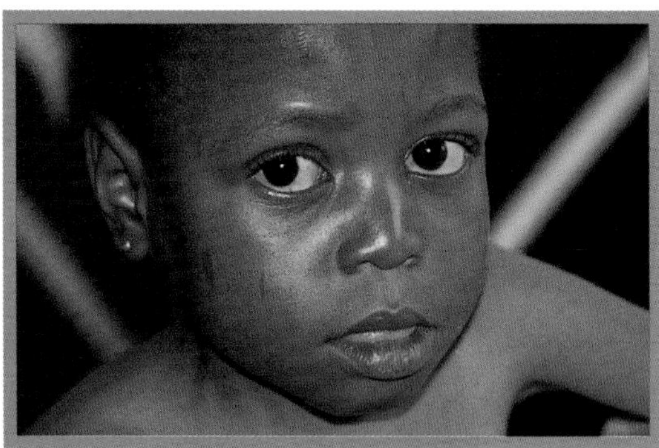

→5.13

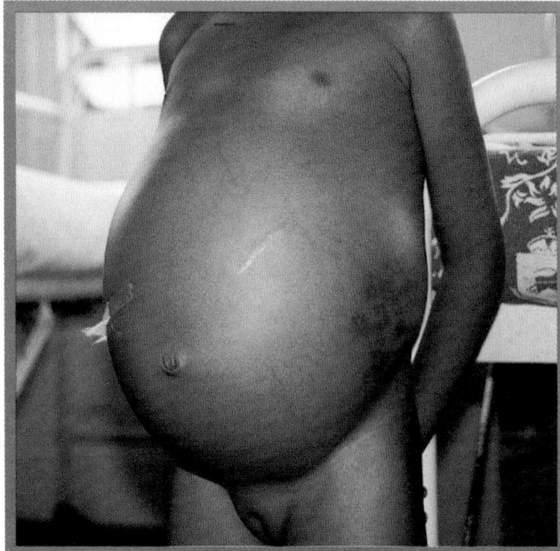

Figure 5.14 Hepatosplenomegaly. The 1-year-old HIV-positive girl shown here had respiratory distress secondary to bronchopneumonia due to tuberculosis. She had had a 1-month history of diarrhoea, resulting in a marasmic appearance. Additionally, she had generalized lymphadenopathy, hepatosplenomegaly, muscle wasting and developmental delay. The cause of her overall condition was vertical transmission of HIV from her mother.

Figure 5.15 Hepatosplenomegaly in a Male Infant. There is a wide differential diagnosis for hepatosplenomegaly, including structural abnormalities, *e.g.*, extrahepatic biliary atresia, infection, hematological disorders including hemoglobinopathies, inborn errors of metabolism, and storage disorders, tumors, and prehepatic and some hepatic causes of portal hypertension. In this child, hepatosplenomegaly is due to HIV infection.

Figure 5.16 Candidal Esophagitis (Endoscopic Photograph). The girl with AIDS discussed here presented with dysphagia and retrosternal discomfort. She also had oral and perianal candidiasis. Treatment consistsed in administration of oral and intravenous antifungals. Systemic spread may occur in immmunocompromised patients and may be life threatening.

Figure 5.17 Extrahepatic Biliary Atresia. This figure shows a 10-month-old Asian boy with massive ascites, jaundice, gross failure to thrive, dilated abdominal veins and jejunostomy. The diagnosis is clinical, and is based on

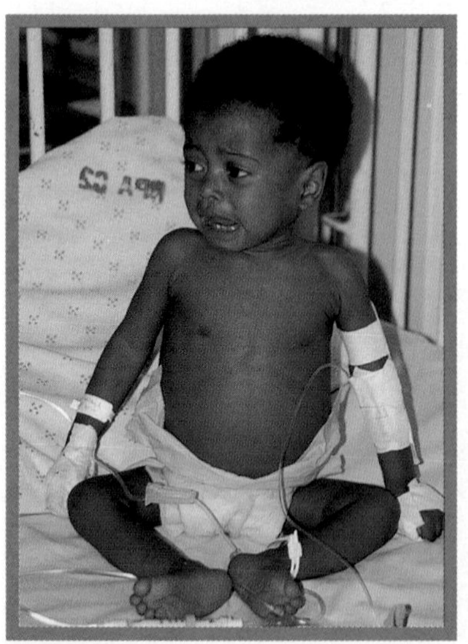

↑5.14

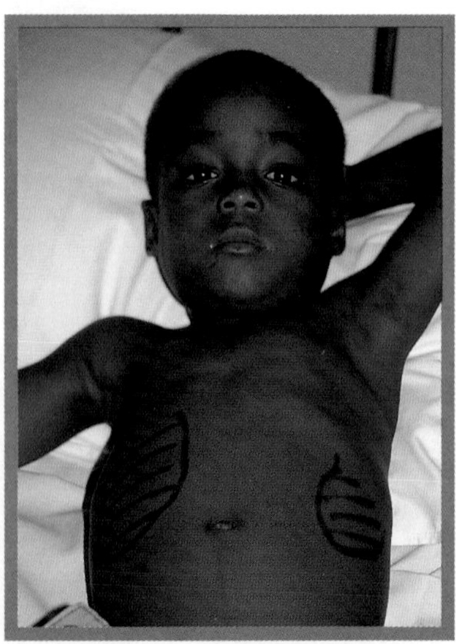

↑5.15

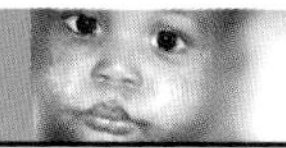

the obstructive pattern of jaundice from 3 weeks of age onwards, with dark 'tea' colored urine and acholic, white stools. Liver function tests showed an obstructive pattern and a radioisotope scan confirmed biliary obstruction. Liver biopsy is recommended after correction of any coagulopathy.

→5.16

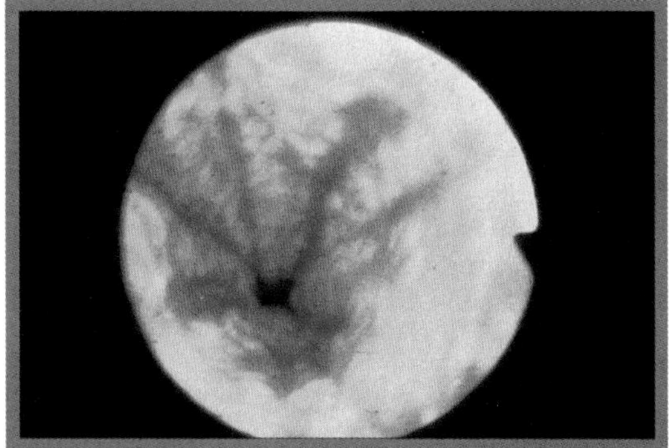

→5.17

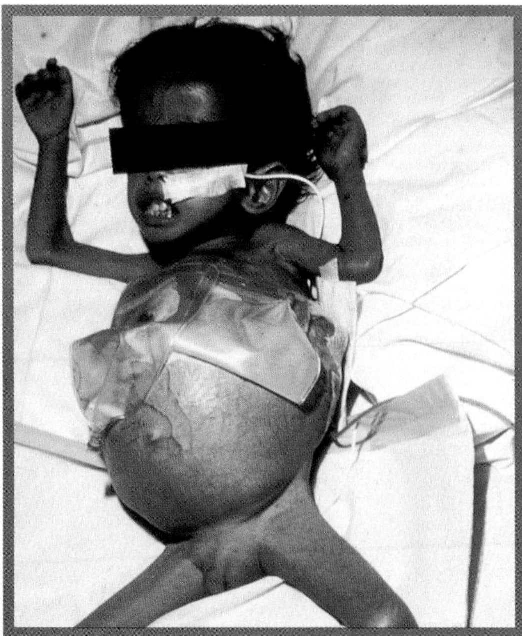

Figure 5.18 Acholic Stools in a Case of Biliary Atresia. Early intervention leads to better results, so treatment should be commenced before 60 days. A surgical drainage procedure (Kasai) may be used, or a transplant in older children where drainage is not possible or fails. Supportive medical therapy consists of dietary manipulation, vitamin supplements and control of sepsis.
Figure 5.19 Jaundice. This figure shows icteric sclerae due to jaundice. The 8-year-old shown here had had a bone marrow transplant. Following the transplant, the child developed cytomegalovirus (CMV) hepatitis.

There is an increased frequency of CMV infection due to immunosuppression, and such infection may be a reactivation of latent disease or may be acquired from the bone marrow donor or blood products. The clinical features were jaundice, lymphadenopathy and hepatosplenomegaly. Investigations revealed atypical lymphocytes, hemolytic anemia, abnormal liver function tests, and a significant rise in complement fixing antibodies to CMV. Liver function tests

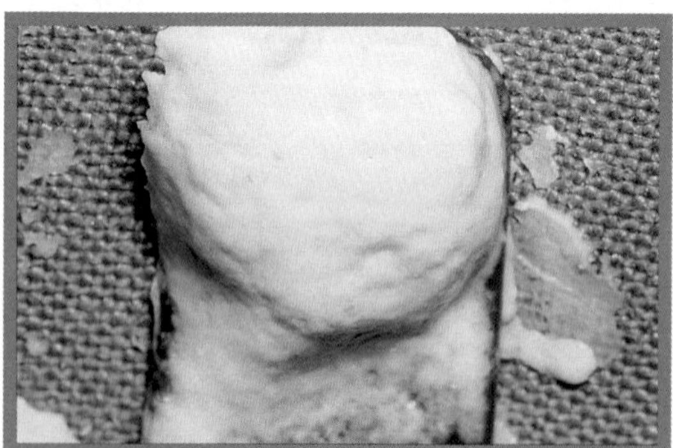

←5.18

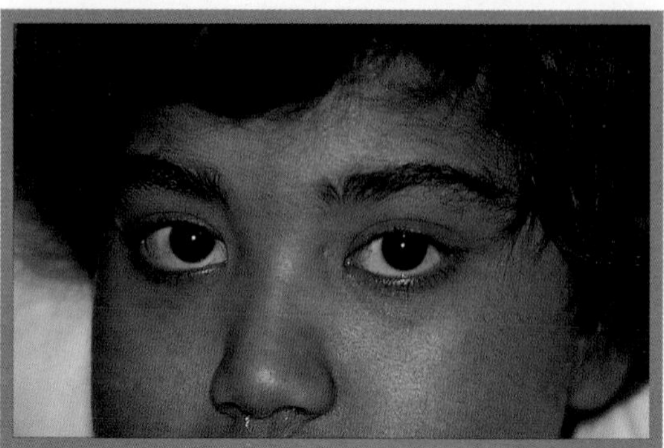

←5.19

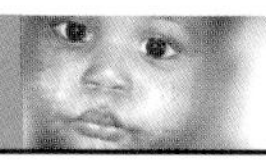

were abnormal and the virus was isolated from the urine. Such patients may develop pneumonitis, retinitis and colitis leading to death. Treatment is with hyperimmune globulin and/or gangciclovir. Relapse may occur in up to 50% of patients after gancyclovir. This is an unusual case.

In older children, the more usual differential diagnosis of jaundice includes:

1. Infection, *e.g.*, viral hepatitis, Epstein–Barr hepatitis.
2. Hemolysis, *e.g.*, due to hemoglobinopathy.
3. Metabolic disorders, *e.g.*, Wilson , Dubin–Johnson, Gilbert disease.
4. Structural disorders, *e.g.*, choledochal cysts, cirrhosis in cystic fibrosis.
5. Autoimmune disorders, *e.g.*, chronic active hepatitis.

Figure 5.20 Pruritus in Obstructive Jaundice. The 7-year-old boy shown here presented with jaundice and hepatomegaly which, in this case, was due to Alagille syndrome. This is a syndrome of intrahepatic bile duct hypoplasia leading to obstructive jaundice. There may be associated cardiac lesions, *e.g.*, peripheral pulmonary stenosis and tetralogy of Fallot. Facial features are a prominent forehead, deep-set eyes, a mongoloid slant, a prominent nasal bridge, a pointed chin and posterior embryotoxin in the lens. Diagnosis is by chromosomal analysis. As shown, obstructive jaundice causing pruritus was a problem in this case. These children often require liver transplantation.

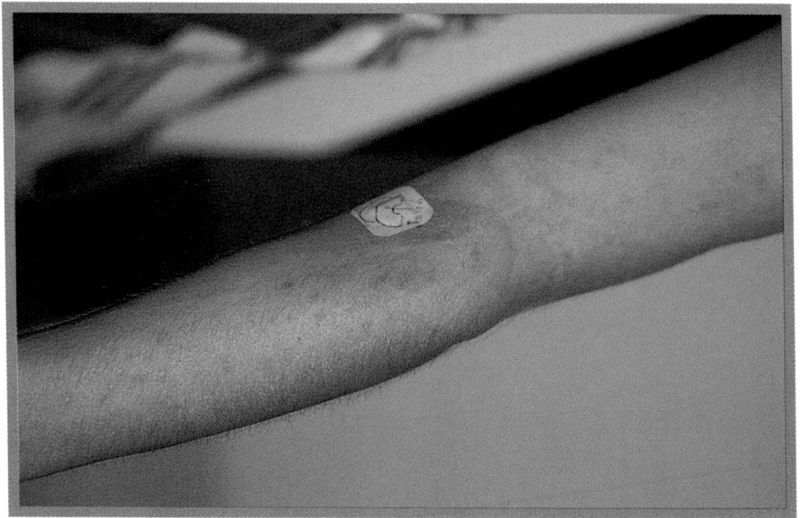

↑ 5.20

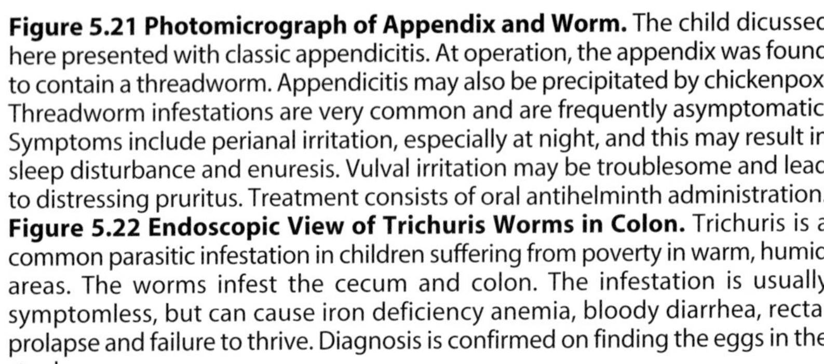

Figure 5.21 Photomicrograph of Appendix and Worm. The child dicussed here presented with classic appendicitis. At operation, the appendix was found to contain a threadworm. Appendicitis may also be precipitated by chickenpox. Threadworm infestations are very common and are frequently asymptomatic. Symptoms include perianal irritation, especially at night, and this may result in sleep disturbance and enuresis. Vulval irritation may be troublesome and lead to distressing pruritus. Treatment consists of oral antihelminth administration.
Figure 5.22 Endoscopic View of Trichuris Worms in Colon. Trichuris is a common parasitic infestation in children suffering from poverty in warm, humid areas. The worms infest the cecum and colon. The infestation is usually symptomless, but can cause iron deficiency anemia, bloody diarrhea, rectal prolapse and failure to thrive. Diagnosis is confirmed on finding the eggs in the stools.

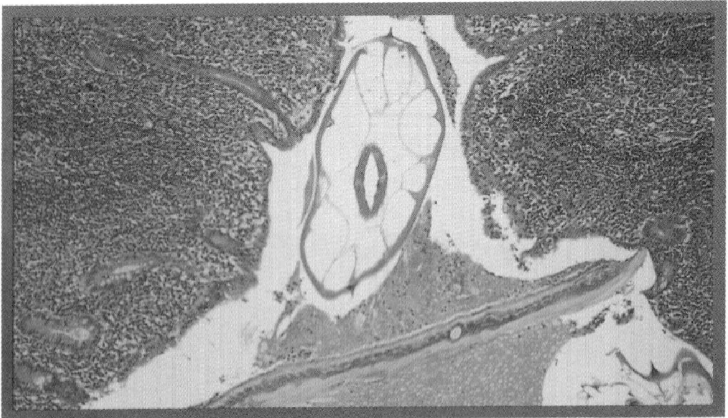

←5.21

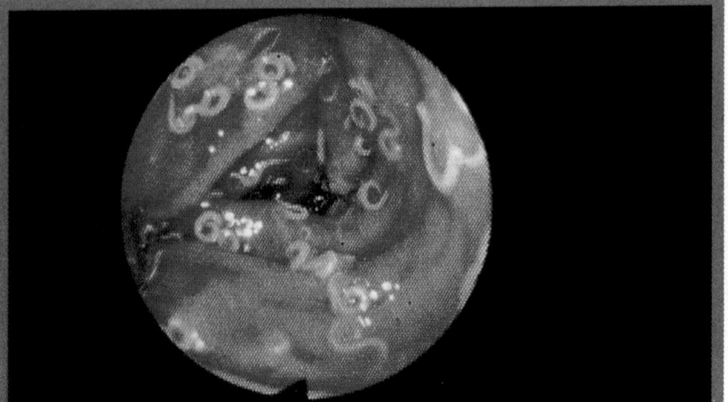

←5.22

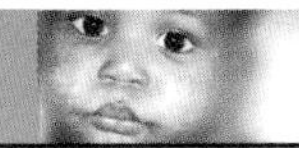

Figures 5.23–5.29 Inflammatory Bowel Disease. Figure 5.23 shows lip swelling in a child with Crohn disease. Note the angular stomatitis. Lip swelling is pathognomonic of inflammatory bowel diseases.
Figure 5.24 Oral Crohn Disease in a 13-year-old Boy with Cystic Fibrosis. Note the lip swelling and oral ulceration. Interestingly, Crohn disease is more common in cystic fibrosis.

→ 5.23

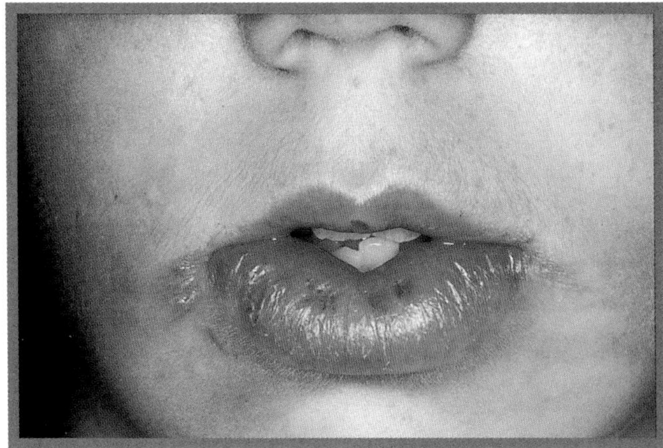

→ 5.24

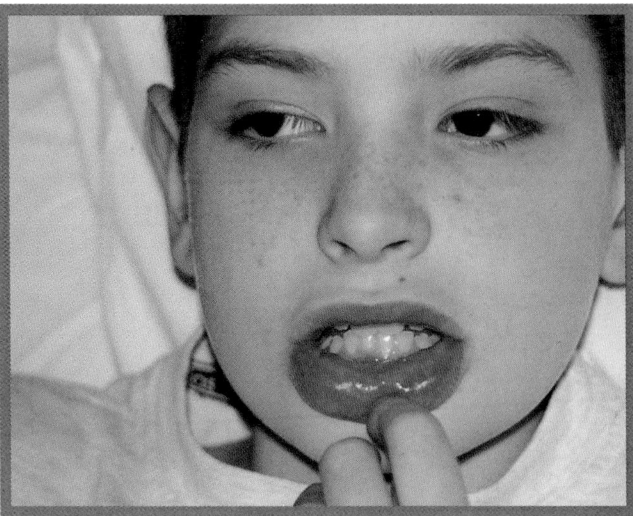

Figure 5.25 Aphthous Ulceration in a Child with Crohn Disease. A large vasculitic ulcer resulting in tissue necrosis from focal vasculitis is shown. This is a common local complication and is a common presenting symptom.
Figure 5.26 Multiple Small Aphthous Ulcers Associated with Crohn Disease. Such ulcers may also be found in ulcerative colitis.
Figure 5.27 Extensive Perianal Crohn Disease. This patient has ulceration, abscess formation and anal fissuring. Fistula formation is common.
Figure 5.28 Severe Colitis in a 1-year-old with Perianal Manifestations of Crohn Disease. The differential diagnosis must include other vasculitic diseases, *e.g.*, Behçet disease and child sexual abuse.

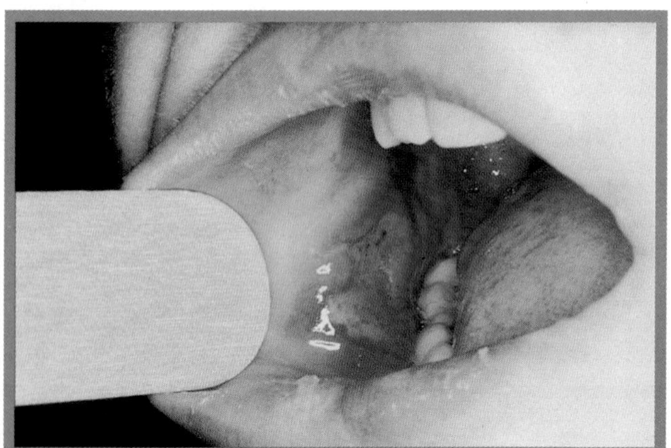

←5.25

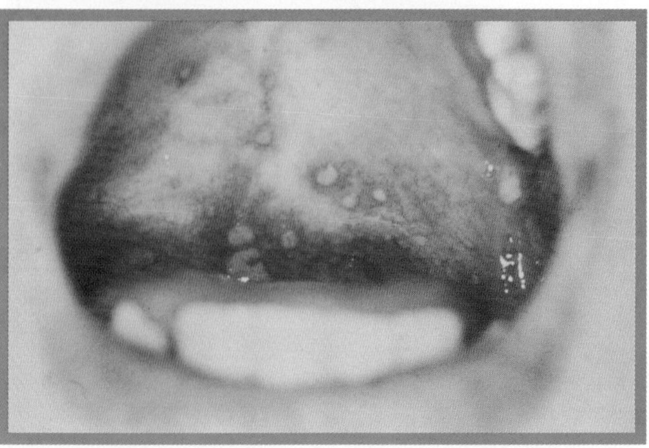

←5.26

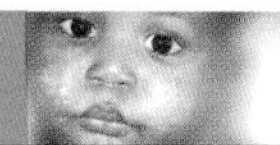

→ 5.27

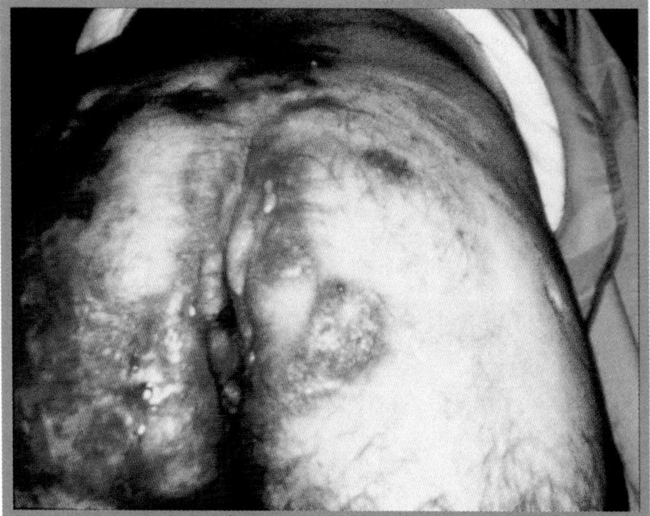

→ 5.28

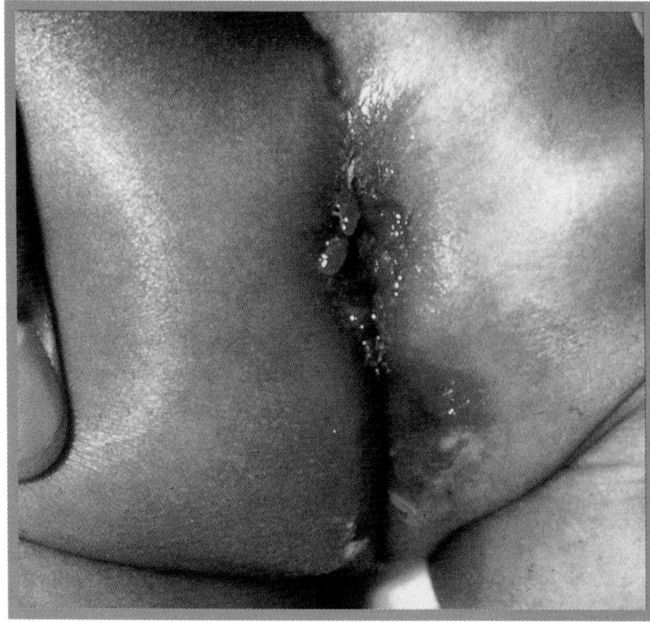

Figure 5.29 Colonoscopic Appearance of Ulcerative Colitis. Erythematous colonic mucosa are shown, with loss of vascular markings and contact bleeding, typical of ulcerative colitis. The diagnosis was confirmed histologically. Investigations may include a barium swallow and follow through, pre- and post-treatment endoscopy, and labelled white cell scans.
Figure 5.30 Chronic Esophagitis on Endoscopy. The baby of 4 months discussed here had severe gastroesophageal reflux, which was investigated with pH monitoring. The baby responded well to antacids, gastric motility agents and a diet free of cows' milk.

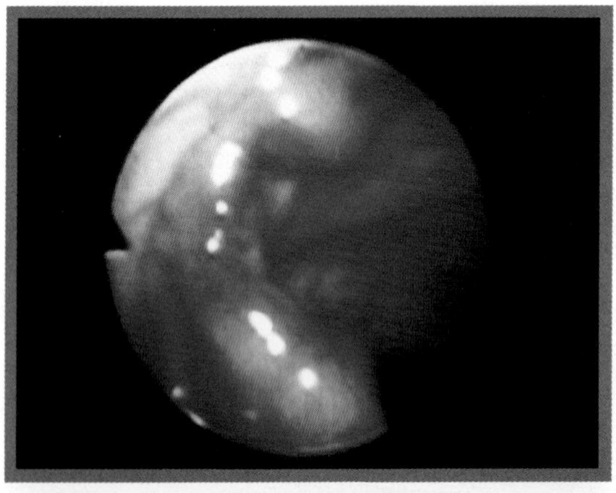

←5.29

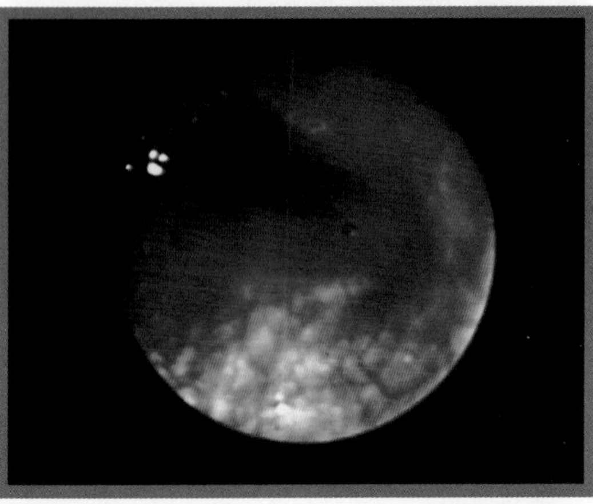

←5.30

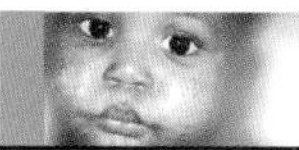

Figure 5.31 Endoscopic Appearance of an Esophageal Ulcer. The esophageal ulceration shown results from chronic gastroesophageal reflux.

Figure 5.32 Endoscopic Appearance of *Helicobacter pylori.* The 6-year-old boy discussed here presented with abdominal pain and vomiting. There was a family history of peptic ulceration. A barium swallow demonstrated multiple, small, peptic ulcers. At endoscopy, gastric lymphonodular hyperplasia was noted. A positive culture result was obtained from mucosal biopsy. The boy was successfully treated with multiple antihelicobacter drug therapy.

→5.31

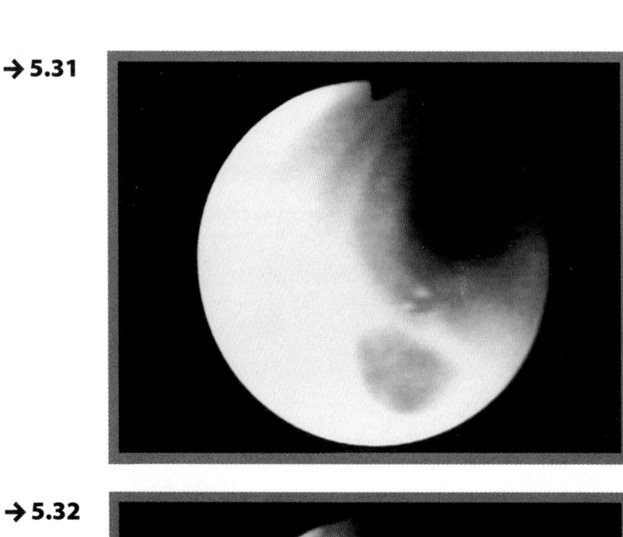

→5.32

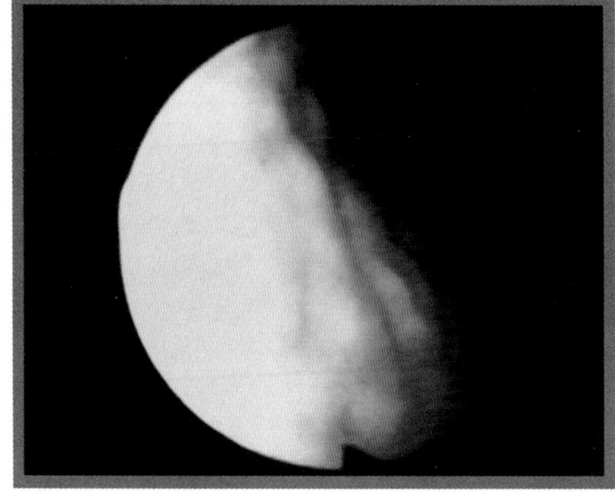

Figures 5.33 and 5.34 Juvenile Colonic Polyp. The 7-year-old child shown here presented with a history of rectal prolapse and bleeding. Colonoscopy was indicated as the prolapse was described as a grape-like structure.

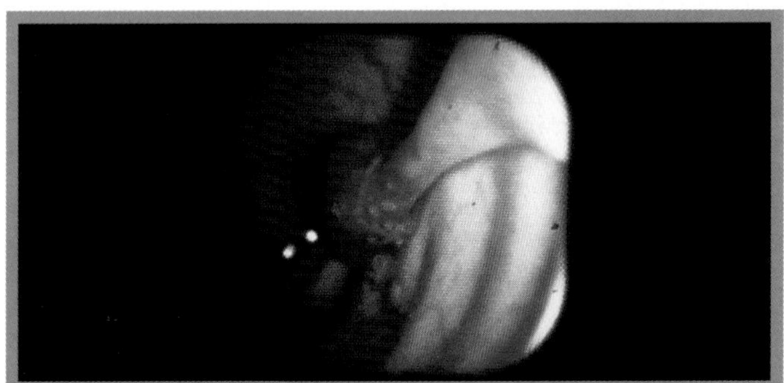

←5.33

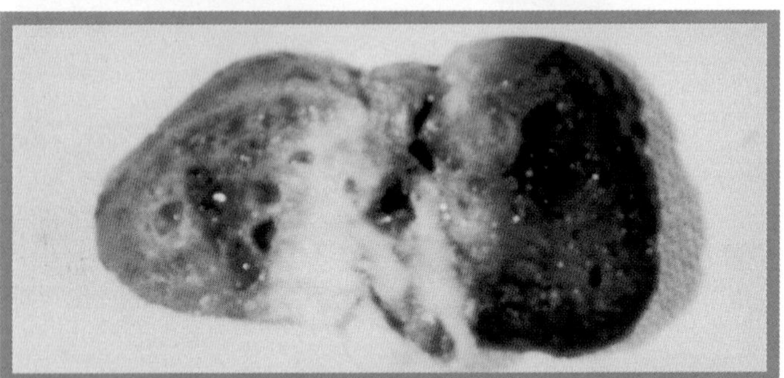

←5.34

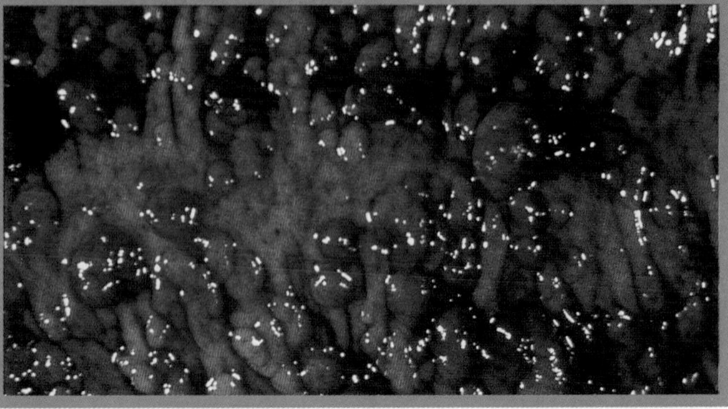

←5.35

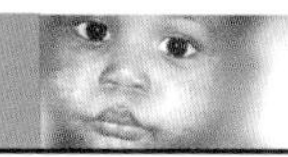

Hamartomatous lesions such as this are found in the rectum or distal colon. As in this case they are pedunculated (mounted on a stalk) and contain mucus-secreting cysts. They may present with recurrent abdominal pain and intussusception. Treatment consists of endoscopic removal.

Figure 5.35 Gross Macroscopic Appearance of Familial Polyposis Coli. Note the multiple polyps in this specimen of colon from a child who presented with blood and mucous in the stools.

This is an autosomal dominant condition, which invariably undergoes malignant change. It requires regular surveillance by colonoscopy from 5 years of age until early adult life when a colectomy will be necessary.

Figures 5.36–5.38 Celiac Disease (Gluten Sensitive Enteropathy). This is a disorder in which a sensitivity to the gliadin fraction of gluten causes predominantly proximal small bowel mucosal damage. This fraction is found in wheat, rye, barley and oats. The boy shown here presented with a 2-year history of bulky, pale, frothy, greasy stools associated with failure to thrive, abdominal distension and abdominal pain.

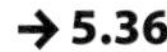

→ 5.36

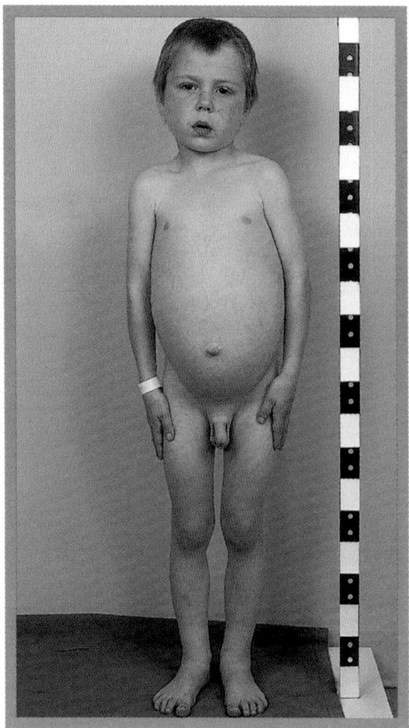

On examination, the boy was found to be of short stature, and had abdominal distension secondary to intestinal accumulation of gas and fluid. There was marked wasting of the buttocks and limbs, with relative sparing of the face. Investigations showed anemia, reduced red cell folate, iron deficiency, hypoproteinemia and prolonged prothrombin time due to vitamin K deficiency. If not IgA deficient, serum IgA endomysial antibodies may be diagnostic. The gold standard, however, remains a jejunal biopsy before starting treatment.

This will show a subtotal villous atrophy, increased lamina propria inflammatory cells and intraepithelial lymphocytes. The differential diagnosis consists of cow- or soya-milk protein intolerance, post enteritis enteropathy, and autoimmune and congenital enteropathies. Cystic fibrosis should be excluded if weight gain is inadequate on a gluten-free diet, and siblings should also be assessed.

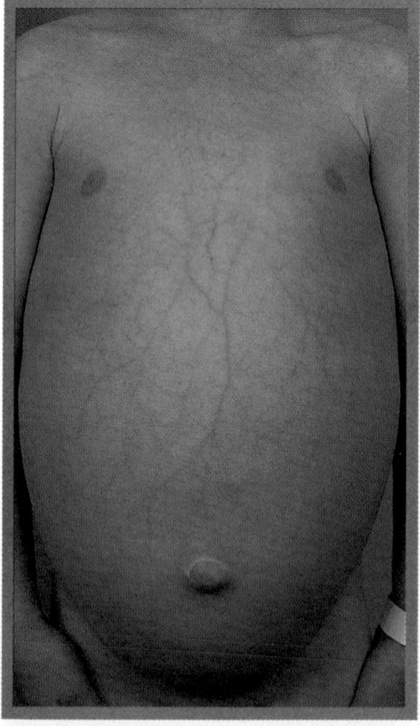

↑ 5.37

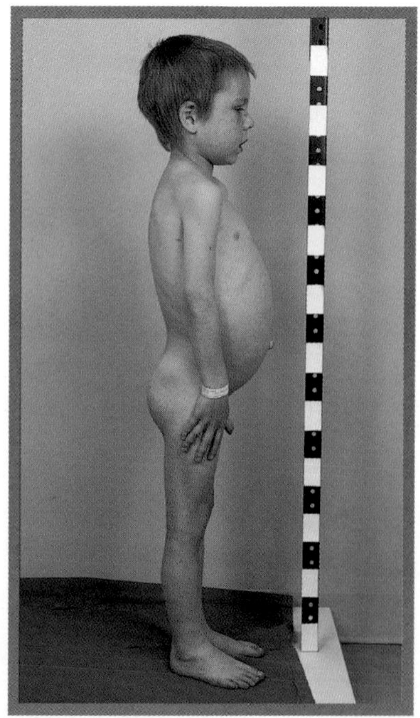

↑ 5.38

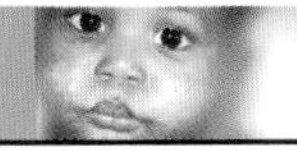

Treatment is effected by giving a gluten-free diet. Re-biopsy is not necessary if the first biopsy was diagnostic and a good clinical response to the new diet is observed. Further challenge may be required if a child is less than 2 years of age at diagnosis, or is anti-endomysial IgA antibody negative. This disorder is linked to HLA-DQ status and is a T-cell mediated disease. Coeliac disease is 10 times more common in diabetes.

Figures 5.39–5.44 Cystic Fibrosis (CF). Figures 5.39 and 5.40 show a 6-year-old boy with severe respiratory and gastrointestinal involvement due to cystic fibrosis. His elder sibling is similarly affected. Both have the common ΔF508 gene abnormality (homozygous ΔF508 in 70–80% of Caucasian CF sufferers). Note the failure to thrive, pallor, loss of muscle bulk, Harrison sulci and barrel chest deformity, with intercostal recession. Compare this to coeliac disease (**Figures 5.36–5.38**), particularly the more marked buttock wasting abdominal, distension, and the absence of chest signs in the coeliac child.

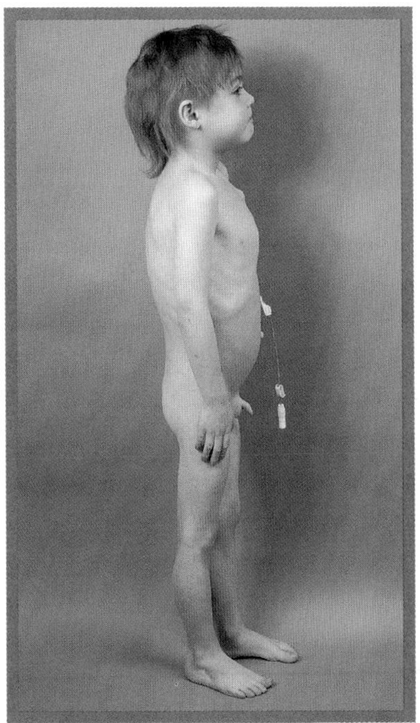

↑5.39

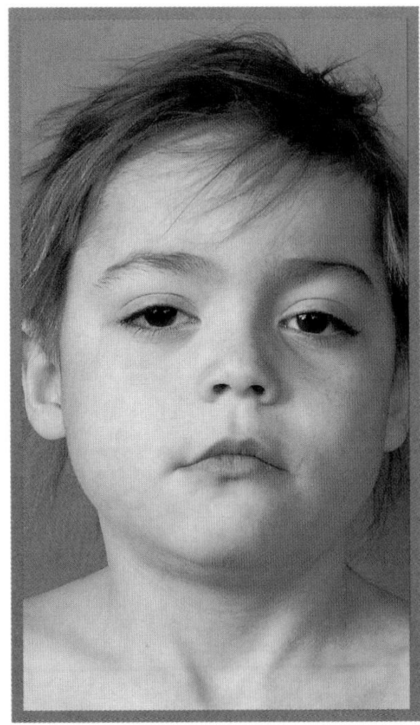

↑5.40

Figure 5.41 shows clubbing and thickening of the proximal interphalangeal joints of hypertrophic osteoarthropathy in cystic fibrosis.
Figure 5.42 Note the gastrostomy feeding tube used to provide extra nutrition in this case of cystic fibrosis. The calorie requirement is approximately 150% above normal. Also shown at the left subclavicular area is the site of an implanted vascular access device (Porta-cath) for regular antibiotic infusions.

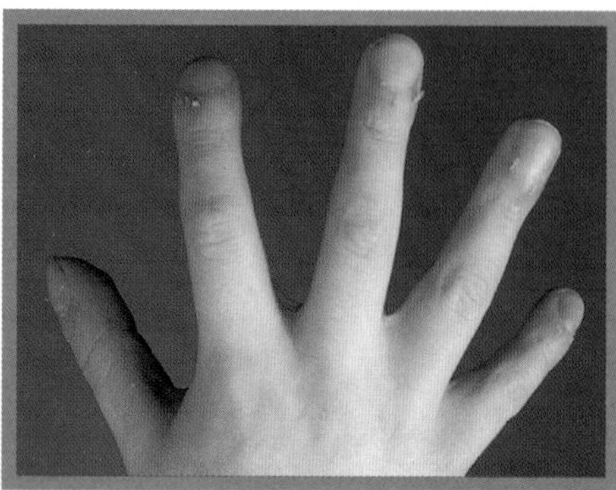

←5.41

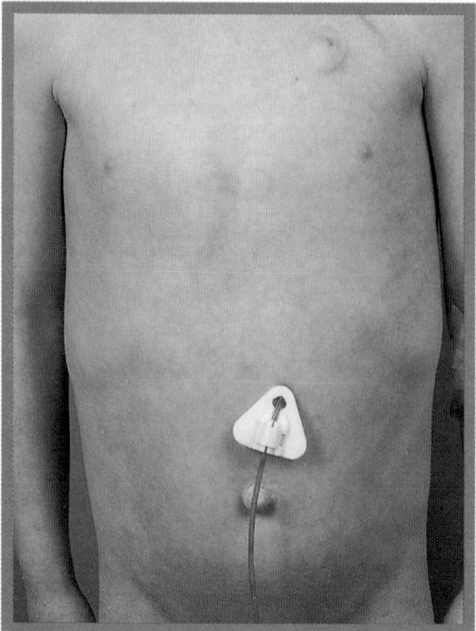

←5.42

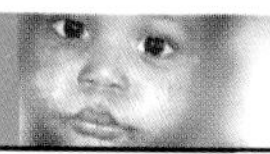

Figures 5.43 and 5.44 Histopathology of the Pancreas. Figure 5.43 shows normal pancreas. **Figure 5.44** shows the pancreas in a patient with cystic fibrosis; it shows flattened epithelium, dilated cyst-like ducts and diffuse fibrosis with fatty tissue.

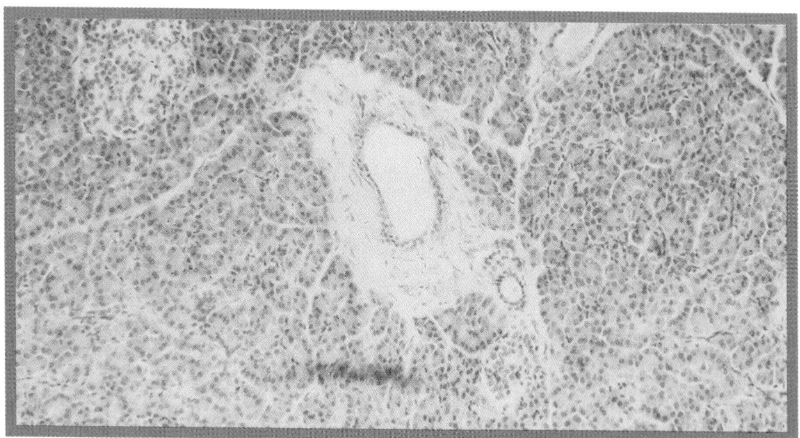

↑ 5.43

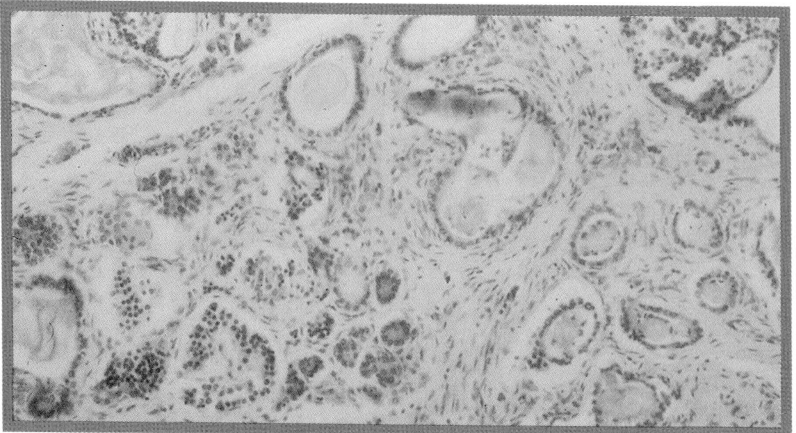

↑ 5.44

Figure 5.45 Kayser–Fleischer Rings of Copper Deposition due to Wilson Disease (Hepatolenticular Degeneration). This is a multi-organ systemic disease caused by defective excretion of copper by the liver. Excess copper deposition in the liver leads to hepatocyte mitochondrial injury, resulting in cirrhosis. As the serum copper levels rise there is deposition in the brain and eye (Kayser–Fleischer rings). Treatment consists of increasing renal excretion using chelating agents.

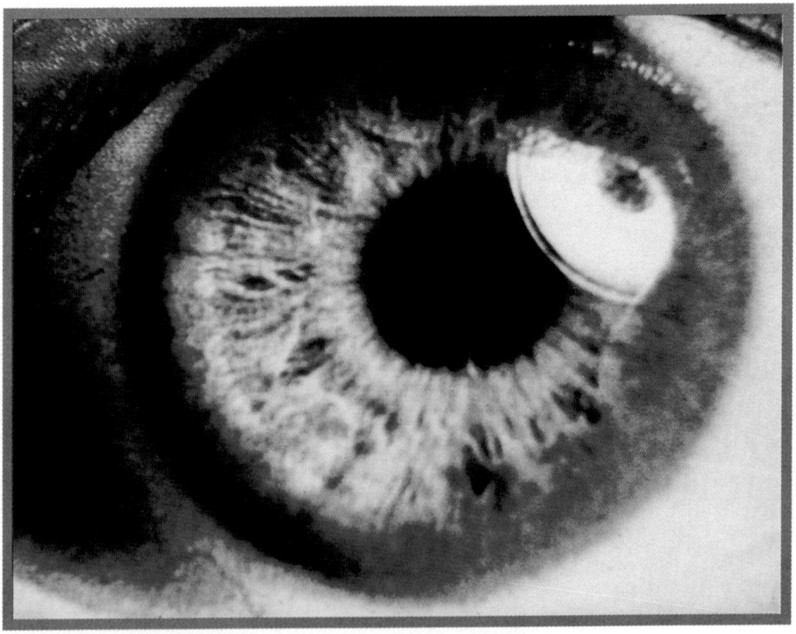

↑5.45

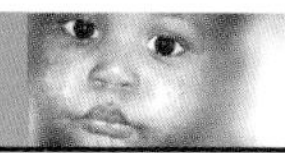

Figures 5.46 and 5.47 Abdominal Distension in a 14-day-old Neonate. This case was due to volvulus, but differential diagnosis includes malrotation, obstruction due to Hirschprung disease, meconium ileus, ilial stenosis, and ileus due to necrotizing enterocolitis and fluid and electrolyte imbalance.

This neonate presented with abdominal distension, bile-stained vomit and irritability. At operation (**Figure 5.47**) it was found to have a mid-gut volvulus, with marked ischemic changes. In this case there was associated malrotation of the mid-gut.

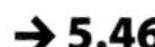

→5.46

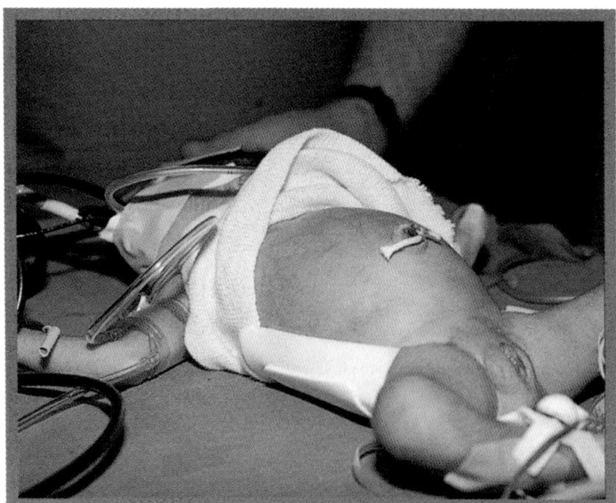

→5.47

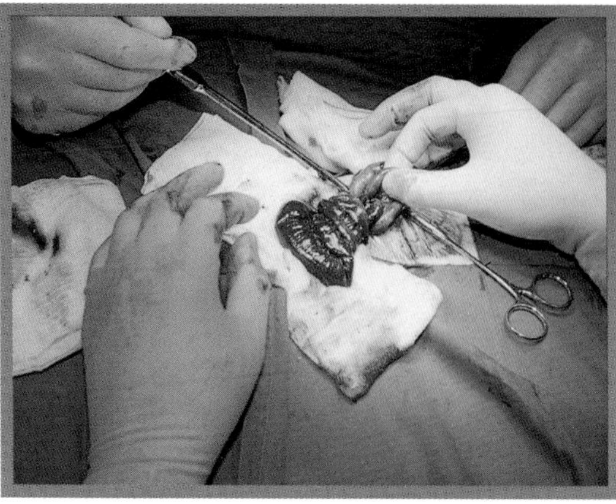

Figure 5.48 Melena Stool – Intussusception. This figure shows the contents of the nappy of an 8-month-old boy who presented with screaming, abdominal discomfort, and a history of a recent upper respiratory tract infection.

An ultrasound scan of the abdomen showed an empty right iliac fossa with a mass in the midline. Attempts to reduce the intussusception by air enema were successful. If the nappy contents had been of mucus and blood ('red-currant stool') then enema reduction would have been contraindicted due to the probability of intestinal ischemia. (see also **Chapter 14, Pediatric Surgery and ENT.**)

Figure 5.49 Meconium Stool. The first stool passed within 36 hours after birth is preceded by the meconium plug. The greenish-black substance consists of swallowed hair, epithelial cells and intestinal secretions high in mucopolysaccharides.

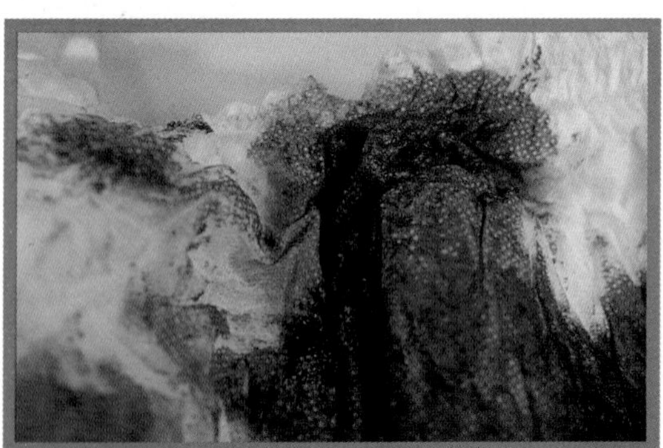

←5.48

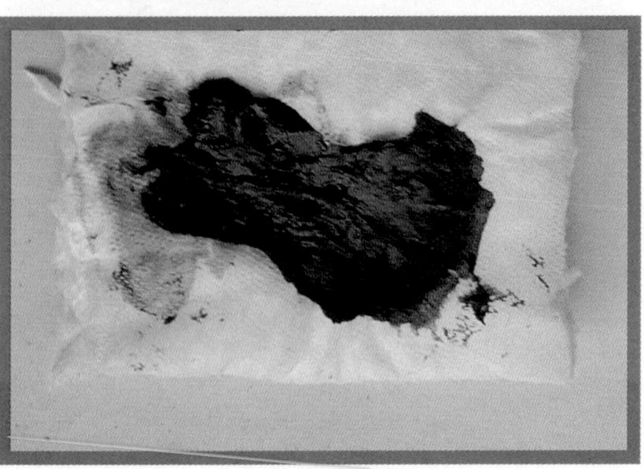

←5.49

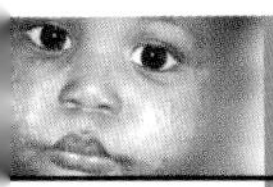

6 Kidney and urinary tract

Figures 6.1 and 6.2 Extrophy of the Bladder. Extrophy of the bladder in this newborn male was diagnosed antenatally. It is more common in males.

This figure shows the classic appearances of: an exposed bladder in the midline, the umbilical cord insertion is toward the head, epispadias of the penis is seen, and there is a broad scrotum with undescended testes.

This child was managed by placing a plastic film over the exposed bladder to prevent dehydration. Intravenous fluids were given and the infant was transferred for specialist pediatric urological surgery. Long-term prognosis depends upon the functioning of the upper urinary tract, especially the degree of vesicoureteric reflux.

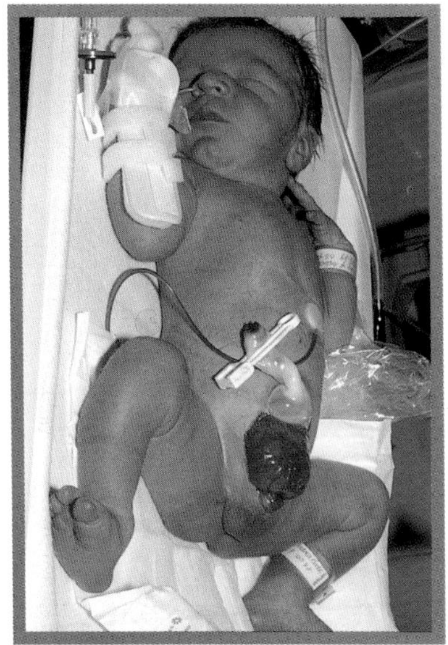

↑6.1

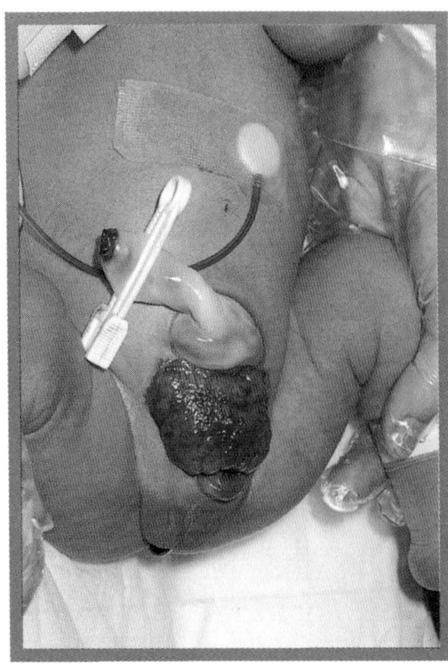

↑6.2

Figure 6.3 ^{99}Tc-DMSA scan of unilateral Multicystic Dysplastic Kidney (MCDK). This case of MCDK was detected antenatally. At birth, a right renal mass was noted and ultrasound confirmed MCDK. A DMSA scan at 6 weeks confirmed that the MCDK was non-functioning. A repeat ultrasound at 1 year showed that the MCDK had resorbed, resulting in left kidney showing compensatory hypertrophy.

There is a risk of an MCDK causing hypertension and neoplastic change. It is important to check that the other kidney is 'normal'. Dysplastic kidneys are more commonly associated with obstruction and reflux and are part of the spectrum of developmental abnormalities. The underlying cause is probably related to abnormal genes and growth factors.

Figure 6.4 Hydronephrosis–Renal Ultrasound. The typical ultrasound appearance of hydronephrosis in a child is shown. The dilated pelvis is indicated. This condition was due to a ureterocele, which was causing an obstruction of the ureter.

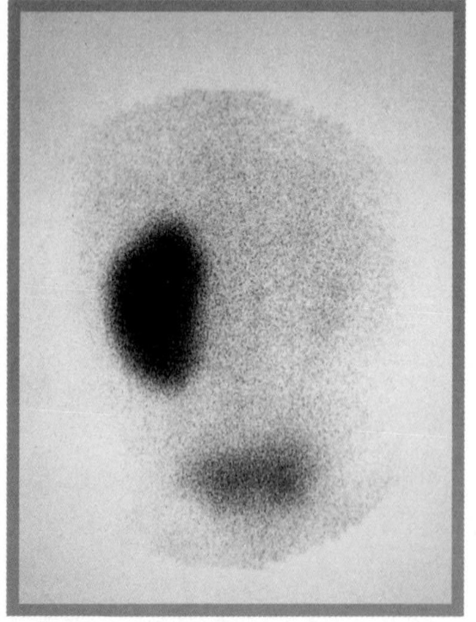

↑6.3

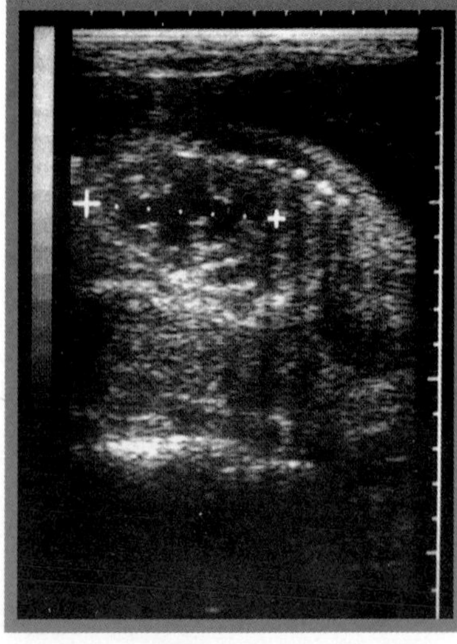

↑6.4

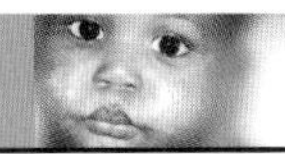

Figure 6.5 Ultrasound–Right ureteric reflux. This infant was diagnosed antenatally with right-sided hydronephrosis. Postnatal ultrasound showed a grossly dilated renal pelvis in (**a**) transverse view and (**b**) longitudinal section. The transverse renal pelvic diameter was 16 mm.
Figure 6.6 Micturating cystourethrogram (MCUG) of the infant whose ultrasound is shown below. Note reflux into a dilated right ureter and pelvicalyceal system on the right. The left side was normal.

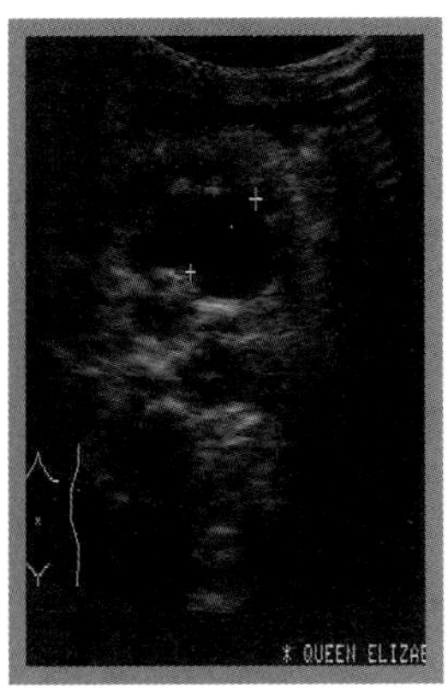

←6.5a →6.5b

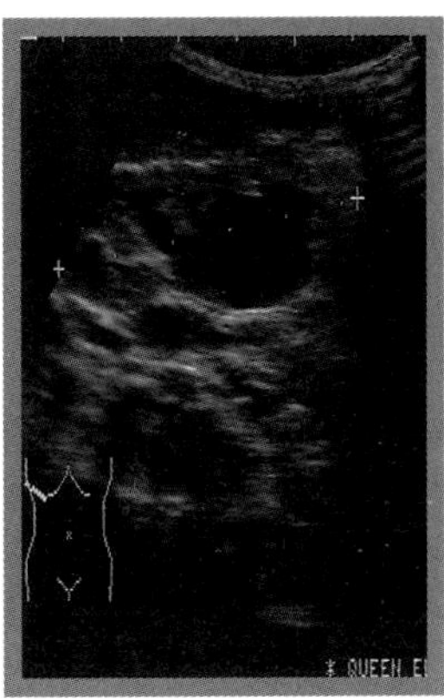

→6.6

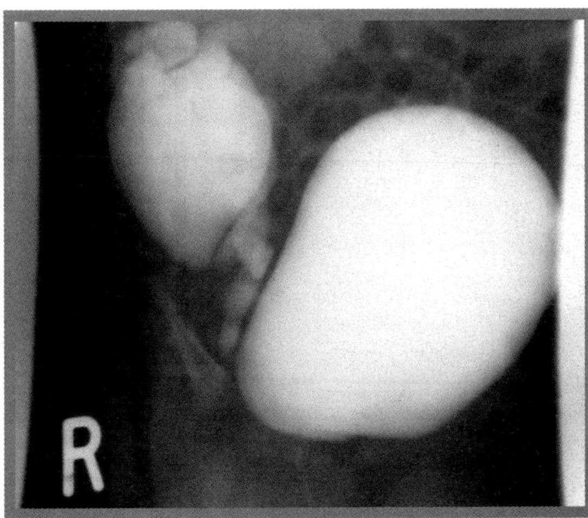

Figure 6.7 Asymmetric Kidneys (^{99}Tc- DMSA Scan). In this case the asymmetry was due to scarring, with a relative uptake on the left of 75%, and on the right of 25%. This child received prophylactic antibiotics. At 5-year follow up there was no deterioration in function and the reflux had resolved. However, blood pressure follow-up is required for life. Two subsequent siblings were investigated for reflux and one was also found to have reflux at birth.

Figure 6.8 Posterior Urethral Valves (MCUG). The late antenatal ultrasound scans of a newborn boy, revealed bilateral hydronephrosis and a thick-walled bladder. Despite antenatal treatment with stents to drain the bladder into the amniotic fluid, chronic renal failure developed.

The figure shows gross, prestenotic urethral dilatation on X-ray, and bladder wall diverticulae. For this important condition to be diagnosed, it is essential that views are obtained with the urethral catheter removed. Treatment consists of endoscopic ablation of the urethral valves.

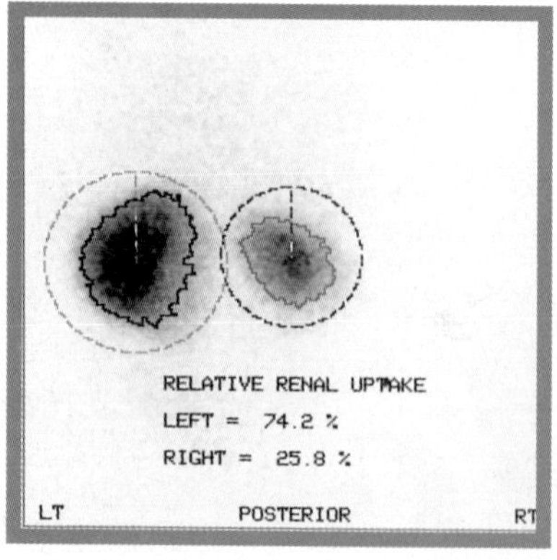

↑ 6.7

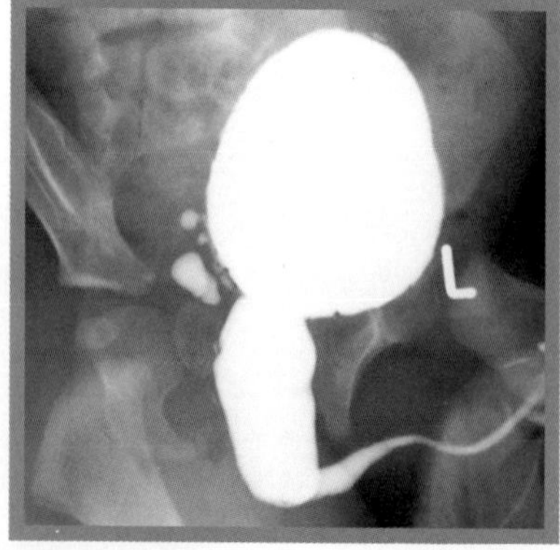

↑ 6.8

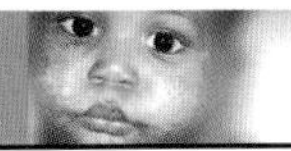

Figure 6.9 Right Ureterocele–Intravenous Pyelogram (IVP). This contrast X-ray shows a congenital cystic dilatation of the distal ureter. The dilated ureter prolapses into the bladder and has a narrow orifice. This produces an obstructive hydronephrosis. The condition is commoner in females than in males. Treatment consists of endoscopic incision of the ureteric orifice, which relieves the obstruction but often results in reflux. Ureteroceles are often associated with a duplex ureteric system. Excision of the duplex system may be required if it is nonfunctioning.

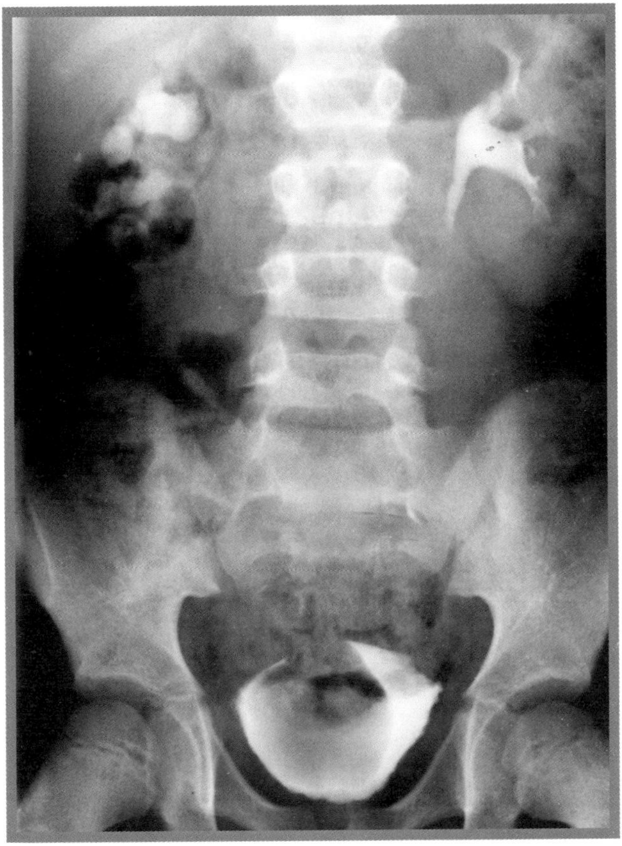

↑ **6.9**

Figures 6.10 Normal indirect cystogram (^{99}Tc- DTPA),in a four-year-old girl. She had presented with a urinary tract infection at age 1 year. Ureteric reflux had been detected on a MCUG at that time. The follow up indirect cystogram was normal. The curve marked (A), is the falling count as the bladder empties, with no increase in count in the ureters (L and R) during this period.
Figure 6.11 Normal ^{99}Tc-DMSA scan in the same patient at age 4 years. No scarring is shown.

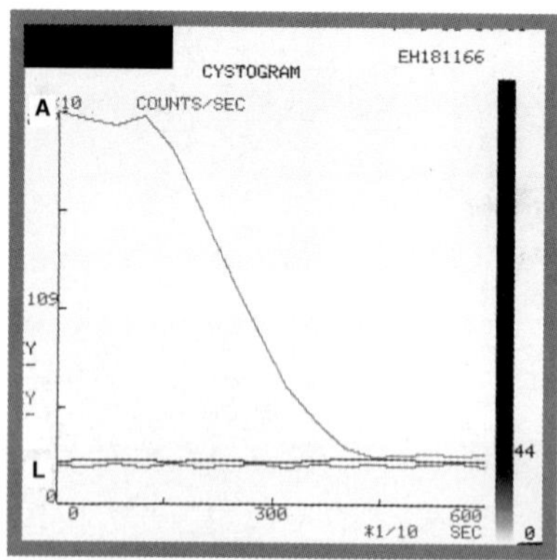

↑6.10

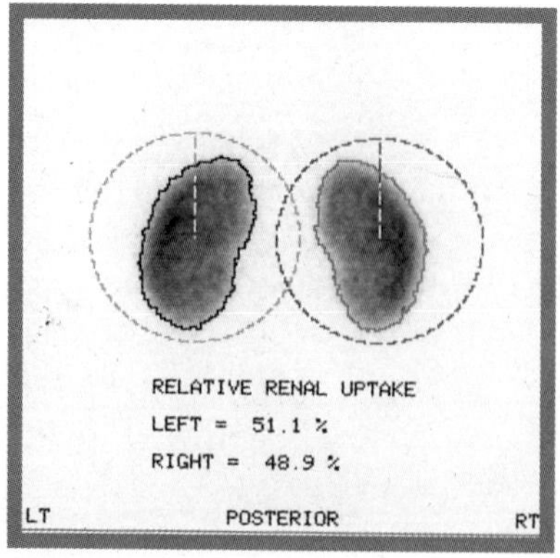

↑6.11

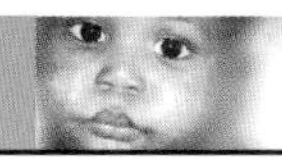

Figure 6.12 Peritoneal Dialysis Catheter (Right Iliac Fossa). The 13-year-old boy shown here required a bilateral nephrectomy for polycystic renal disease. He has received two transplants, both of which have been rejected, and is currently receiving continuous ambulatory peritoneal dialysis. This is carried out by his mother at home.

He is of short stature and is receiving growth hormone. His anemia is treated with erythropoetin injections. He is thin due to his catabolic state, and has a marked proximal myopathy related to his chronic renal failure.

Figure 6.13 Nephrotic Syndrome. The 3-year-old child shown here has steroid-sensitive nephrotic syndrome. Note the distended abdomen and minimal edema of the extremities. The child is managed using a no-added-salt diet, penicillin prophylaxis and oral steroids. Diuresis occurred after 10 days of steroid treatment.

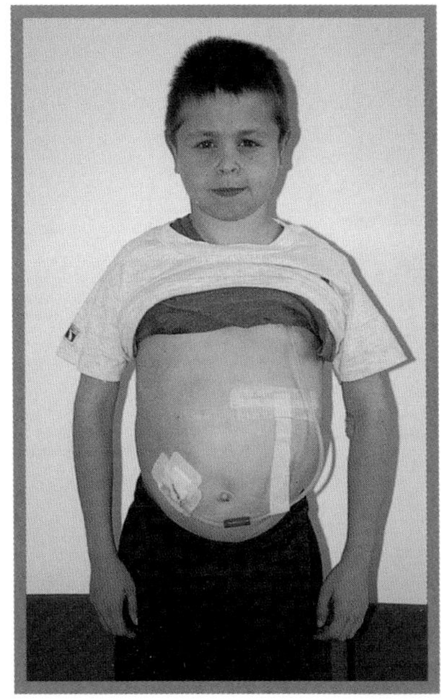

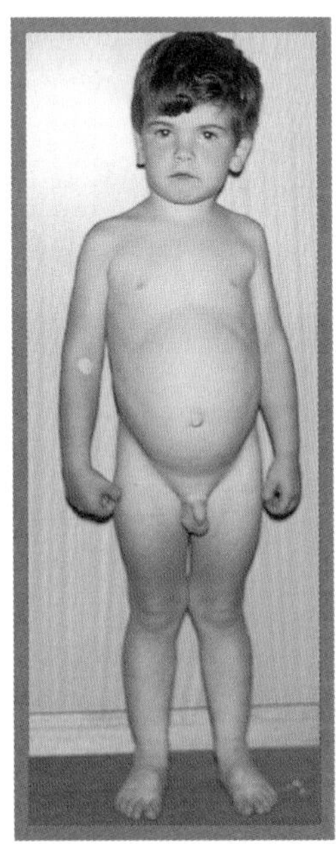

↑6.12

↑6.13

Figures 6.14 and 6.15. A 4-year-old Girl with Nephritic Syndrome. The girl shown here presented with a 1-month history of a cough with yellow sputum. On examination, she was found to have gross ascites, basal crepitations and a raised jugular venous pressure. A chest X-ray showed cardiomegaly and a pleural effusion. She was moderately hypertensive due to fluid overload, with a creatinine level of 120 µmol/l, and her urine had a large amount of blood and protein in it. Her serum complement (C3) level was low. The underlying cause was a streptococcal infection. Diuresis occurred at 14 days, and she made a complete recovery.

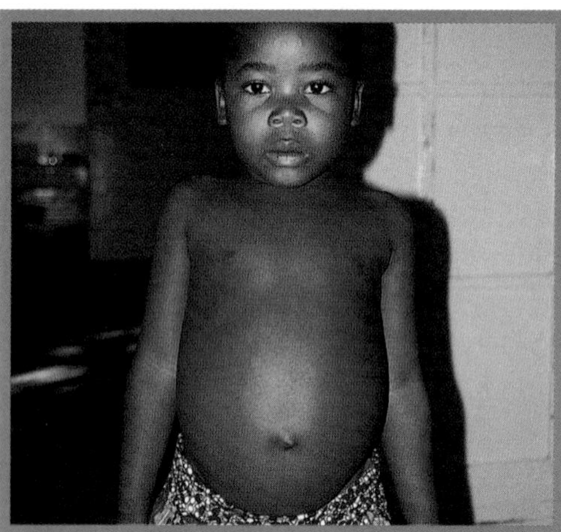

←6.14

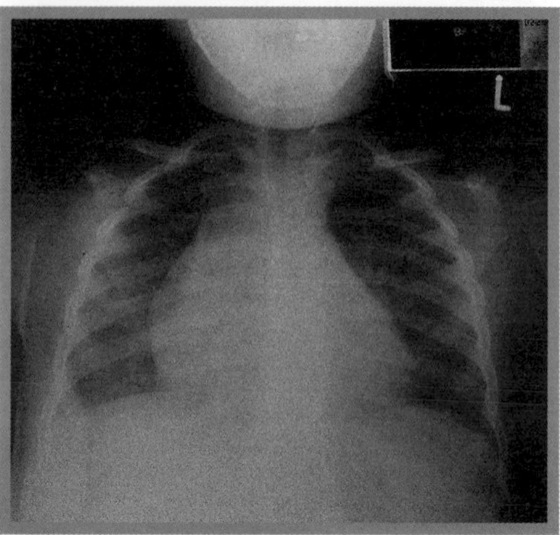

←6.15

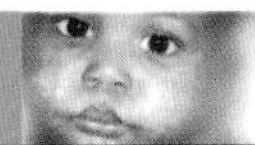

Figure 6.16 Left Scrotal Abscess. This 4-year-old presented with a painful scrotal swelling. The differential diagnosis is torsion of the testes. This abscess was treated by incision and drainage.
Figure 6.17 Left Inguinal Hernia. The 11-year-old shown here had a long history of painless swelling in the groin. The testes were both readily palpable in the scrotum. Treatment consists of surgical herniorrhaphy. There is commonly an associated undescended or maldescended testes if the hernia is indirect.

→6.16

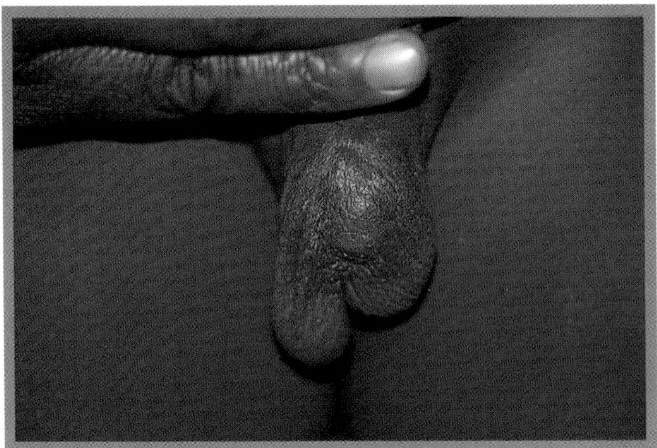

→6.17

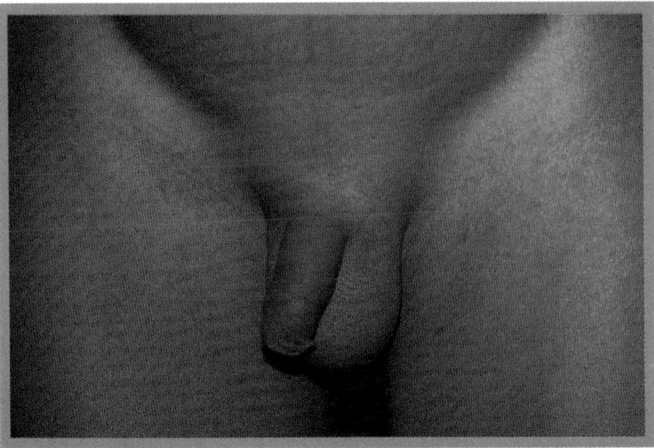

Figure 6.18 Phimosis. The 6-year-old shown here with a long foreskin has a non-retractile prepuce, and ballooning occurred on micturition. Ninety percent of male infants under 3 years of age will have a non-retractile foreskin. The inability to retract the foreskin under the age of 3 years is not abnormal, and is not an indication for circumcision.

Figure 6.19 Renal Mass – Neuroblastoma. The 6-month-old infant shown here presented with a palpable mass in the right flank. The differential diagnosis includes Wilm tumor (nephroblastoma), nephroblastomatosis, mesoblastic nephroma and neuroblastoma. On ultrasound, the infant was found to have a mass separate from and above the right kidney.

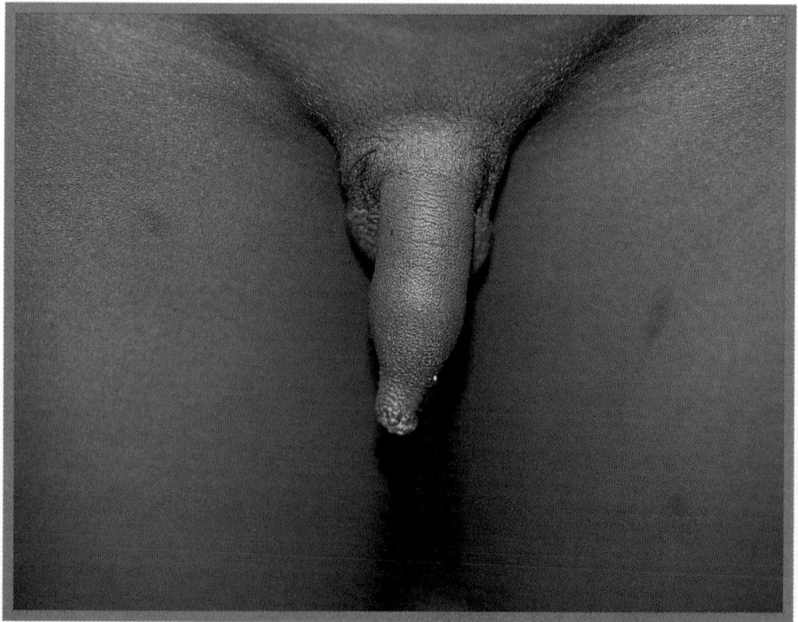

↑6.18

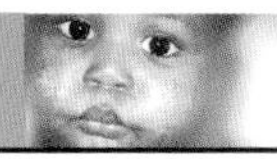

CT showed this mass to extend into the chest.Investigations showed a raised urinary vanillylmandelic acid (VMA) level.

Note the thin limbs from the secondary effects of the tumor, which cause suppression of appetite. The diagnosis was confirmed on biopsy. An MIBG (meta-iodo benzylguanidine) scan, which is a catecholamine analogue, taken up by catecholamine-producing cells, confirmed secondary spread to the bone marrow.

Figure 6.20 Neuroblastoma (IVP). A right-sided suprarenal mass is shown with distortion of the normal calyx and displacement of the kidney.

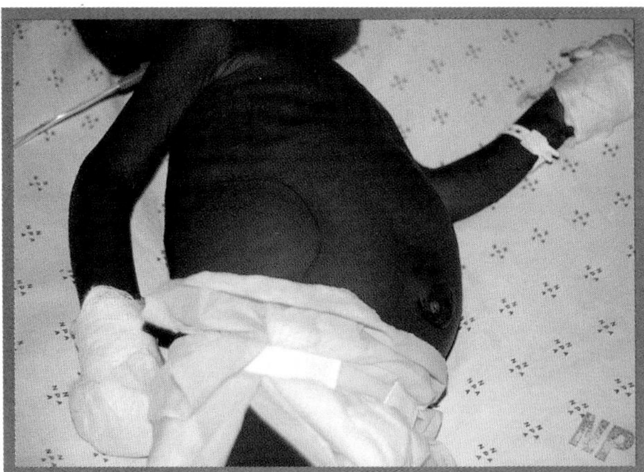

←6.19

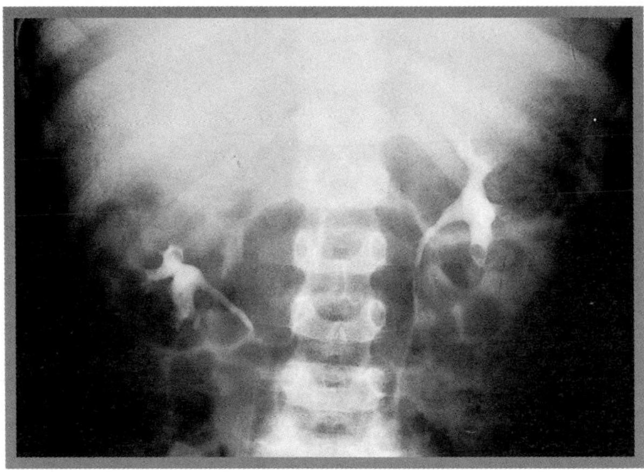

←6.20

Figure 6.21 Wilms Tumor. The figure shows an IVP of a left-sided unilateral Wilms tumor. A large, opaque shadow is seen on left flank, distorting the left ureter (arrowed). The tumor was first noted as a mass in the abdomen on routine examination of a 3-year-old boy who had presented with abdominal pain.

On CT scan the mass appeared to be intrarenal and did not invade the renal vessels. Treatment consisted of excision and chemotherapy. Chest X-ray and CT of the chest confirmed the absence of metastatic spread.

The median age of diagnosis is 3 years, and staging is essential in assessing the prognosis. Optimal treatment requires the referral of all cases to a pediatric oncologist.

Figure 6.22 Bladder Calcification. Bladder and ureteric calcification from *Schistosomiasis hematobium* infection is shown. The chronic inflammation in the urinary tract associated with this infection may result in obstructive uropathy, stones, secondary infection, bladder cancer, fistulae and anemia from hematuria.

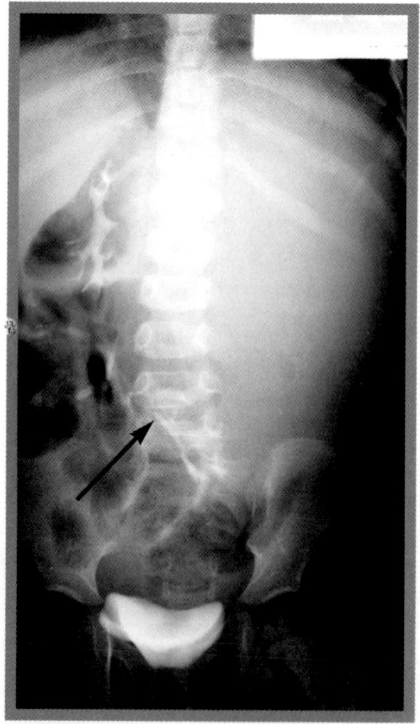

↑6.21

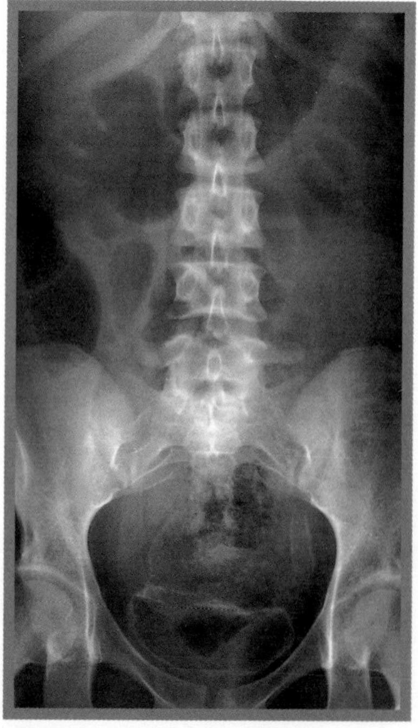

↑6.22

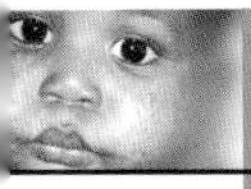

7 Neurological disorders

Figure 7.1 Hydrocephalus – Shunted. This figure shows a 6-month-old girl with hydrocephalus. The head is enlarged (macrocephaly) with visible sclerae above the cornea (the 'sun-setting sign') – this is indicative of a long-standing process. Note the depressed fontanelle due to excessive drainage of CSF in this shunted case.

Hydrocephalus can be categorized as *communicating,* where CSF absorption is impaired and *non-communicating,* where the CSF circulation is blocked within the ventricular system or from passing from the ventricular system into the subarachnoid space. There are a number of etiologies, including infection, hemorrhage, tumor and congenital malformations.

→7.1

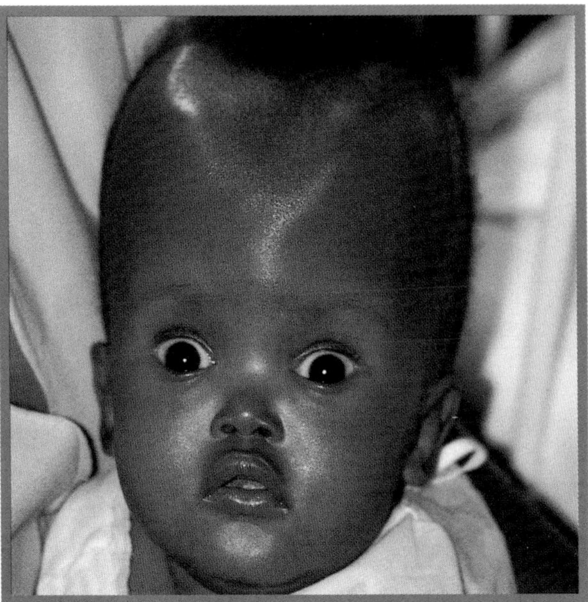

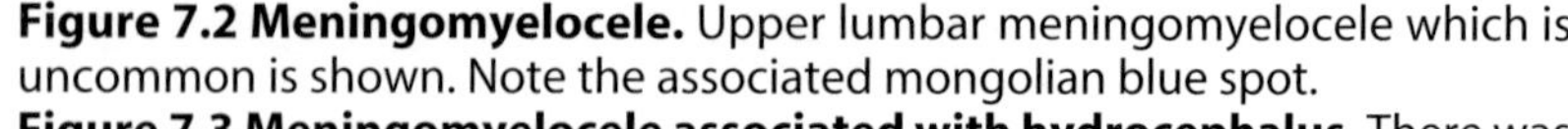

Figure 7.2 Meningomyelocele. Upper lumbar meningomyelocele which is uncommon is shown. Note the associated mongolian blue spot.
Figure 7.3 Meningomyelocele associated with hydrocephalus. There was no associated paralysis of the lower legs.

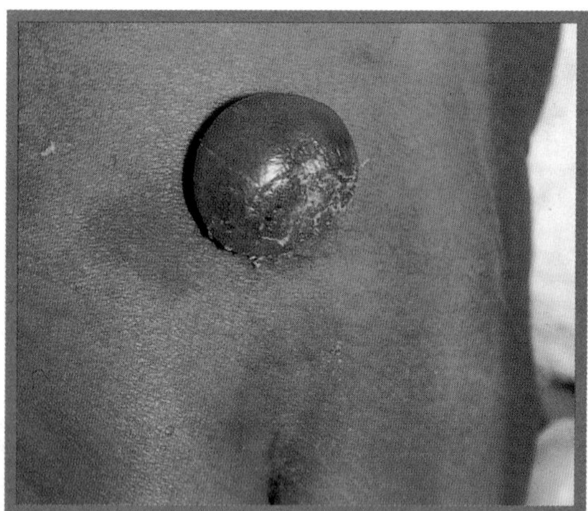

←7.2

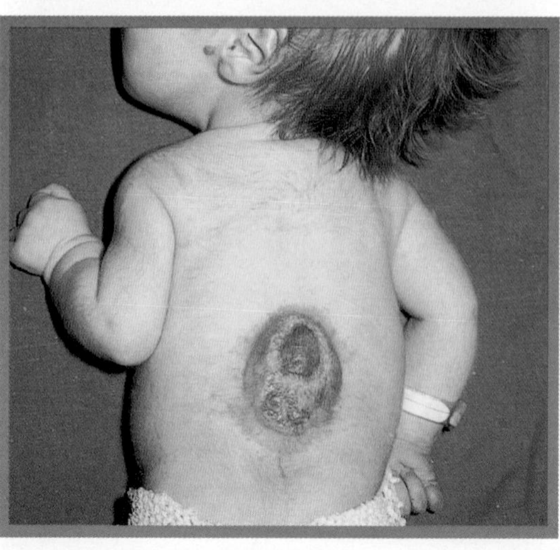

←7.3

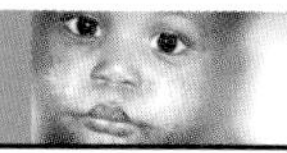

Figure 7.4 Meningomyelocele in 5-month-old boy with paralysis of the legs and an associated Arnold–Chiari malformation, resulting in hydrocephalus. Spina bifida with meningocele (meningomyelocele) is less commonly seen than previously due to antenatal ultrasound, Alpha-Feto-Protein measurements (raised in spina bifida) and preconceptual folic acid supplements, and a possible spontaneous fall in incidence.

Problems encountered are urinary retention with overflow, nephropathy from Vesico-Ureteric Reflux, fecal incontinence, lower limb weakness and hydrocephalus.

Figure 7.5 Sacral Sinus with a Vascular Nevus and Café-au-Lait Spot. Sacral sinuses are commonly seen in healthy newborn infants. If the sinus becomes infected then excision may be necessary. Midline vascular nevi may be associated with underlying spinal cord abnormalities.

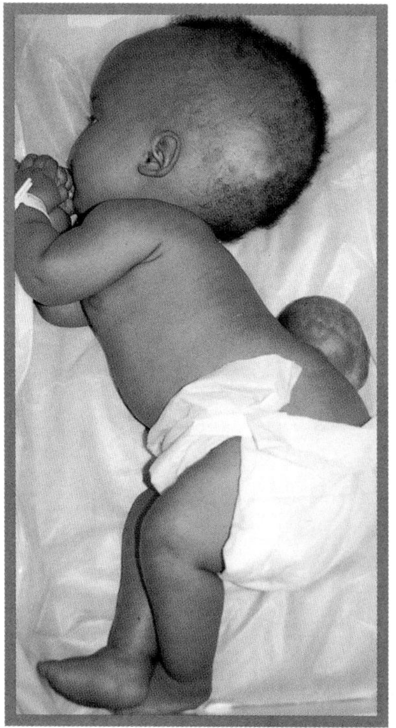

↑ 7.4

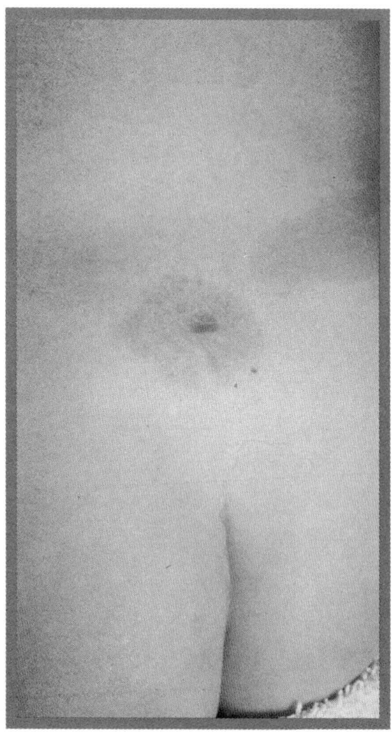

↑ 7.5

Figure 7.6 Frontal Encephalocele and Preauricular Skin Tag. These are usually associated with other abnormalities and syndromes. X-ray, ultrasound and MRI are used to assess the degree of bone loss and associated brain abnormality. Large lesions are associated with hydrocephalus and significant disability.
Figure 7.7 Hydranencephaly (Transilluminated Skull). This probably arises as a result of a vascular accident affecting blood supply to the brain, causing infarction of both cerebral hemispheres. Diagnosis requires ultrasound and CT scanning. In some cases a rudimentary dysplastic brain is found surrounded by large amounts of fluid external to the brain.

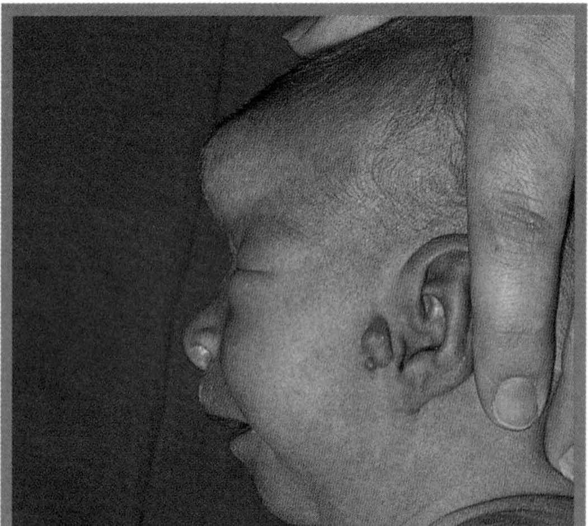

←7.6

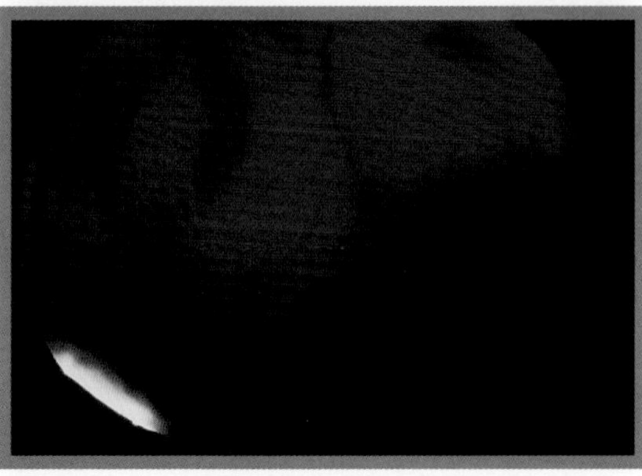

←7.7

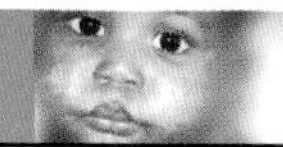

Figure 7.8 Opisthotonic Posture. This figure shows an opisthotonic posture due to the development of ventriculitis following shunt insertion for hydrocephalus. Note the extension of the neck and scissoring of the legs.
Figure 7.9 Cerebral Palsy. This figure shows a 10-month old boy with cerebral diplegia as a result of intraventricular hemorrhage following a premature delivery. The infant showed extensor hypertonus maximal when lying supine, arching into opisthotonos on contact with a hard surface, as displayed. There is extension of the neck, fisting of the hands, the arms are internally rotated and flexed, the legs are extended with plantar extension of the feet. Pain or noise enhanced the tone and resulted in opisthotonic posturing. Note the dressing covering a recent gastrostomy insertion.

→7.8

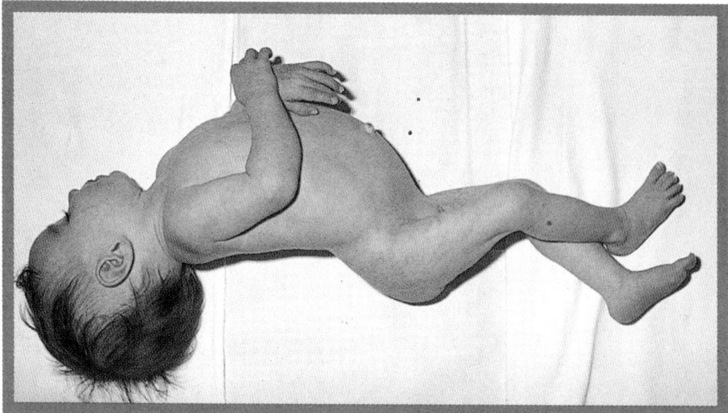

→7.9

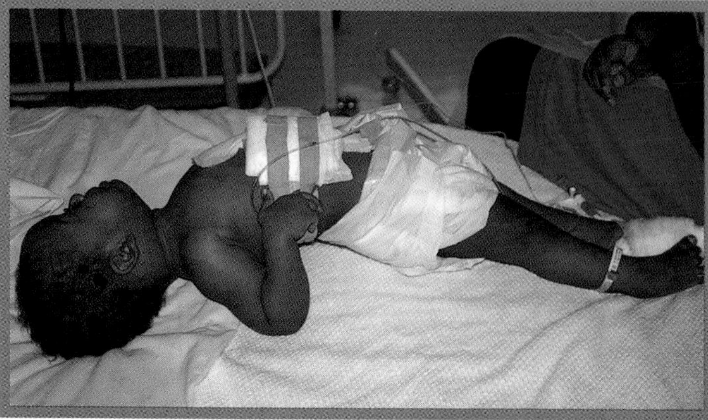

Figure 7.10 Spastic Diplegia. All four limbs are affected in spastic diplegia, but the lower limbs dominate. There is scissoring due to adductor spasm, there is plantar extension of the feet and internal rotation of the legs.
Figure 7.11 Microcephaly and Spastic Tetraplegia. The patient shown has microcephaly as a result of birth-related cerebral injury. The child is also visually impaired with roving eye movements. Visible here are the upper limbs flexed at the elbow, and the fingers flexed across the adducted thumbs (fisting) with spasticity of the pronators.

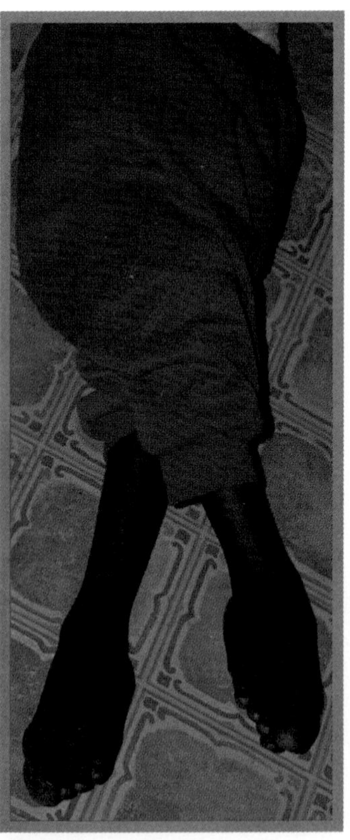

↑7.10

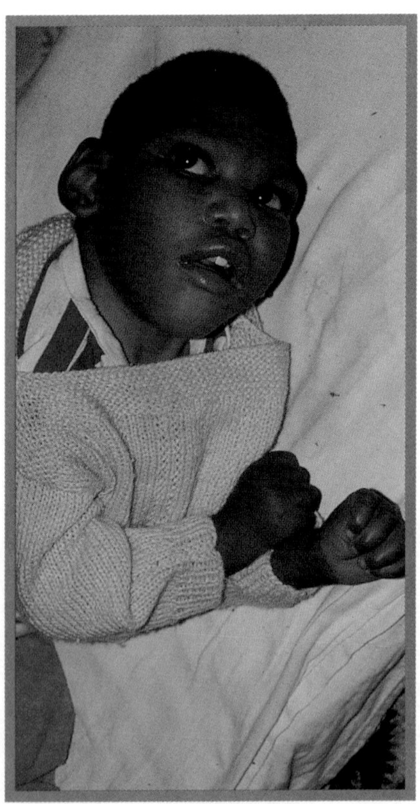

↑7.11

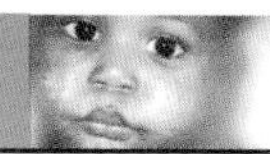

Figure 7.12 Hemiplegic Posture in a 15-year-old Girl. Note the flexed posture of the left arm and leg. The hemiplegia presented soon after birth. Investigations should include CNS imaging to exclude treatable lesions.

Figure 7.13 Anencephalic Infant. Anencephaly results from the failure of closure of the rostral part of the neural tube. It is rarely seen nowadays because of the antenatal use of folate supplements, and selective termination of antenatally diagnosed cases.

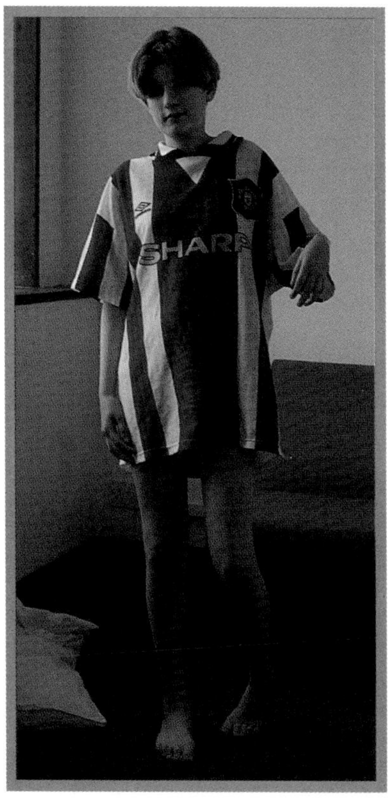

↑7.12

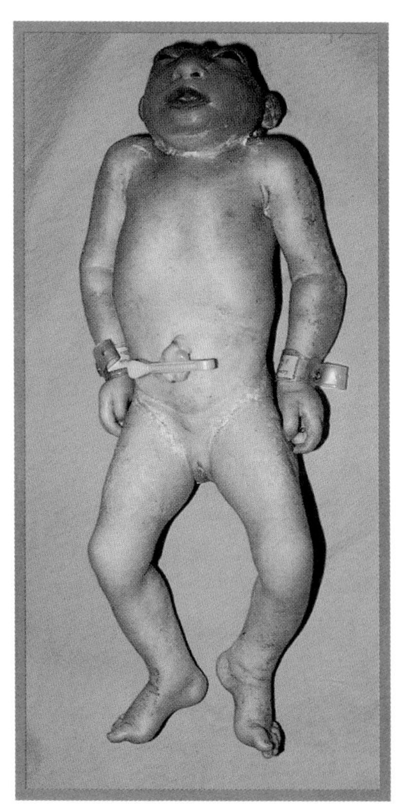

↑7.13

Figure 7.14 Hydrocephalus. The 6-year-old shown here presented to child psychiatrists with a fear of descending stairs. She was noted to have a large head circumference (61 cm – well above the 97th centile). On review of her health record, she was noted to have had a large head circumference for some years. No intracranial lesions were seen on CT scaning. Her condition was due to congenital aqueduct stenosis. Her visual perception improved after the insertion of a shunt. Note the horizontal surgical abdominal scar where the lower end of the shunt is located.

Figures 7.15 and 7.16 Facial Palsy. Seventh nerve palsy is shown in both figures on the left side in these newborns. Note that the babies are unable to close their eyes completely on the affected side. The mouth is drawn over towards the non-affected side. It has recently been recognized that only a minority of cases are due to obstetric trauma. Many cases are congenital. When the eye lid is not affected, then hypoplastic muscles around the mouth may be responsible. Referral for plastic surgery is indicated.

Figure 7.17 Bell Palsy. The child shown here had right lower motor neurone involvement of the facial nerve, and could not close the right eye when asked. This palsy is usually due to viral infection but can be associated with hypertension and lymphoreticular diseases. The underlying cause should be treated, and steroids may be beneficial if given early.

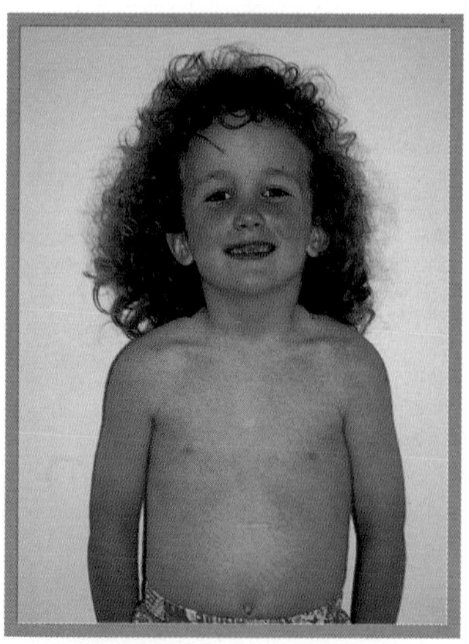

↑7.14

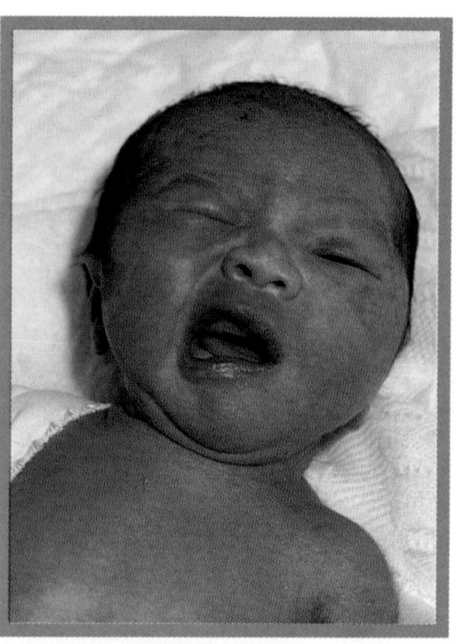

↑7.15

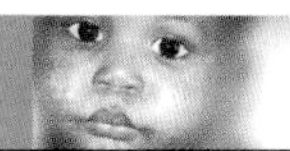

→7.16

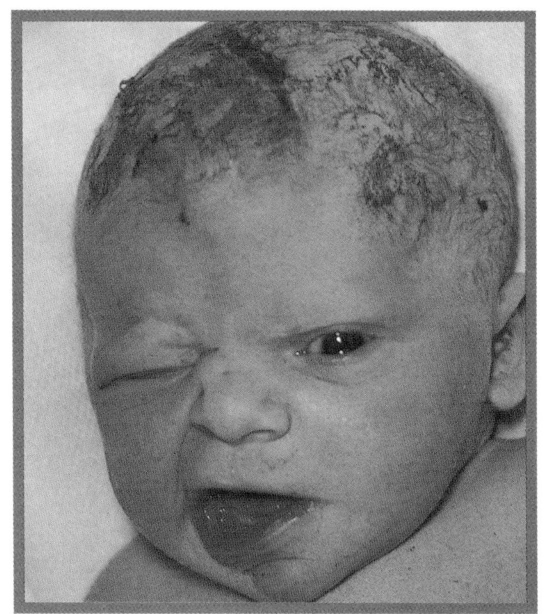

→7.17

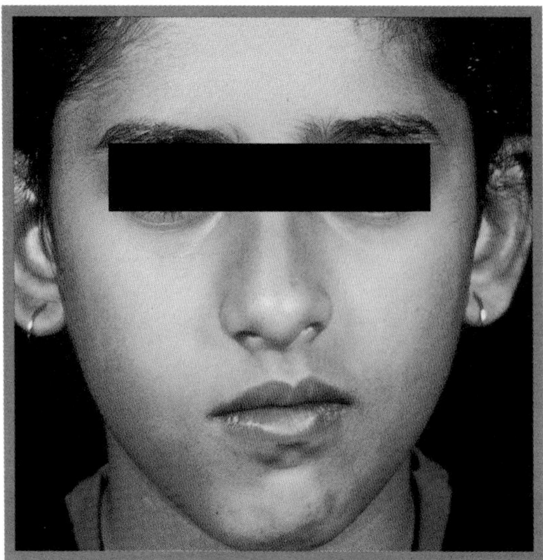

Figures 7.18–7.22 Neurofibromatosis. Neurofibromatosis is a neuro cutaneous condition with autosomal dominant inheritance. It is characterized by multiple café-au-lait spots, tumors and skeletal, neurological and other abnormalities.

Figure 7.18 Café-au-lait spots are usually greater than five in number and more than 1.5 cm in diameter in post-pubertal patients (or more than 5mm in pre-pubertal patients). They are mostly found on the trunk but, as in this case of neurofibromatosis, can occur on the limbs.

Figures 7.19 and 7.20 show axillary freckling which usually develops during adolescence.

Figure 7.21 shows neurofibromata. These can cause significant deformity and may be associated with a mass effect on the spinal cord, *e.g.*, plexiform neurofibroma. Rarely, malignant change may occur in neurofibromas.

Figure 7.22 shows keloid formation with neurofibromata in the scar tissue.

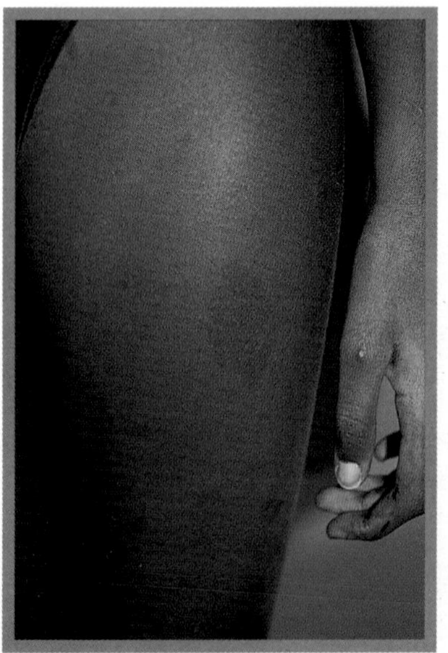

↑7.18

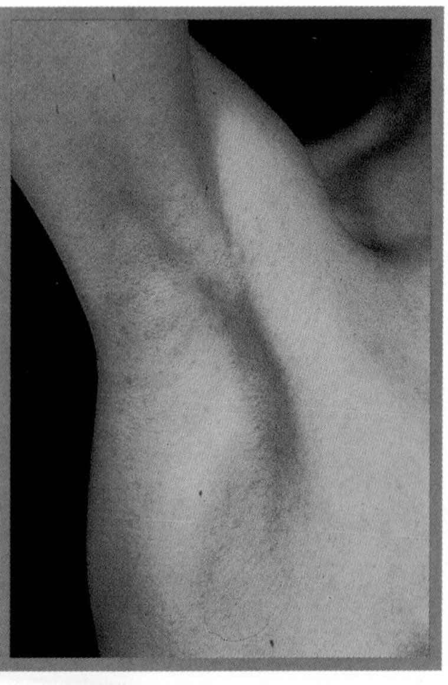

↑7.19

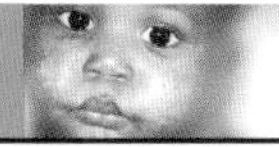

→7.20

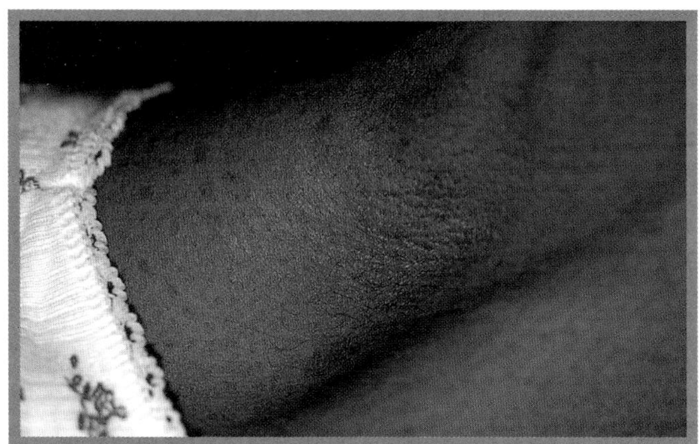

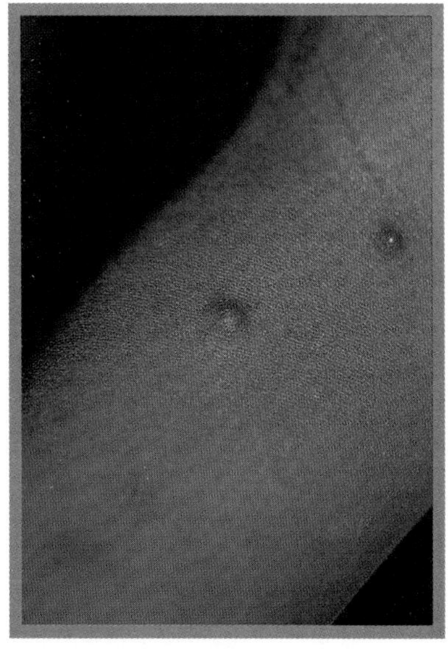

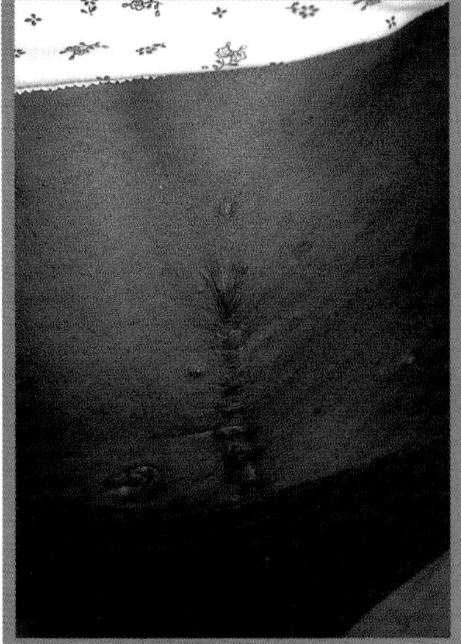

↑7.21

↑7.22

Figures 7.23–7.28 Tuberous Sclerosis. Tuberous sclerosis is a condition with autosomal dominant inheritance. It affects structures arising from the neuroectoderm, and its main clinical manifestations are neurocutaneous features, epilepsy, and learning difficulties.

Figure 7.23 shows the face of a 4-year-old with a typical rash of adenoma sebaceum localized to the cheeks, and a shagreen patch over the right upper forehead.

Figure 7.24 shows adenoma sebaceum in an older child who had presented in infancy with salaam attacks. This was shown on EEG to be due to a hypsarrhythmia.

Figure 7.25 shows the rash in an adolescent with epilepsy and learning difficulties.

Figure 7.26 shows a shagreen patch in the classic position of the lumbosacral region.

Figure 7.27 shows an ash-leaf-shaped depigmented macule on the upper arm.

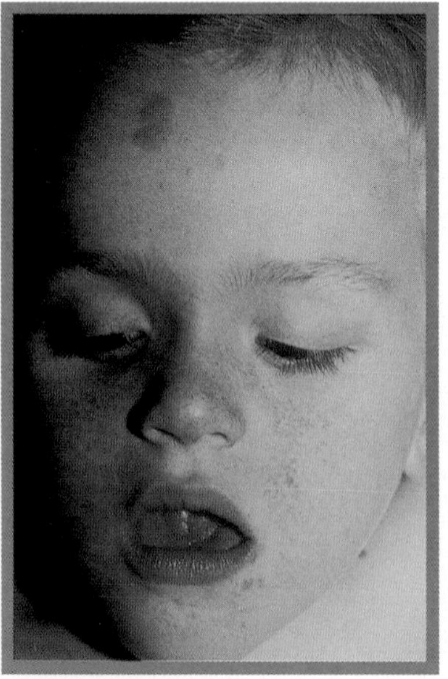

↑7.23

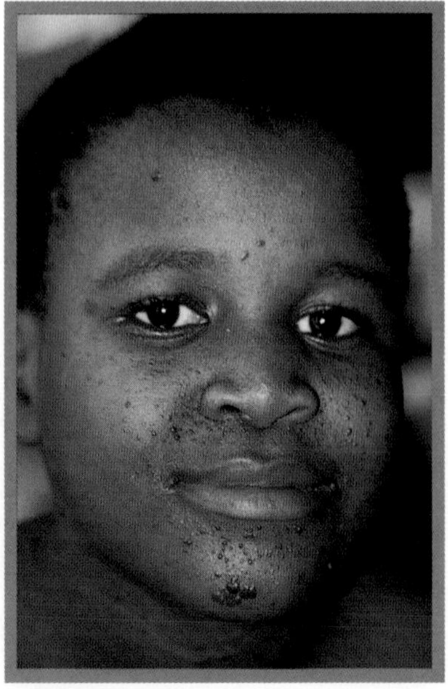

↑7.24

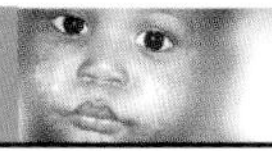

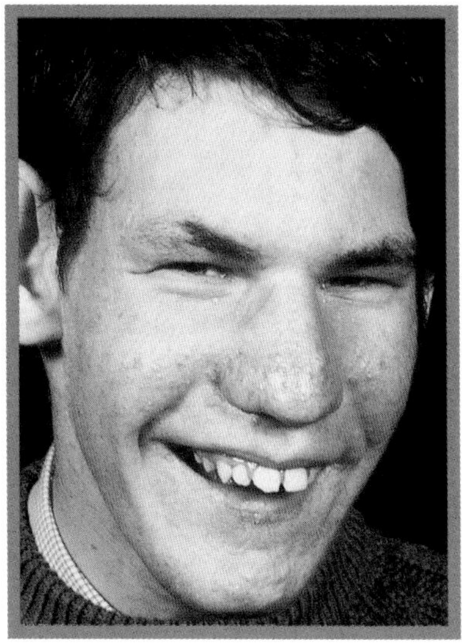

↑ 7.25

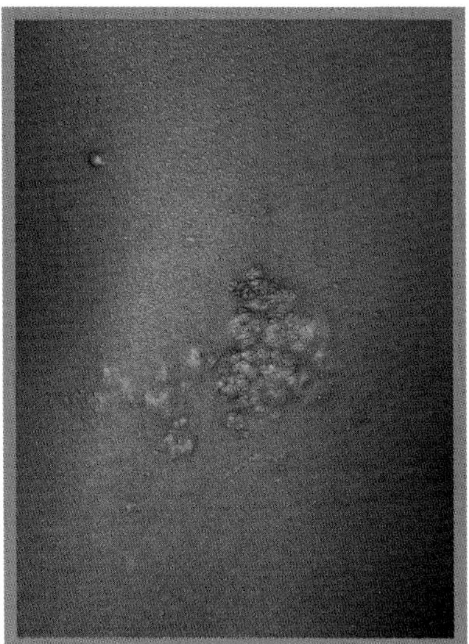

↑ 7.26

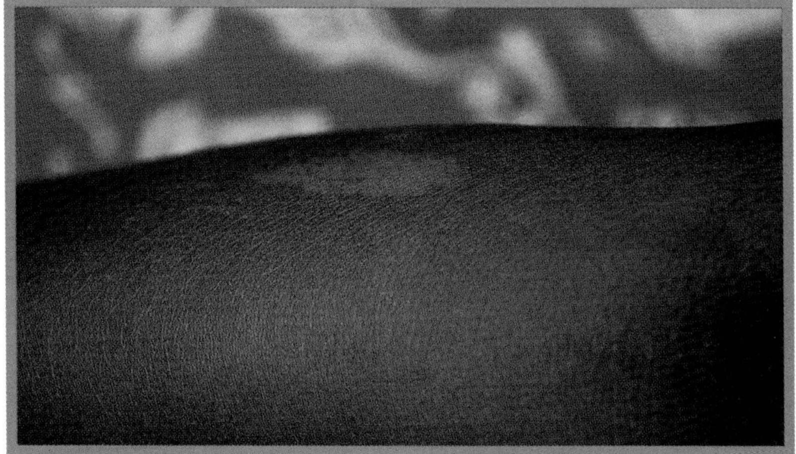

↑ 7.27

Figure 7.28 shows an ash-leaf-shaped macule on white skin. Examination under ultraviolet light (Wood's light) is required to demonstrate these.

Figure 7.29 CT Scan Appearance of Periventricular Intracranial Calcification caused by Tubers. This disorder has a very variable course, with incidental diagnosis in many elderly people. However, the disease may present in infancy with salaam attacks and gross, severe, neuro-developmental delay. The paraventricular and cerebral nodules may enlarge and lead to obstructive hydrocephalus, and rarely, may undergo malignant change.

Other associated findings are abnormalities of the nails and teeth, with subungual fibromas being quite common. Renal angiomyolipomas and cardiac rhabdomyomas are also found. In newly diagnosed cases, genetic counselling is recommended as well as renal, cardiac and CNS imaging.

Figures 7.30 and 7.31 Ataxia Telangiectasia. This is an autosomal recessive disorder, identified on special chromosomal radiosensitivity analysis where DNA repair is faulty (11q22–q23). It results in the appearance of telangiectasia over the bulbar conjunctivae (**Figures 7.30 and 7.31**), and is often visible in the pinna of the ear. There is an associated immunodeficiency and a progressive cerebellar ataxia and choreoathetosis. Clinically, the children are late in achieving gross motor skills and tend to have an ataxic gait. There is a progressive dysarthria, nystagmus, intention tremor and oculo motor apraxia. The immune abnormality affects immunoglobulin production and T-cell function, resulting in increased susceptibility to infections. Lymphomas are more common in affected children.

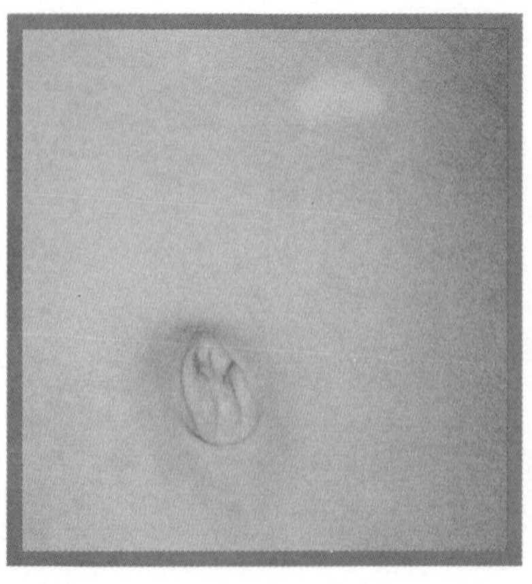

↑7.28

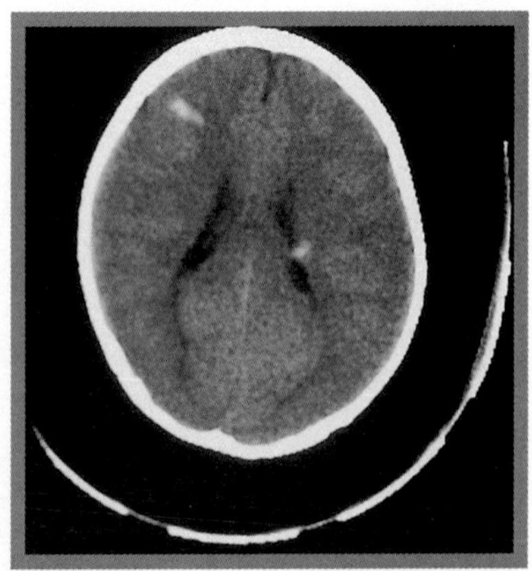

↑7.29

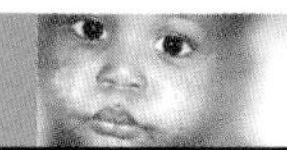

Differential diagnosis includes Friedreich ataxia.

Diagnosis consists of the demonstration of increased chromosomal breakage after exposure of cells to ionizing radiation, abnormalities of the immunoglobulins, and a raised serum alphafetoprotein level.

→7.30

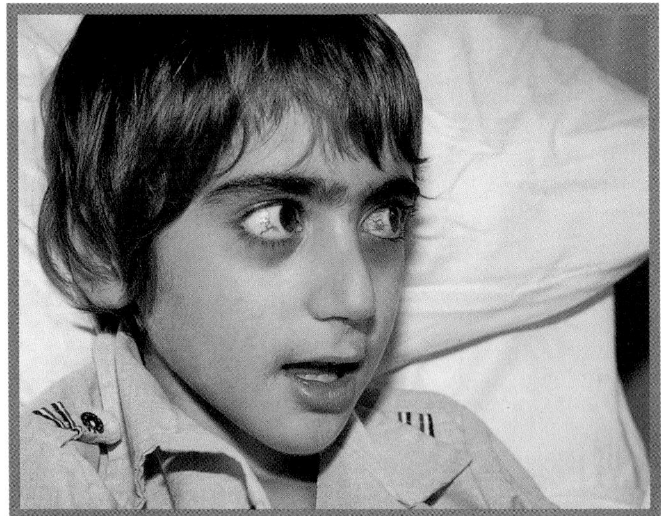

→7.31

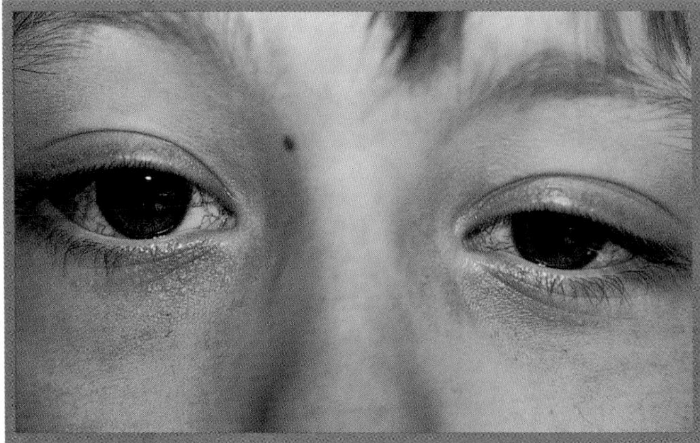

Figure 7.32 Angelman Syndrome. The boy shown here had a jerky, unsteady, wide-based gait resembling the step of a marionette. He often had outbursts of laughter with hand flapping and generally a happy disposition. He displays a typical facial appearance, with a prominent chin, fair hair, microcephaly, and maxillary hypoplasia with a large mouth. In addition he had a profound speech deficit with hydrophilia. In 60% of cases Angelman syndrome results from deletions or rearrangements of the long arm of chromosome 15 at 15q11–q13. A small percentage of cases have paternal disomy for chromosome 15, and at least 20% have normal chromosomes.

Figures 7.33–7.34 Peripheral Neuropathy. Figure 7.33 shows clawing of the hands with wasting of the small muscles in a child with a peripheral neuropathy.

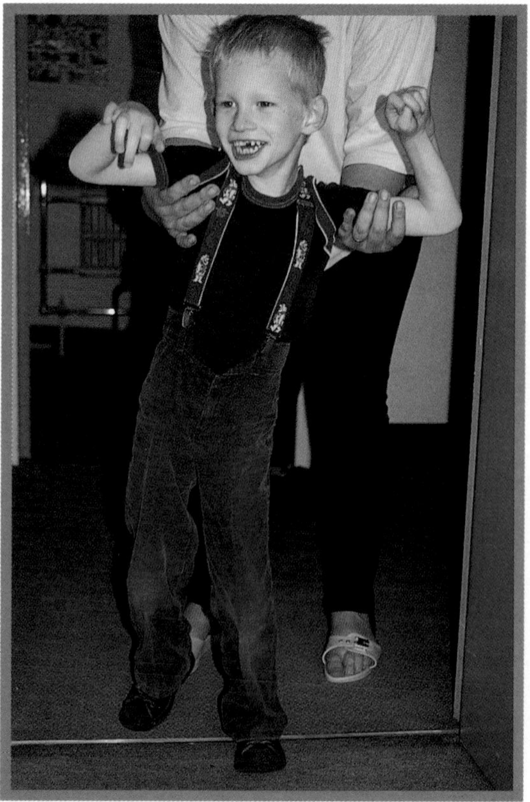

←7.32

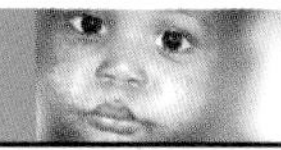

Figure 7.34 shows the early wasting of the peroneal and gastrocnemius muscles, giving rise to the so-called champagne stem sign.

Peripheral neuropathies may affect many peripheral nerves (polyneuropathy) or only one (mononeuropathy). Polyneuropathies may be drug induced, *e.g.*, by vincristine and isoniazid, in which case they tend to improve upon withdrawal of the drug, or may, as in this case, be due to an inherited disorder, the commonest of which is peroneal muscular atrophy (Charcot–Marie–Tooth disease). This is one of the hereditary motor and sensory neuropathies (HMSN Type I). Genetic testing in combination with nerve conduction tests are used to make the diagnosis. HMSN Type I is a progressive disease, but it may have very little overall efffect on an individual. Treatment predominantly consists in physiotherapy and occupational therapy.

→7.33

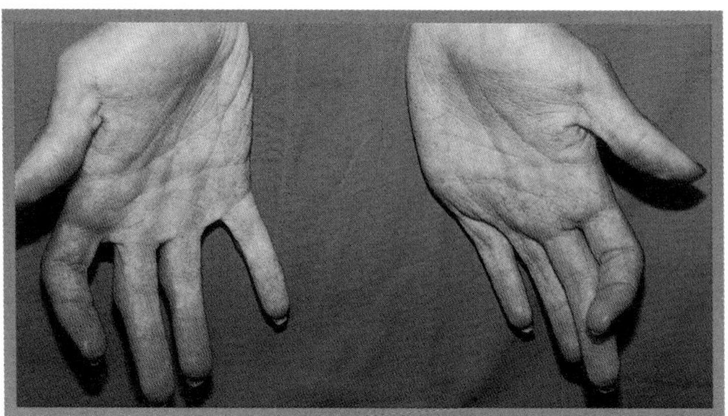

→7.34

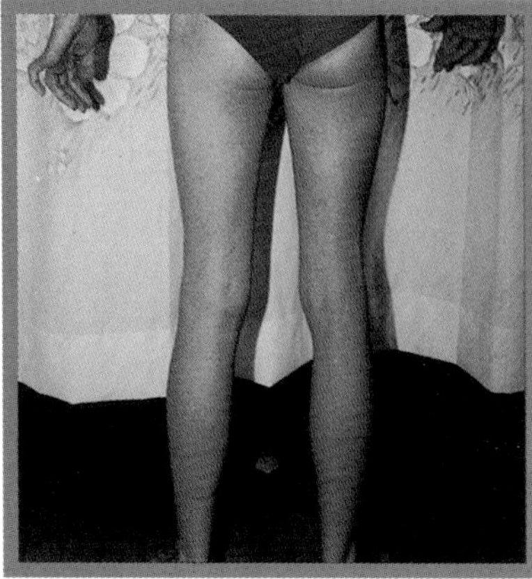

Figures 7.35–7.37 Tuberculosis (TB). Figure 7.35 shows an infant with a classic opisthotonic posture due to TB meningitis. This infant had not received BCG immunization, which is effective in preventing TB meningitis in very young infants. This infant died despite treatment.

Figure 7.36 shows TB meningitis in a 1-year-old, which is due to spread from miliary TB of the lung. Note the left third nerve palsy, with ptosis. This infant developed a left-sided hemiplegia and epilepsy with hydrocephalus, all secondary to TB meningitis.

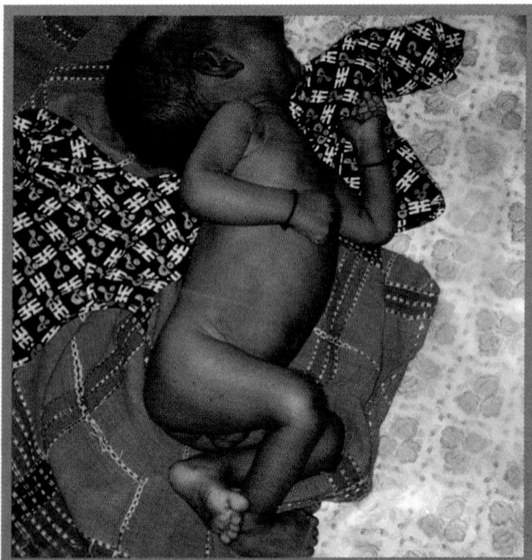

←7.35

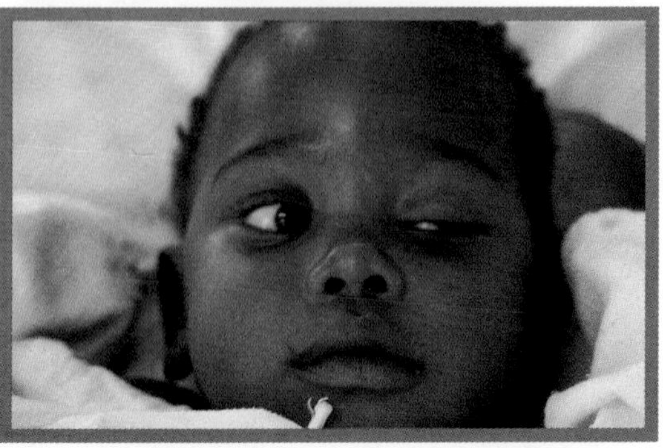

←7.36

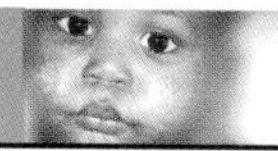

Figure 7.37. The X-ray shows a tuberculous osteitis of the skull bones. Note the clearly demarcated lytic region in the vertex of the skull. Differential diagnosis would include a lytic lesion secondary to malignancy or histiocytosis.
Figure 7.38 Plagiocephaly. This figure shows a child with plagiocephaly, which is a very common normal variant and needs no treatment. It is characterized by occipital flattening on one side with a parallel change in the frontal bones. This results in the head shape being that of a parallelogram. This resolves spontaneuosly when the child adopts an upright posture. Intrauterine moulding gives rise to an asymmetrical head, and the asymmetry is increased due to the infant lying persistently on the affected side.

→7.37

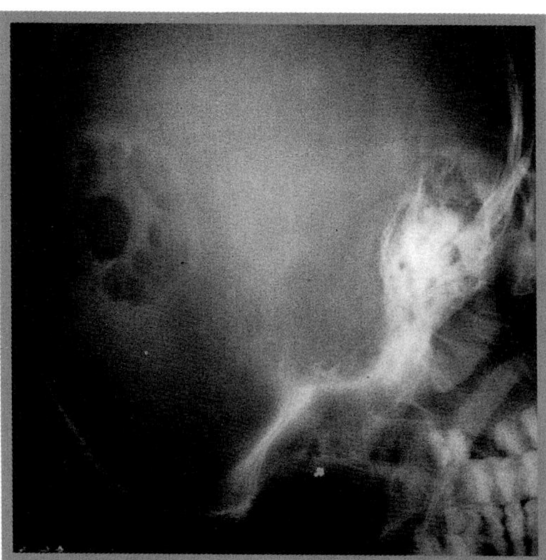

→7.38

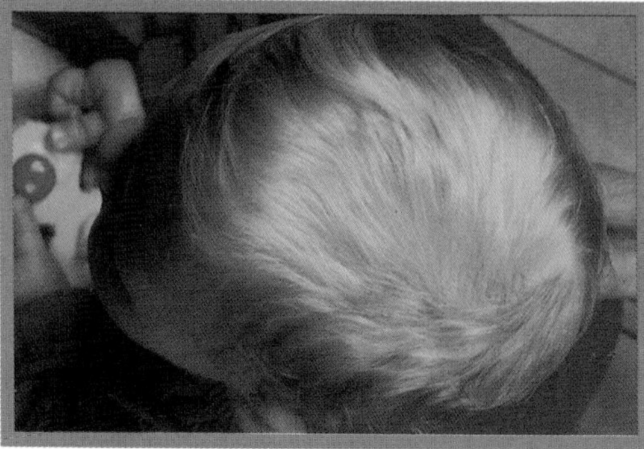

Figures 7.39 and 7.40 Cerebellar Astrocytoma. This 4-year-old girl presented with a history of clumsiness and tremor, with the signs predominating on the left. Note that prominent veins can be seen on her forehead, which is a sign of hydrocephalus. An urgent CT scan demonstrated a large, partly cystic mass in the left cerebellum (see **Figure 7.40**). Treatment consisted in surgical excision and shunting. Adjuvant chemotherapy and radiotherapy are indicated if there is metastatic spread or secondary recurrence. Differential diagnosis would include medulloblastoma, which has a worse prognosis, and ependymoma, which arises from the floor of the fourth ventricle.

Figure 7.41 Apert Syndrome. The 3-year-old girl shown here has Apert syndrome. Her facial features show acrocephaly, slight prominence of the eyes, hypertelorism, an antimongoloid slant to the eyes, crowding of the teeth with

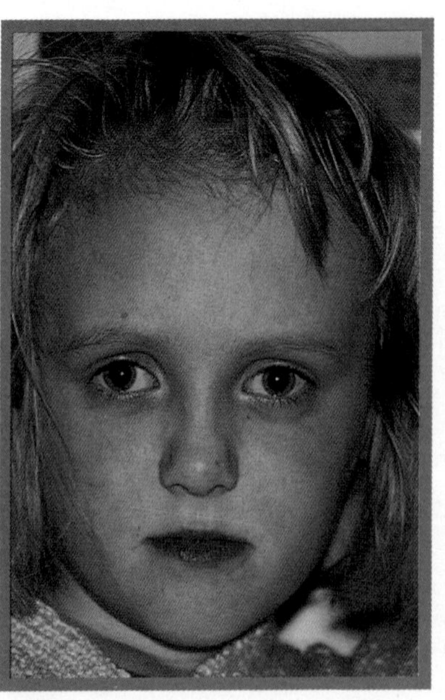

↑7.39

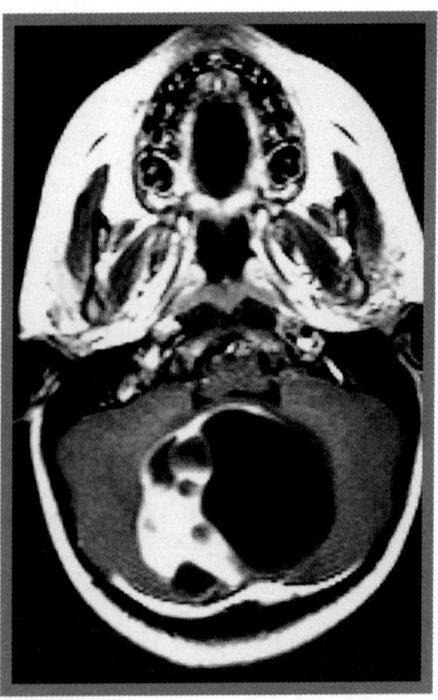

↑7.40

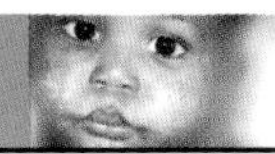

a prominent mandible, and mid-facial hypoplasia. There is also syndactyly of all fingers giving a 'base-ball glove' appearance, with bony syndactyly of the third and fourth digits. Her toes are similarly affected. There is no family history, so this case was considered to be a fresh mutation. Apert syndrome accounts for 4.5% of all cases of craniosynostosis.

Figure 7.42 Porencephalic Cyst. This is a plain CT scan of a 7-month-old boy who had presented with a left hemiplegia. He had been born at term with no complications. Investigations of the causes of hemiplegia should include a CT scan.

The child had a family history of a thrombophilic tendency, *i.e.*, CVA and myocardial infarction in young adults. This was due to protein C deficiency.The CT scan shows a large cystic area occupying the region of the right cerebral hemisphere.

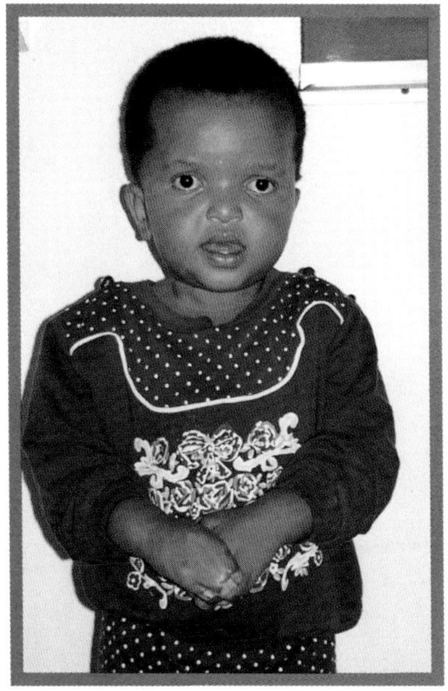

↑7.41

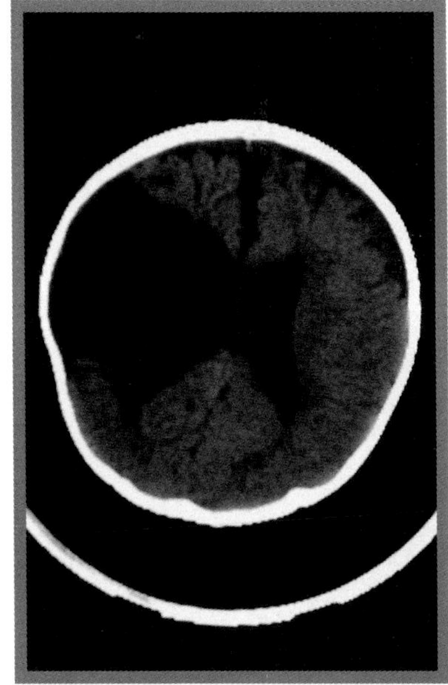

↑7.42

Figures 7.43–7.47 Spinal Muscular Atrophy (Type II). The 6-year-old girl shown here has type II spinal muscular atrophy. It was diagnosed at 11 months of age when, despite sitting at 7 months, she had failed to weight bear. Now she is wheelchair bound.

She suffered from recurrent chest infections and esophageal reflux. Note the profound scoliosis. She is only able to sit unaided if she is wearing a brace (see F**igures 7.43 and 7.44**). On examination, she was generally hypotonic with muscle wasting. There was no antigravity movement in either upper or lower limbs and reflexes were absent. Her chest is bell-shaped with a prominent sternum (see **Figure 7.45**), and she had paradoxical breathing with intercostal recession (see **Figure 7.47**). Note that, in contrast, she has an alert facial expression as a result of normal facial muscles. Electromyelography showed changes of denervation, and muscle biopsy displayed group atrophy of fibers. She required overnight oxygen through a masked facial Continuous Positive Airway Pressure (CPAP) (see **Figure 7.46**).

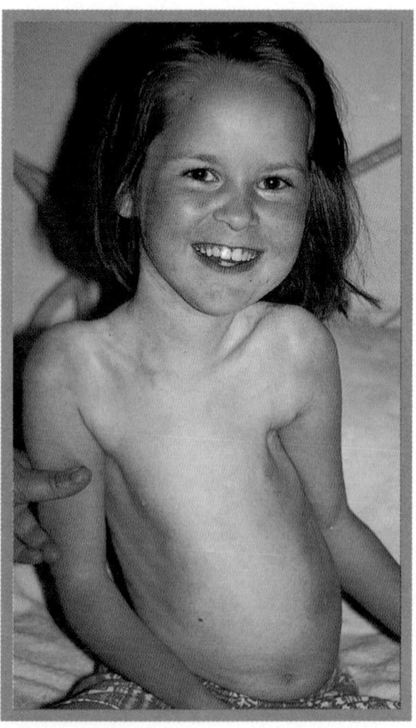

↑7.43

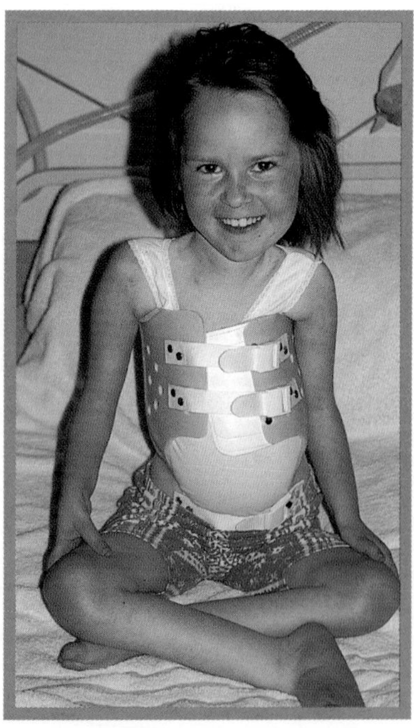

↑7.44

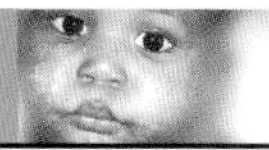

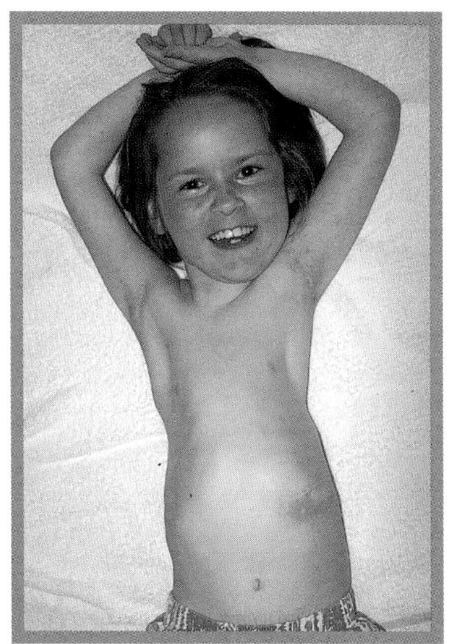

↑ 7.45

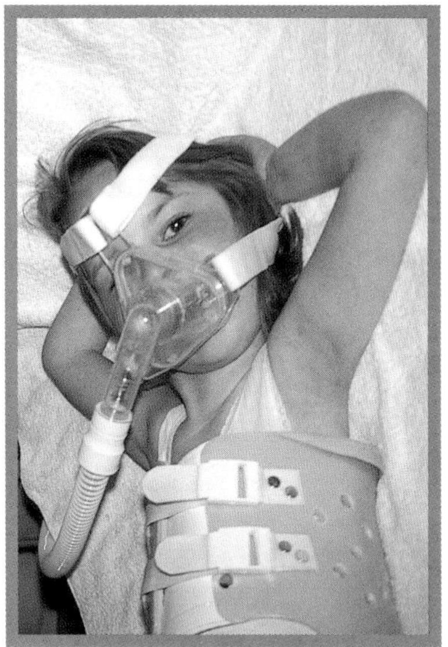

↑ 7.46

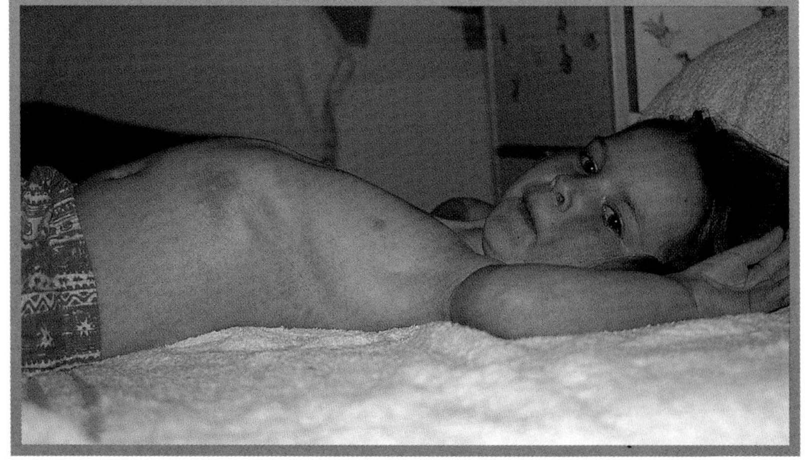

↑ 7.47

Figure 7.48 MRI Scan of Lipomyelomeningocele. An MRI scan of a 4-month-old boy is shown. Clinically, the child had a fatty lump on his back. A small hydromyelic cavity adjacent to the tethered cord can be seen.

Figure 7.49 Cerebellar Agenesis. The 20-month-old male infant shown here has cerebellar agenesis. Note the hypotonic posture with the legs being grossly abducted. He also demonstrated other cerebellar signs of nystagmus, intention tremor and hyporeflexia. Cerebellar agenesis may have an underlying genetic cause. This child had a sibling with the same problem.

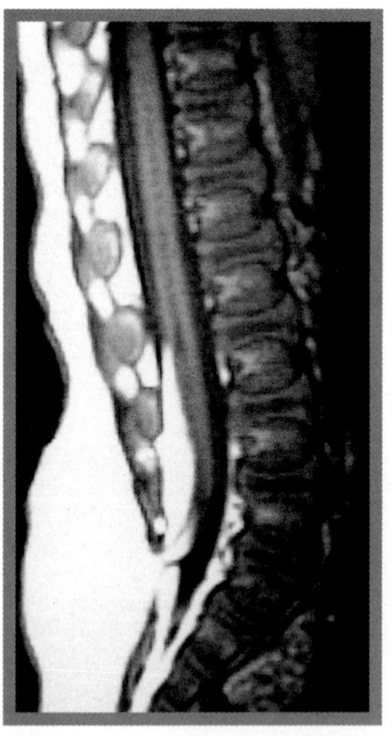

↑7.48

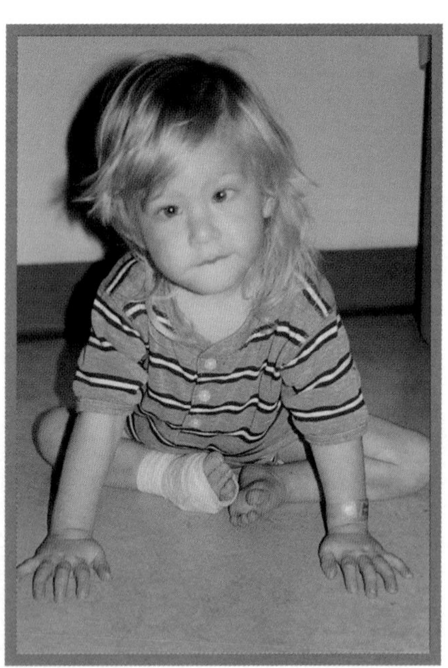

↑7.49

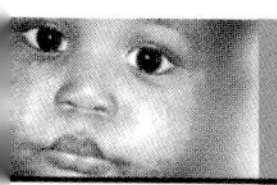

8 Hematological disorders

Figure 8.1 Anemia. The child discussed here has a smooth, painful, beefy-red tongue. This is glossitis in a child with megaloblastic anemia. The child was also pale with increased fatigueability, but had a normal neurological examination.

Megaloblastic anemia is a macrocytic anemia usually caused by deficiencies of vitamin B^{12} or folic acid. In this case the child had intestinal malabsorption resulting in B^{12} deficiency. In this age group, congenital vitamin B^{12} malabsorption and defects of B^{12} utilization must be considered.

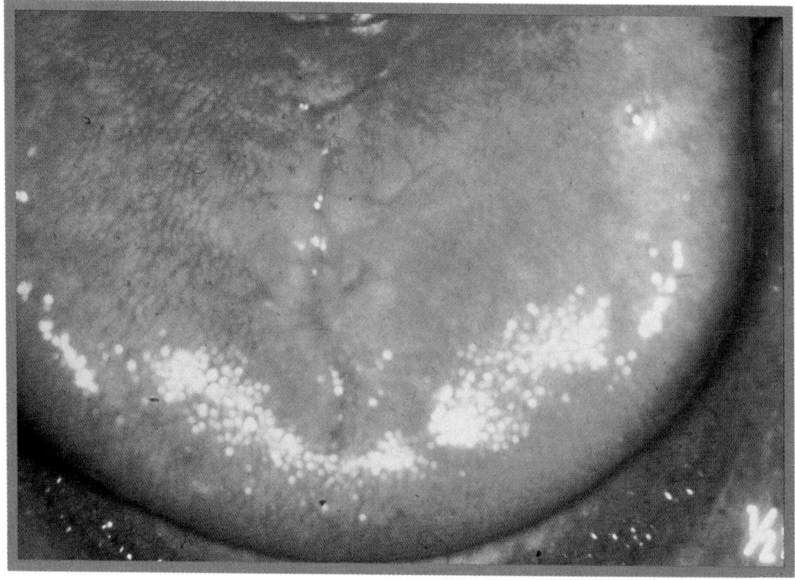

↑ **8.1**

Figure 8.2 Occipital Bossing due to Extramedullary Hemopoesis. The 4-year-old African child shown here has occipital bossing from severe iron-deficiency anemia due to a deficient diet of iron. A history of unusual dietary cravings (pica) was elicited (**Figure 8.3**), as well as one of delayed motor development. On examination he was thin and looked anemic. The blood film showed a microcytic, hypochromic anemia. There was a low serum ferritin confirming iron deficiency.

Differential diagnosis includes thalassemia, sickle-cell disease and other hemolytic anemias, and hemoglobinopathies should be considered, as should lead poisoning. The anemia of chronic disease or infection can also be microcytic. Any child over 2 years of age presenting with a diagnosis of iron deficiency should also be investigated for blood loss.

Iron deficiency anemia is a very common problem, especially in areas of urban deprivation and where early introduction of cows' milk (before 6 months of age) is frequent. The significance of iron deficiency (with or without anemia) lies in the adverse effects on neuro-developmental progress, particularly in cognitive functioning. The treatment of iron deficiency is recommended as it appears to reverse these neuro-developmental changes.

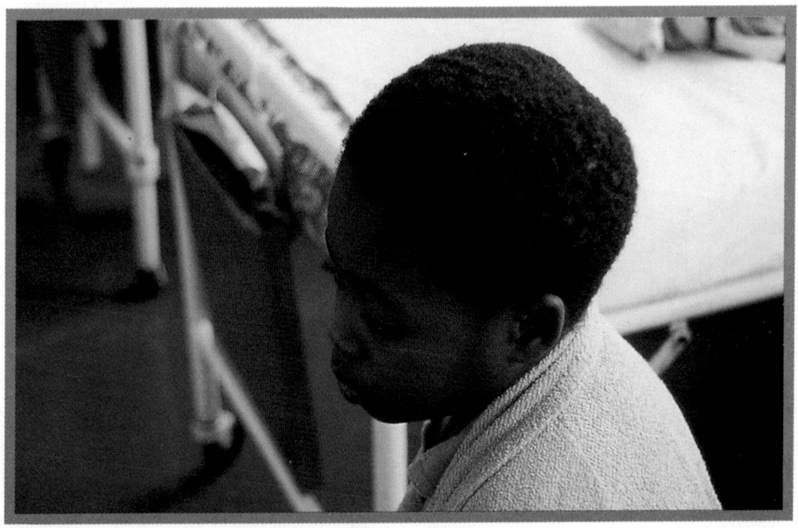

↑8.2

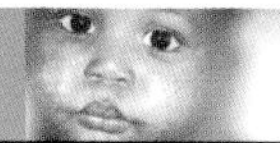

Figure 8.3 Abdominal X-ray shows Pica and Air Surrounding Roundworms. Dense mineral flecks are seen throughout the bowel, with serpigenous air shadows signifying roundworm infestation.

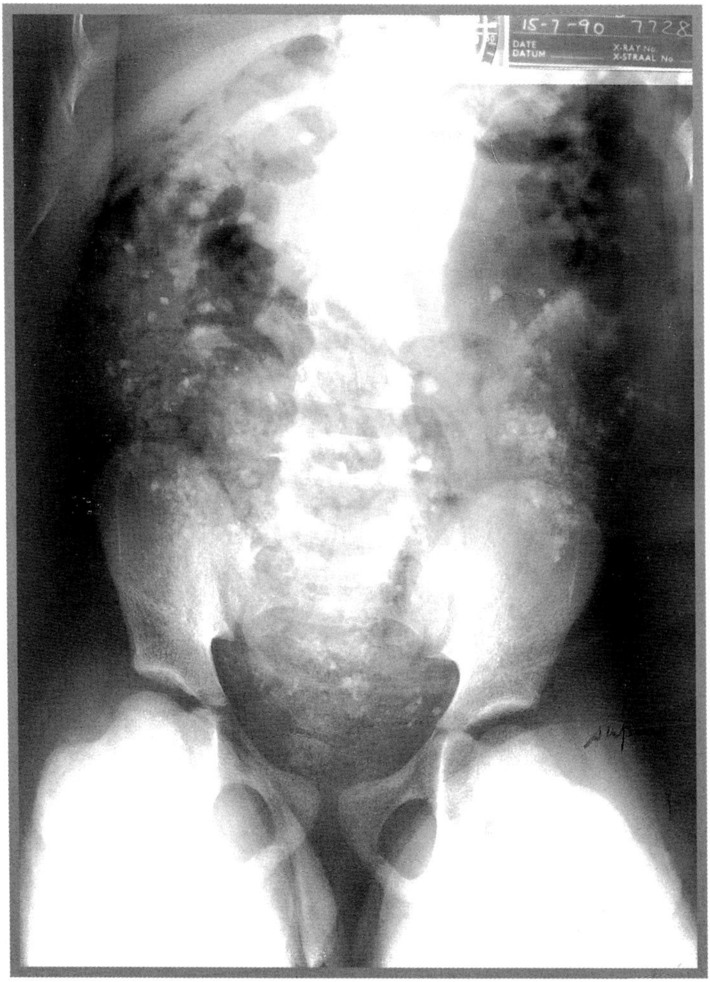

↑8.3

Figures 8.4–8.8 Idiopathic Thrombocytopenic Purpura. Figures 8.4–8.5 show extensive purpura in a 4-year-old girl who was otherwise well. There were petechiae, ecchymoses, and buccal mucosal and gingival hemorrhages present, following an acute upper respiratory tract infection. On examination no splenomegaly or lymphadenopathy was found. In **Figures 8.6 and 8.7** a 12-year-old girl presented with epistaxis and gastrointestinal bleeding in addition to the above features. Her platelet count was 20×10^9/l (normal range 220–450 $\times 10^9$/l).

The diagnosis rests on expert examination of the blood film (**Figure 8.8**) to exclude other causes. The film shows the almost total absence of platelets.

The choice of treatment is controversial. In view of the very low incidence of serious complications and the high chance of spontaneous resolution, some authorities recommend conservative management. Alternative strategies currently recommended are a 5-day course of intravenous immunoglobulin or oral prednisolone, and splenectomy should be offered to non-responders

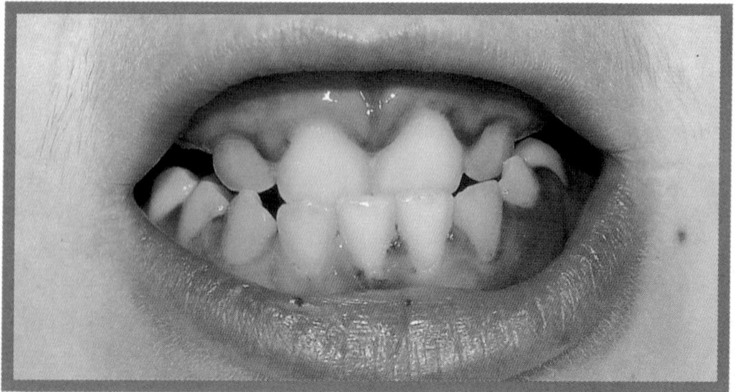

←8.4

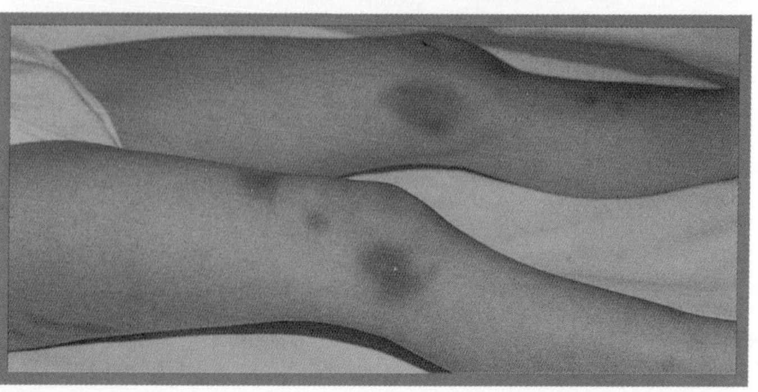

←8.5

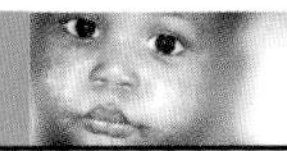

of medical management. Low platelet counts alone do not require treatment. Possible complications are severe generalized purpura, bleeding from the oral mucosa and gastrointestinal tract, fundal hemorrhage and intracranial hemorrhage.

Differential diagnosis includes; non-accidental injury and bleeding diathesis.

Other causes of thrombocytopenia are:

1. Failure of platelet production due to congenital causes, *e.g.*, primary hematophagic processes associated with trisomies 13 and 18, metabolic abnormalities and acquired disorders of the marrow, *e.g.*, infiltration, hypoplasia and aplastic anemias.
2. Platelet sequestration, *e.g.*, hypersplenism, hypothermia.
3. Increased destruction from other primary platelet consumption syndromes, either immunological or non-immunological, *e.g.*, disseminated intravascular coagulopathy.

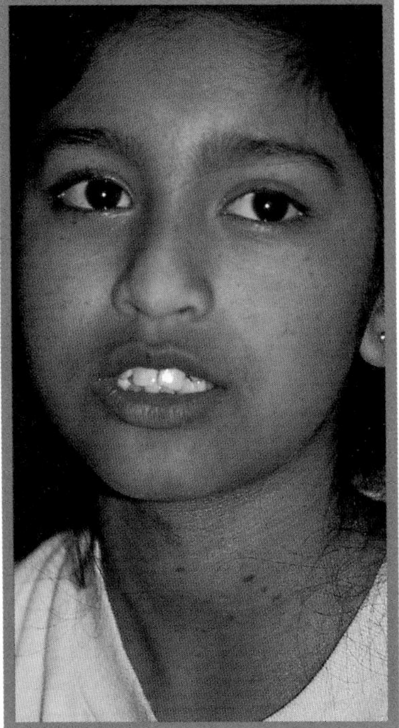

↑**8.6**

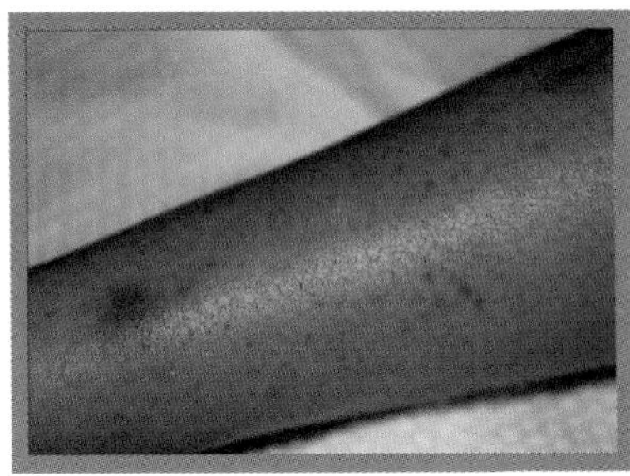

↑**8.7**

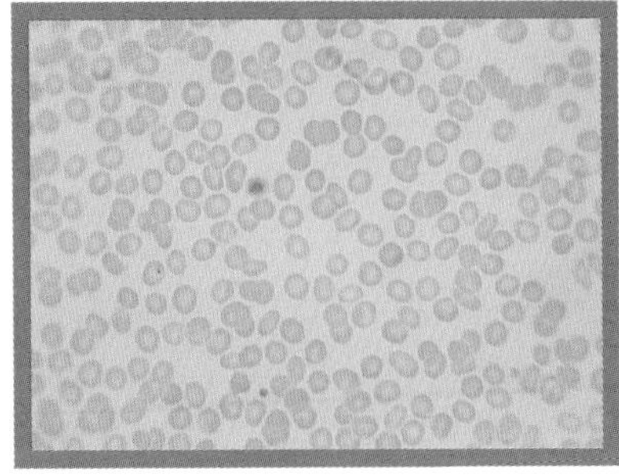

↑**8.8**

Figures 8.9 and 8.10 Leukemia. These figures respectively show hepatosplenomegaly and cervical lymphadenopathy in a 12-year-old girl. There was a 4-week history of a triad of symptoms associated with bone marrow failure, *i.e.*, anemia, bleeding and infection.

Clinically, glandular fever was suspected, but a blood count revealed pancytopenia and a blood film showed lymphoblasts to be present. Initially the anemia was corrected and broad-spectrum intravenous antibiotics and fluids were given. Bone marrow confirmed a diagnosis of acute lymphoblastic leukemia, immunocytochemistry confirming it to be of the 'common' type. Treatment consisted in high-dose intensive chemotherapy to induce remission, followed by maintenance chemotherapy for 2 years. Current prognosis for this type of leukemia is 90% remission, and 70% for being long-term disease-free at 5 years.

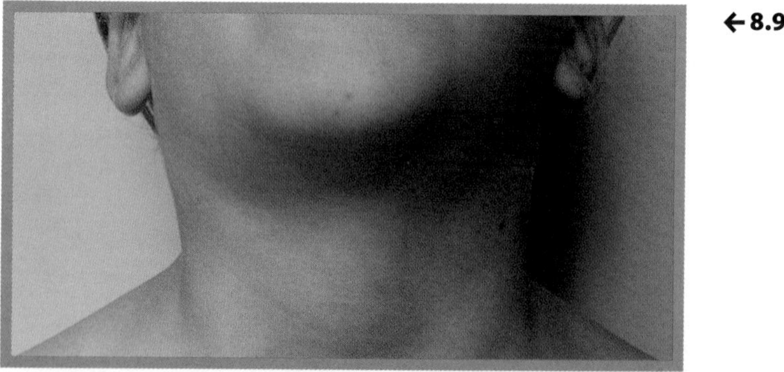

←8.9

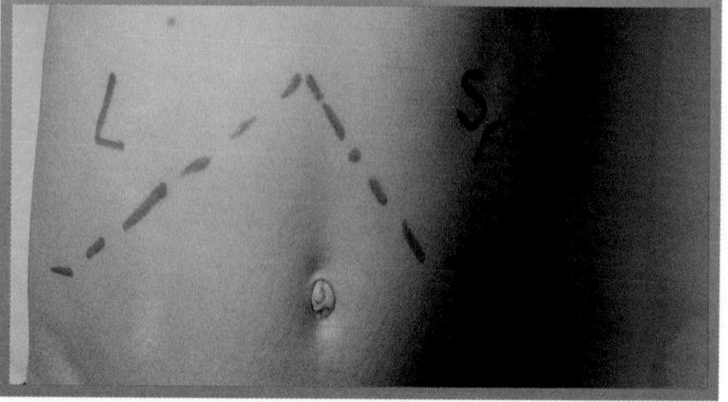

←8.10

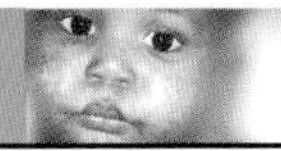

Figure 8.11 T-Cell Acute Lymphoblastic Leukemia (ALL). The x-ray shows massive thymic enlargement obscuring the mediastinal structures. This type of ALL occurs often in young males with a high white-cell count.

Figure 8.12 Neuroblastoma in the Chest. Note the rib abnormality, indicating a large, posterior mediastinal mass in the chest cavity impinging upon the ribs and causing distortion, thinning and splaying of the right ribs posteriorly with adjacent vertebral abnormalities. Other chest X-ray abnormalities may be seen in primitive tumors arising from the mediastinum, including effusions. CT and MRI will help differentiate the origin of these masses. Biopsy is required.

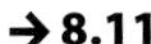

→8.11

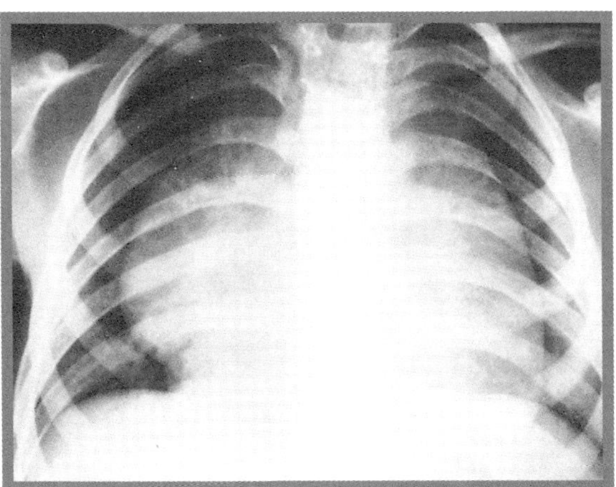

→8.12

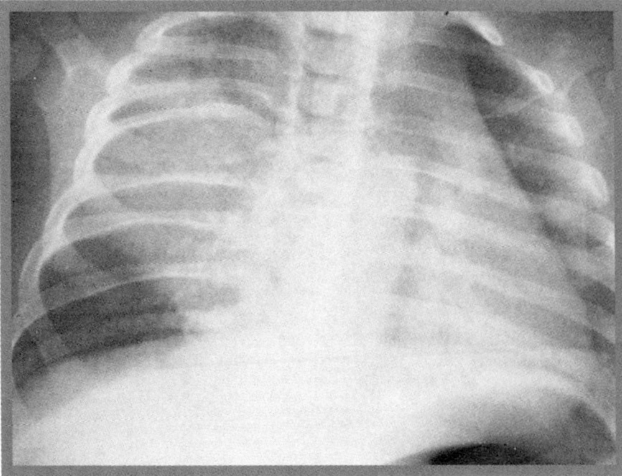

Figures 8.13 and 8.14 Langerhans Cell Histiocytosis. Maculopapular, non-pruritic, reddish-brown lesions are shown on the trunk. In areas the rash was scaly. In this case there was no evidence of pituitary insufficiency (polydypsia/polyuria) but there were osteolytic lesions in the skull, petechia, hepatosplenomegaly, mucous membrane involvement, generalized lymphadenopathy and pulmonary infiltration (Letterer–Siwe syndrome).

Skin biopsy revealed Langerhan cells containing Birbeck granules (CD1 markers).The differential diagnosis includes seborrheic dermatitis.

Figure 8.15 Kasabach–Merritt Syndrome. The girl shown, aged 22 months, has a giant cavernous hemangioma over the right shoulder and neck. Consumptive coagulopathy within such a hemangioma leads to peripheral depletion of platelets and coagulation factors.

Investigations revealed thrombocytopenia and fragmented red cells; coagulation screening tests were prolonged with increased amounts of

↑8.13

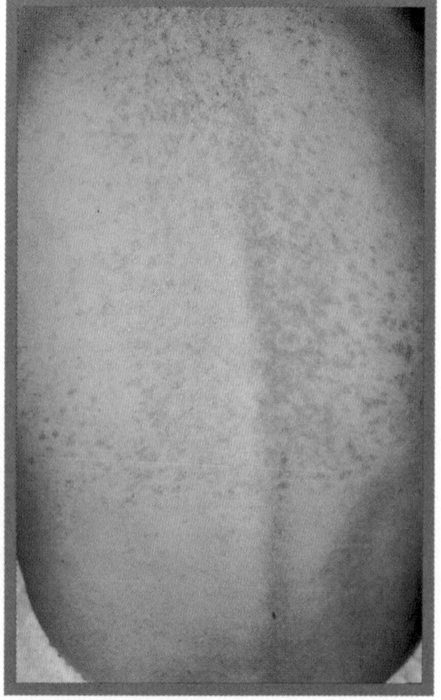

↑8.14

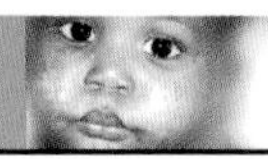

fibrinogen degradation products. Treatment consists in first, correcting the coagulopathy, followed by the use of steroids, embolization, and administration of interferon.

Figure 8.16 Alkaptonuria. This figure shows a urine specimen from a child whose mother had noted that the urine in the nappy became progressively darker the longer the nappy was left on. The defect is in the conversion of homogentisic acid to acetoacetic acid.

The urine discolors on exposure to oxygen and sunlight as the excess homogentisic acid in the urine becomes oxidized. A similar reaction in the exposed areas of cartilage, *e.g.*, ears, nose and sclerae leads to a gradual darkening of these structures. A degenerative arthritis is the result of the deposition of homogentisic acid in the cartilagenous surfaces of joints. Sweat will stain clothing. There is no intellectual impairment.

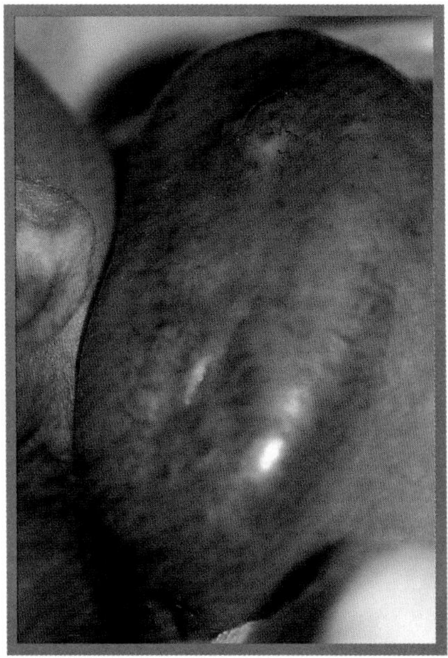

↑8.15

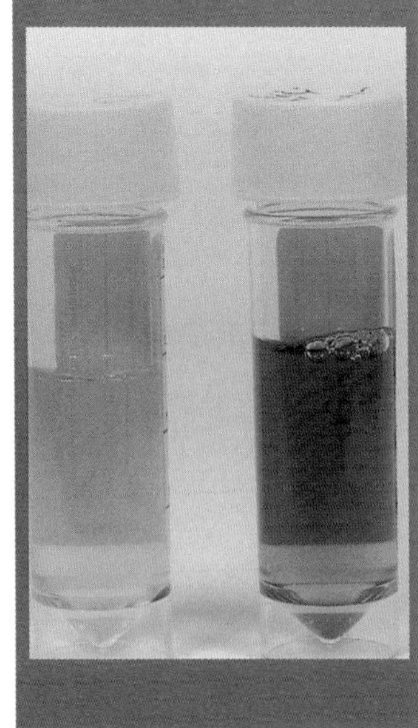

↑8.16

Figure 8.17 Di George Syndrome. The figure shows a 5-year-old boy, whose parents are first cousins. The typical facial features shown are low-set, abnormally formed ears, hypertelorism, micrognathia, a short philtrum of the upper lip and a high, arched palate.

He presented initially with intractable hypocalcemia in the neonatal period, which was due to hypoparathyroidism. Due to the absence of the thymus he has an abnormality of cell-mediated immunity, with recurrent respiratory tract infections, diarrhea and candidiasis. Chest X-ray demonstrated an absence of the thymic shadow.

Figure 8.18 Absent Radius. The child shown here displays bilateral absence of the radii. The absence or hypoplasia of the radii occurs in a number of conditions:

1. VATER/VACTERL associations: vertebral anomalies, imperforate anus, cardiac abnormalities, tracheoesophageal fistulae, radial and renal dysplasia, and limb abnormalities.
2. Fanconi syndrome: pancytopenia, multiple congenital anomalies, short stature, ear anomalies, café-au-lait spots.

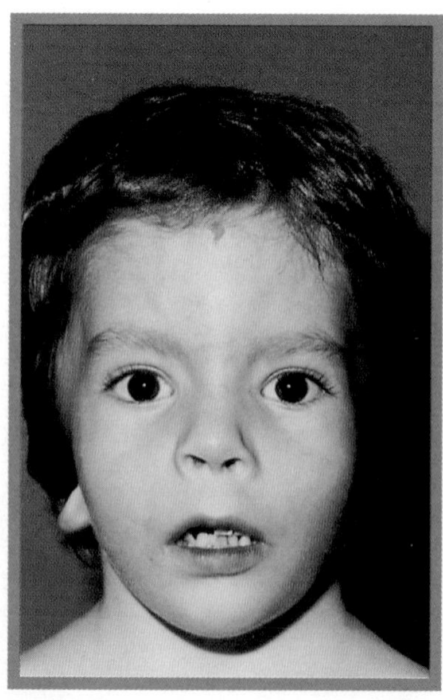

↑8.17

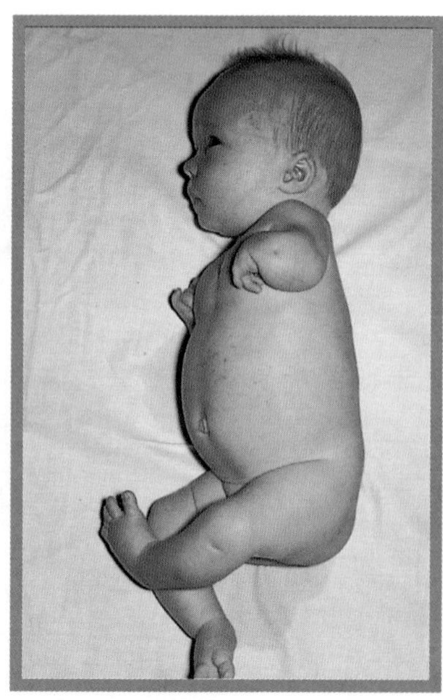

↑8.18

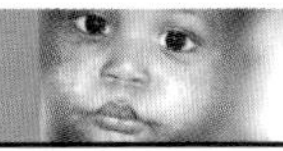

3. Holt–Oram syndrome: atrial or ventricular septal cardiac defects.
4. Thrombocytopenia absent radii (TAR) syndrome with immune deficiencies.
5. Thalidomide embryopathy.

Figures 8.19 and 8.20 Hodgkin Lymphoma. Figure 8.19 shows cervical lymphadenopathy in a 10-year-old African boy. This was a Hodgkin lymphoma. The child presented with non-tender cervical lymphadenopathy and B symptoms: fever, night sweats, malaise and weight loss. He had associated hepatosplenomegly. The diagnosis was established by histology of the infected node (see the scar on the right lateral neck in **Figure 8.20**) of the nodular sclerosis category.

Hodgkin disease is rare in childhood, usually occurring in late adolescence. It should be considered in children with persistent lymphadenopathy. With modern therapy, long-term disease-free survival is 90%.

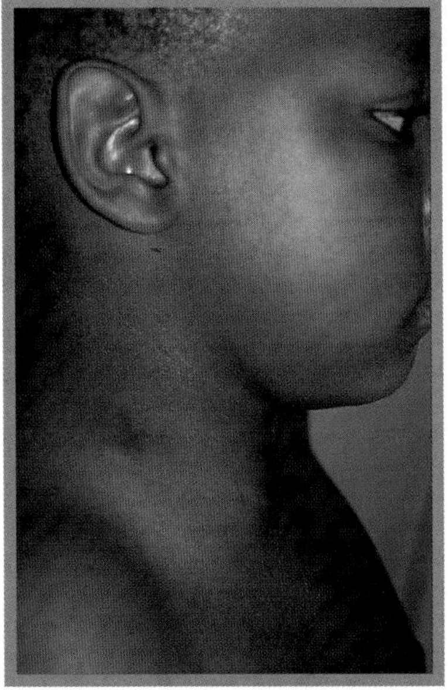

↑ 8.19

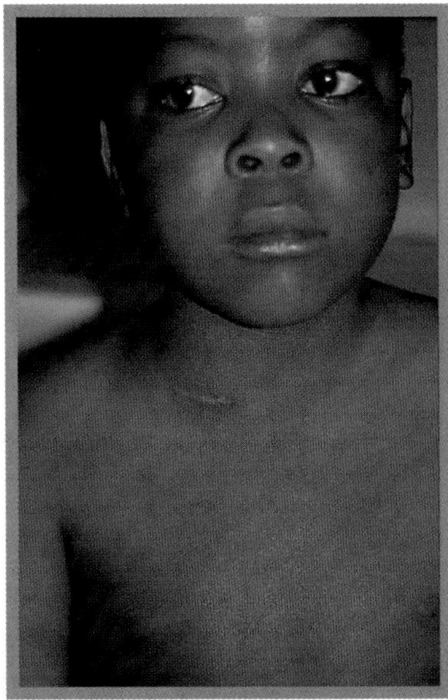

↑ 8.20

Figure 8.21 Burkitt Lymphoma. The 4-year-old boy shown here presented with unilateral enlargement of right part of the jaw, and associated hepatosplenomegaly and loss of weight. He also developed mesenteric lymph node involvement, which resulted in a perforated terminal ileum.

Burkitt lymphoma is a subtype of B-cell lymphoma, characterized on histology by small, non-cleaved cells. It has a predilection for jaw lesions and extranodal abdominal involvement in young African children. The nodes are firm and non-painful. Prognosis is dependent upon the histological appearance. Treatment consists in chemotherapy and radiotherapy, and is dependent upon the staging. The Epstein–Barr virus appears to play an important role in the tumor's development.

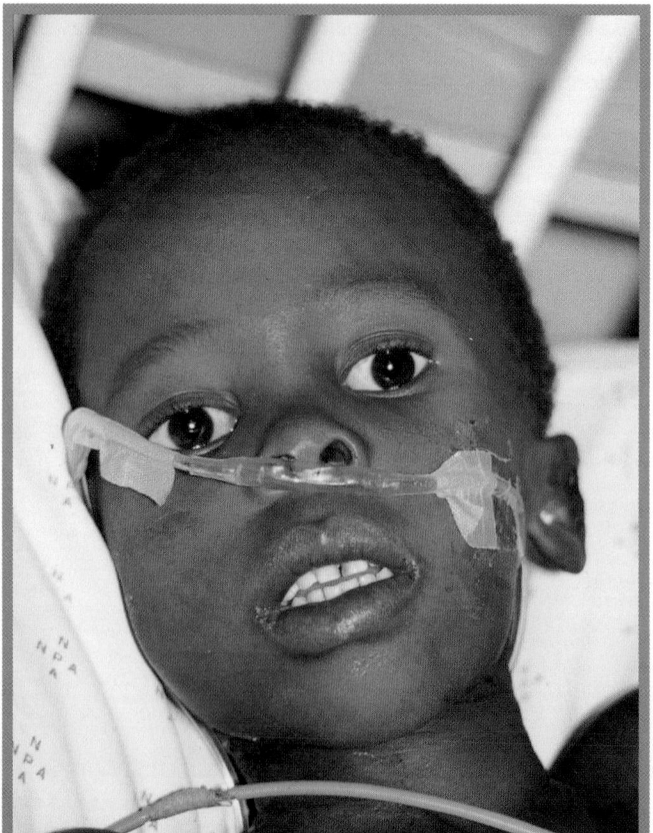

←8.21

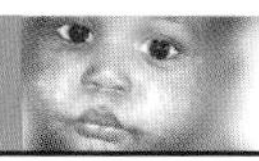

Figures 8.22 and 8.23 Hereditary Spherocytosis. Hereditary spherocytosis is shown in an 11-year-old African boy. Note the splenomegaly and jaundice. Hereditary spherocytosis may present as anemia in the newborn or as prolonged jaundice. The anemia may be mild or severe, and may require transfusion. Diagnosis is made upon the blood film showing spherocytes and a negative direct Coombs' test. The reticulocyte count will be raised. Long-term folate therapy is indicated. In older children, gallstones may be the presenting feature in unrecognized cases. In children with moderate-to-severe anemia, splenectomy and cholecystectomy may be necessary. In these cases, immunization with pneumococcal vaccines is indicated, as is life-long penicillin therapy.

→8.22

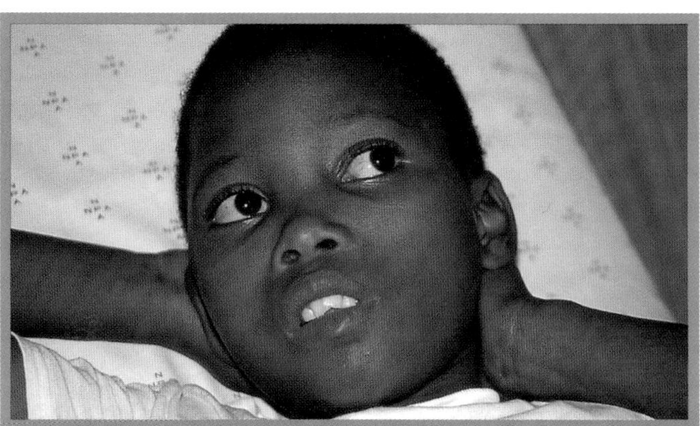

→8.23

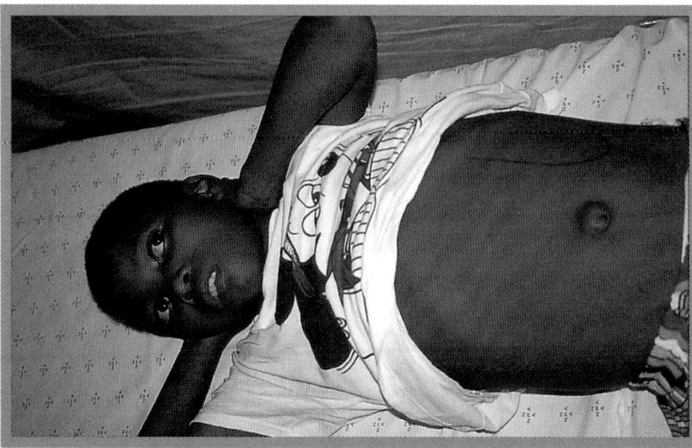

Figure 8.24 and 8.25 β-Thallassemia Major. The 6-year-old boy shown here, of mediterranean origin, presented in the first year of life with pallor, failure to thrive and hepatosplenomegaly due to extra-medullary hemopoieses, associated with poor hemoglobin synthesis. Investigations revealed severe hypochromic, microcytic anemia with raised reticulocyte count, nucleated red blood cells and basophilic stippling in the blood film.

Figure 8.25 The figure shows an X-ray of the tibia, fibula and femur of a child with β-thalassemia major. Expansion of marrow cavity with thinning of the cortices can be seen. When this is *in extremis* it forms an Ehrlenmeyer-flask deformity.

Hemoglobin electrophoresis showed an almost complete absence of HbA, that most hemoglobin was HbF, and that there was a slightly raised HbA_2.

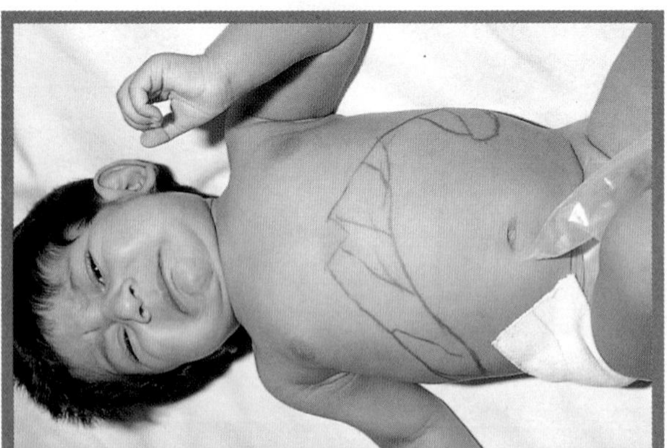

←8.24

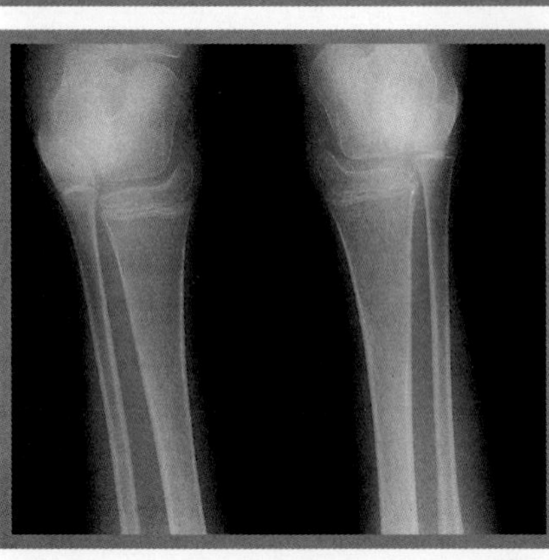

←8.25

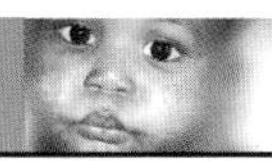

The child was being treated with regular blood transfusions, maintaining a hemoglobin above 11 g/dl. There were daily subcutaneous infusions of desferrioxamine (as an iron chelator) and oral vitamin C to increase the excretion of iron and to improve the immune status. Bone marrow transplantation has been successfully carried out from HLA-matched siblings.

Children with β-thalassemia major are at an increased risk of infection for a number of reasons: anemia in infancy predisposes to bacterial infection, splenectomy,results in increased susceptibility to encapsulated bacteria and gastrointestinal infection is more common, particularly in iron-loaded patients on desferrioxamine.

Figures 8.26–8.28 β–Thalassemia Major. This hemoglobinopathy is relatively common throughout the Mediterranean delta, despite the possibility of antenatal diagnosis. The 10-year-old boy shown here was diagnosed with the disease at 1 year of age. He had chronic anemia and hemolysis leading to extramedullary hemopoiesis. The typical facies show frontal bossing.

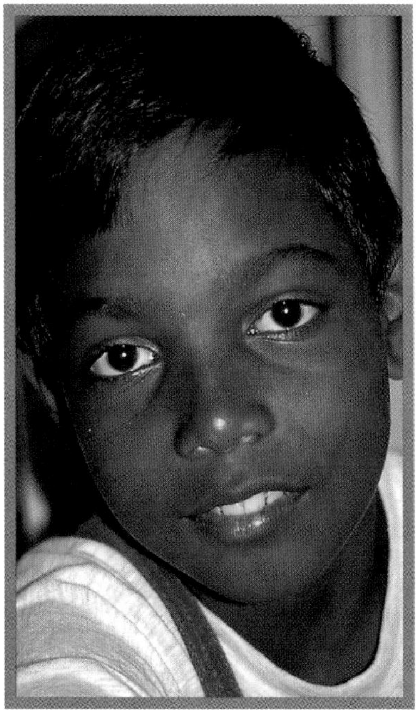

↑8.26

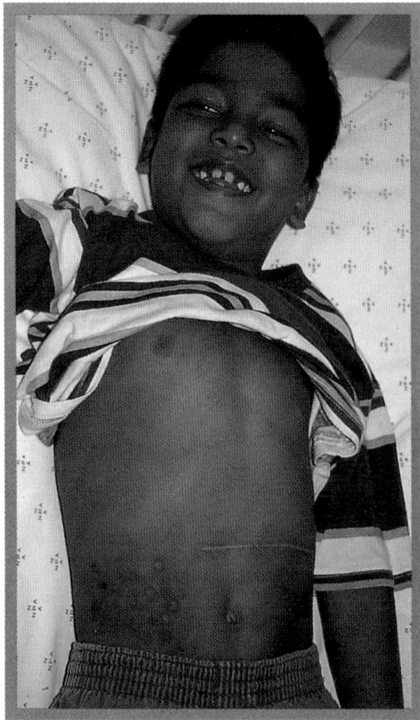

↑8.27

Management of the anemia by transfusion therapy leads to iron overload, which can be managed by subcutaneous infusions of the chelating agent desferrioxamine. Note the scarring due to reactions to the infusion on the anterior abdominal wall (**Figure 8.28**).

Splenomegaly may be enormous. If splenic sequestration, infarct or rupture occur, splenectomy may be necessary as shown (note the abdominal scar).

Figure 8.29 Sickle-cell Anemia Blood Film. Note the deeply stained sickle cells and target cells. Sickle-cell anemia is most common in Afro-Caribbeans. On deoxygenation, sickle hemoglobin forms reversible fibrils leading to sickling of red cells and subsequent increased blood viscosity and capillary obstruction. Sickling is exacerbated by dehydration, infection, acidosis and hypoxia. The cause of sickle-cell anemia consists in ongoing hemolysis punctuated by crises which may be both painful and life threatening.

The main complications are splenic sequestration crisis, overwhelming sepsis, aplastic crisis, vaso-occlusive (infarctive) crisis, chronic hemolysis and anemia, hemolytic crisis and hyposthenuria.

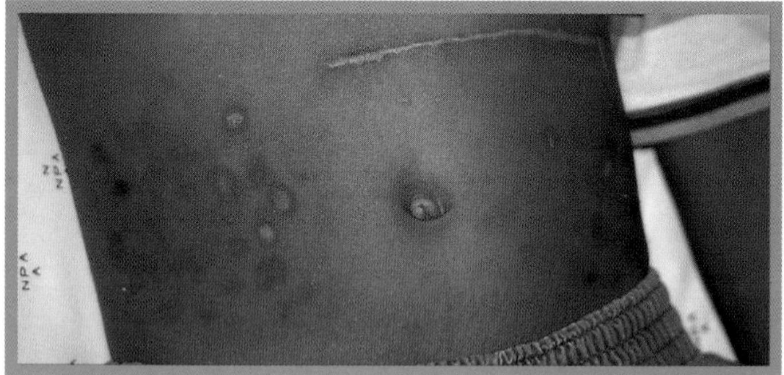

←8.28

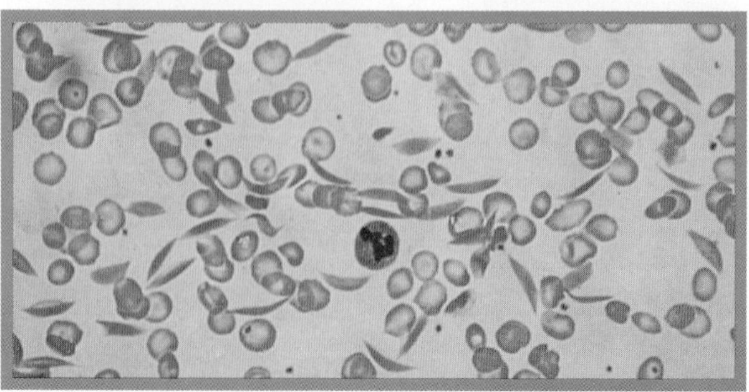

←8.29

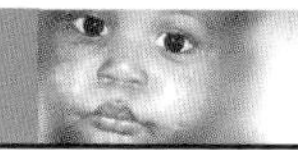

Figure 8.30 Hemophilia A (Classic Hemophilia) Factor VIII Deficiency. The 3-year-old boy shown here has hemorrhaging in to the breast tissue on the right and in to the right hip. This is a severe case in view of the age of presentation. There may be no family history in about 20% of cases. The probability of carrier status can be determined by assay of factor VIII in carrier females. Hemarthroses, as shown here, are the hallmarks of the disease, and these are painful and require prompt treatment with replacement factors. Hemorrhaging into the joints results in degenerative changes in the connective tissues.

Diagnosis consists in assay of factor VIII levels, and treatment in regular infusions of factor VIII. Recombinant factor VIII is now given to newly diagnosed patients to avoid the risk of viral transmission from blood products. Twenty percent of patients develop resistance to conventional therapy due to the appearance of factor VIII inhibitor. In up to 50% of cases the hemorrhagaes disappear spontaneously. In mild cases of hemophilia A, the use of DDAVP may control hemorrhaging.

Figure 8.31 Hereditary Lymphedema. Primary lymphedema caused by congenital hypoplasia of the lymphatics in an 8-year-old male is shown. The swelling was firm but pitted. Differential diagnosis is elephantiasis due to filariasis infection.

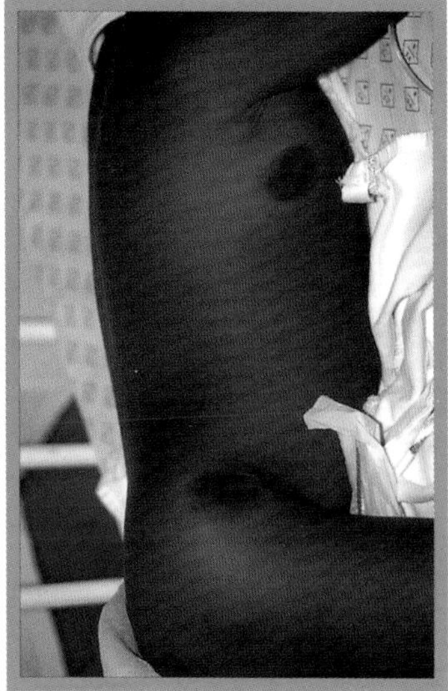

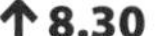
↑ **8.30**

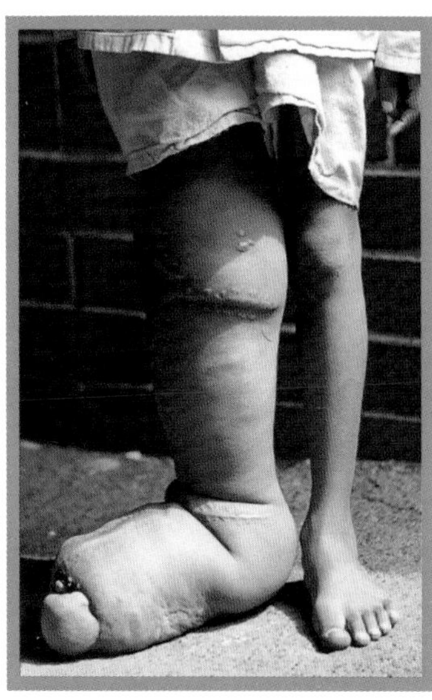

↑ **8.31**

Figure 8.32 Lead Poisoning (Blood Film). Basophilic stippling due to degenerate microsomes and siderosomes is shown in this case of lead poisoning. This is also found in severe infections and thalassemia. Hypochromic anemia is also present.

Figure 8.33 Knee showing Lead Lines (X-ray). Dense horizontal metaphyseal lines are seen on both sides of the knee at the line of the growth plate. Involvement of the fibula metaphysis is pathognomonic of metallic poisoning.

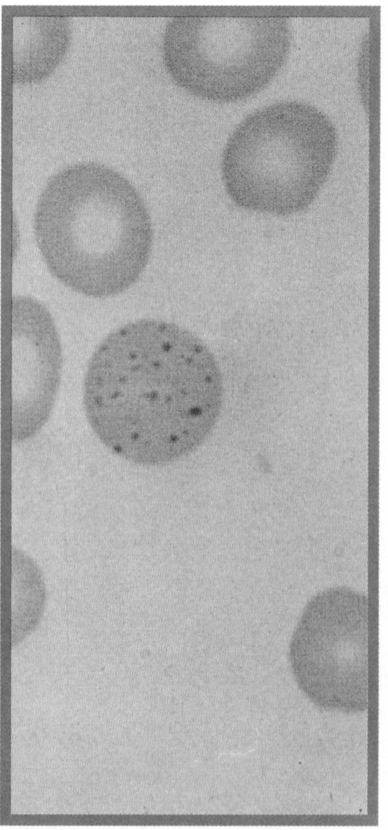

↑8.32

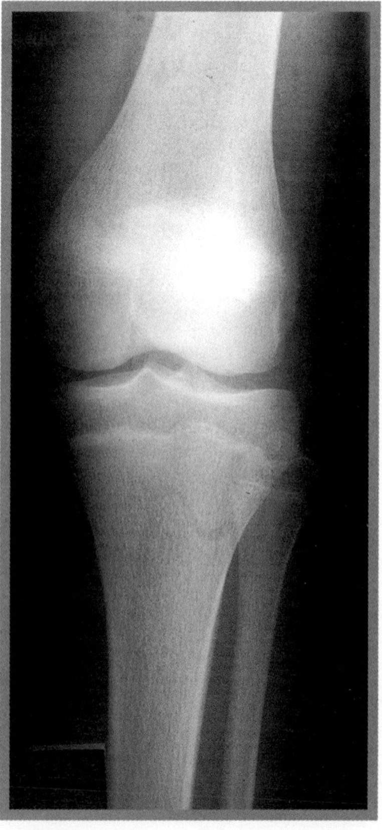

↑8.33

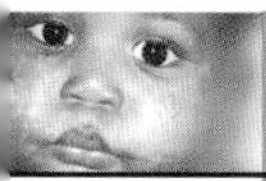
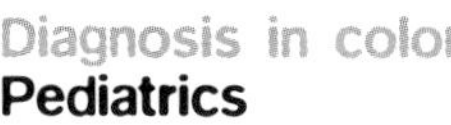

9 Endocrine and metabolic disorders

Figure 9.1 Diabetes – Necrobiosis Lipoidica Diabeticorum. Multiple yellowish-brown, atrophic, plaque-like lesions with raised borders can be seen around the shins bilaterally. This painless condition is extremely rare in childhood diabetes, and is commoner in female patients. Ulceration of the lesions may occur.

→9.1

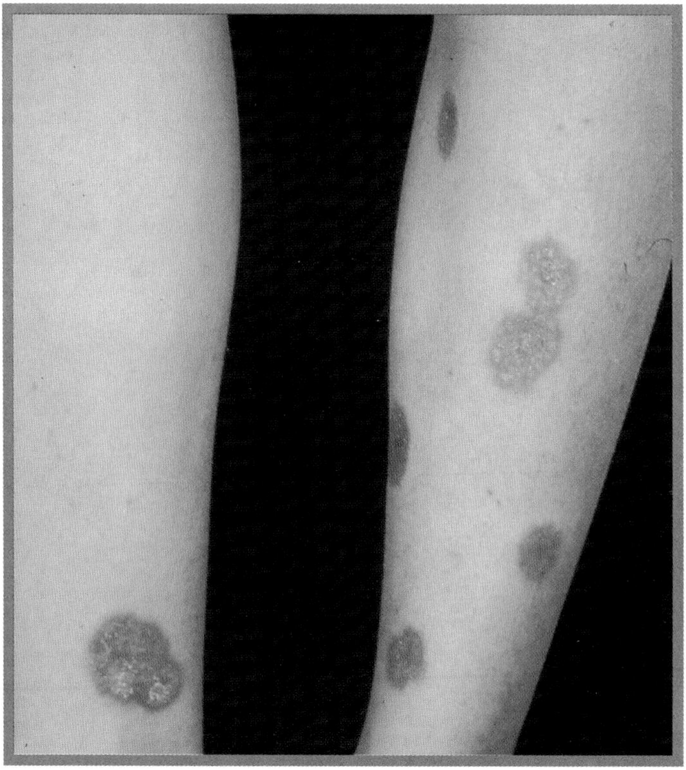

Figure 9.2 Peripheral Neuropathy in Diabetes. This figure shows the 'prayer sign'—the loss of full flexion at the wrist—in a young diabetic. The patient is unable to oppose the finger tips or the palmar surface of the hand.

There are flexion contractures in the metacarpal–phalangeal and proximal–interphalangeal joints. This is a good screening test for limited joint mobility, which has been reported to occur in up to 33% of diabetics after 10–15 years.

Figures 9.3–9.5 Lipodystrophy. Lipodystrophy is relatively common in childhood diabetes, especially if the injection sites are not rotated. **Figures 9.3 and 9.4** show lipohypertrophy, and **Figure 9.5** shows lipoatrophy. Rotating the injection sites usually results in resolution of the problem. It is suggested that human insulins are less prone to causing this problem, but both of the children shown here were on human insulin.

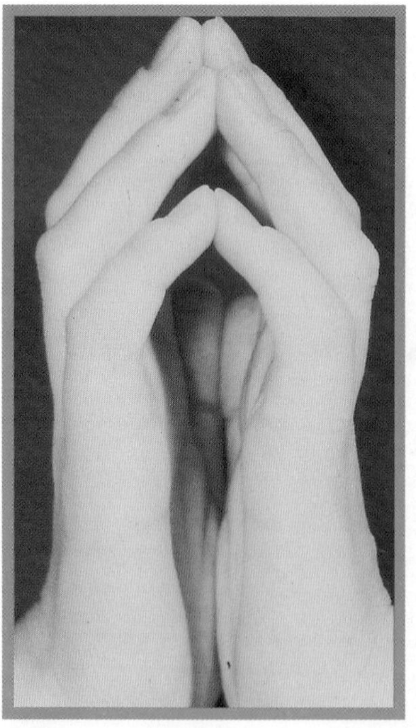

↑**9.2**

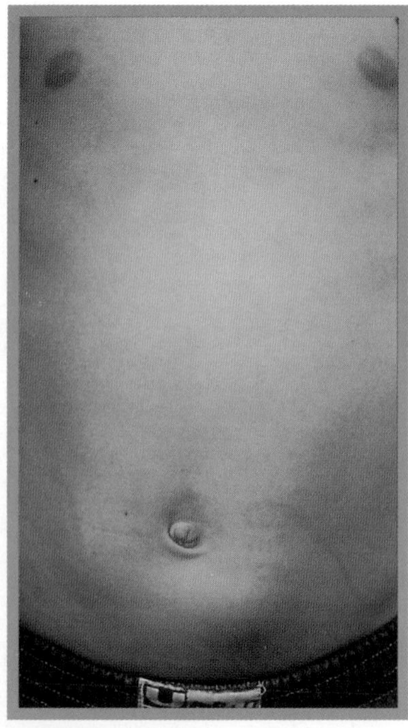

↑**9.3**

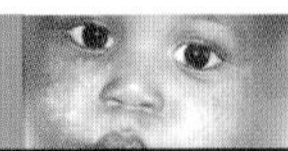

→9.4

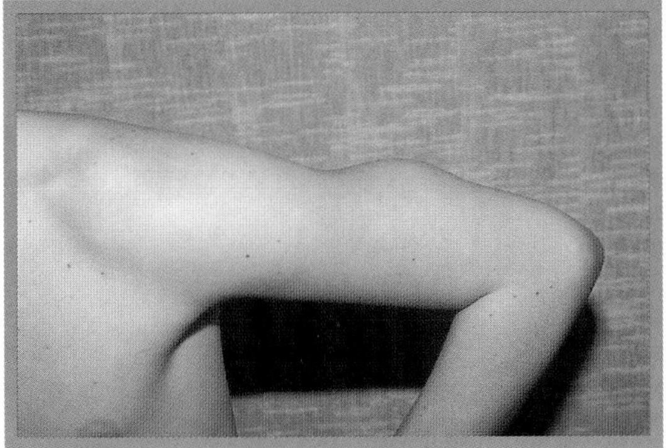

→9.5

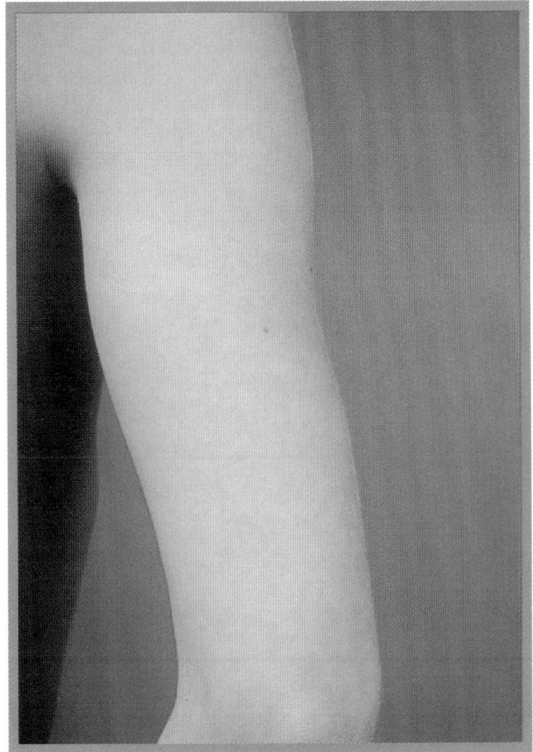

Figure 9.6 Retinopathy. Eye signs in pediatric diabetes are relatively rare. The occurrence of retinopathy is related to glucose control, the duration of the diabetes and genetic predisposition.

The retinal changes can be classified into three main groups:

1. Background retinopathy: this is characterized by microaneurysms (tiny red dots), capillary occlusion, blot hemorrhages, and hard exudates.
2. Preproliferative retinopathy: this type shows cotton-wool spots indicating ischemia, venous loops and beading, and arterial abnormalities.
3. Proliferative retinopathy: in this type, new peripheral or optic disk vessels develop. These result in visual complications if hemorrhage occurs, and also in retinal detachment due to traction. Vessel proliferation leads to rubeosis iridis and glaucoma.

This figure shows late adolescent proliferative retinopathy involving the optic disk.

Figure 9.7 Infant of a Diabetic Mother. This figure shows a typical infant of a diabetic pregnancy. The child is macrosomic with polycythemia. Once delivered, such infants have problems with transient hyperinsulinemic hypoglycemia, hyaline membrane disease, hyperbilirubinemia, feeding difficulties and apneic episodes. There is an increased incidence of thrombosis (particularly of the renal vein), hypocalcemia and transient cardiomyopathy. Management should be expectant, with early and regular enteral feeding and,

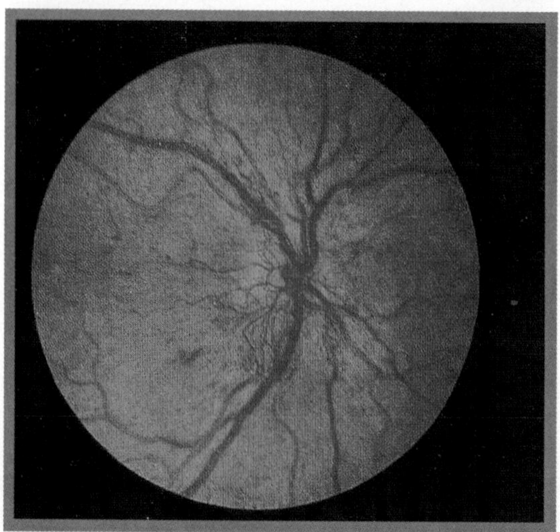

←9.6

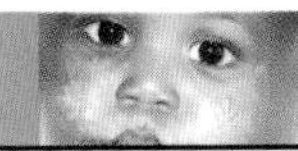

when necessary, intravenous glucose infusion. Problems of hyperinsulinemia in the infant can be avoided via the strict control of maternal glucose regulation duing pregnancy. *In utero* consequences of hyperinsulinism include macrosomia with teratogenesis, cardiac, central nervous system and skeletal anomalies and fetal death.

Figure 9.8 Diabetic Embryopathy. This figure shows **sacral agenesis** in a 2-month-old boy. The mother had previously been a non-insulin dependent diabetic, but during pregnancy a deterioration in her diabetic control resulted in insulin therapy being started in the second trimester. Sacral agenesis is most usually found in association with diabetes in pregnancy.

→9.7

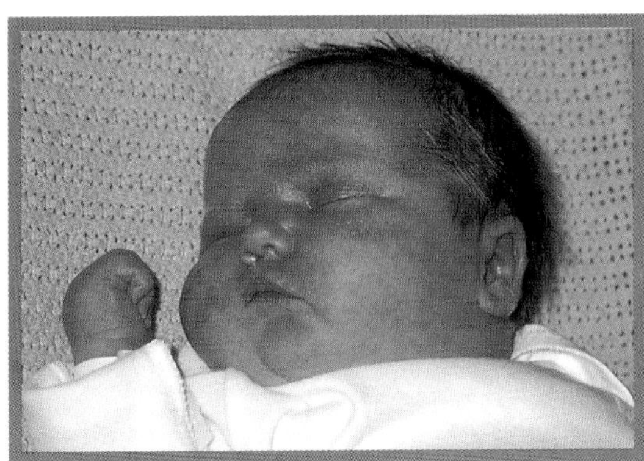

→9.8

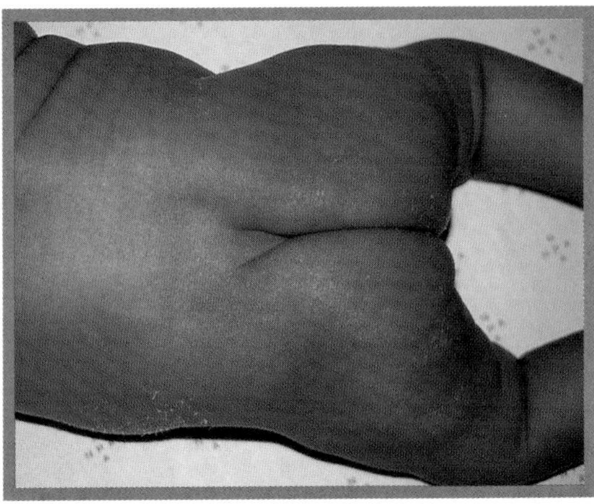

Figure 9.9 Diabetic embryopathy: Radial hypoplasia. Note the medially angulated forearm with an additional skin crease. In addition there is abnormal development of the metacarpals with an abnormal dimple visible on the dorsal aspect of the hand. Other congenital abnormalities are also relatively more common in infants born to mothers with diabetes in pregnancy, *e.g.*, gastroschisis, duodenal and anorectal atresias, and congenital heart disease, particularly transposition of the great vessels.

Figure 9.10 Congenital Hypothyroidism in a Neonate. This baby presented with prolonged jaundice on the same day that the neonatal screening laboratory reported an abnormal TSH on the dried-blood spot test. The classic signs evolve progressively during the first few months of life. Typical facies and a slight protrusion of the tongue are shown. The tongue is thickened and protuberant, the facies are coarse, there is an enlarged muscle mass of the eyelids, and the lips are swollen. Note the protuberant abdomen due to

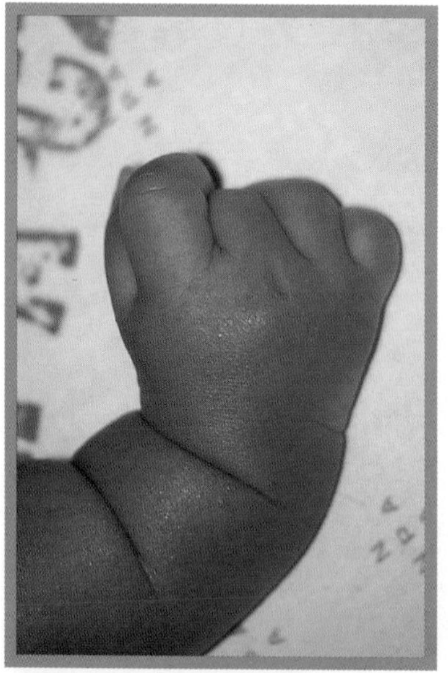

↑9.9

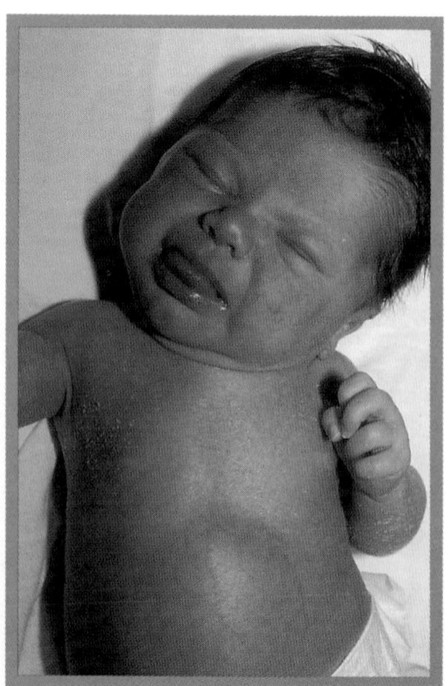

↑9.10

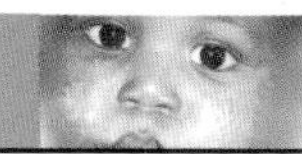

constipation. Prenatal hypothyroidism causes neuro-developmental delay, which is not cured but prevented from progressing by early-onset treatment. Differential diagnosis does not usually present a problem if thyroid function screening in the newborn has been undertaken. Alternative diagnoses are Beckwith–Wiedemann syndrome, Down syndrome, glycogen storage disease (Type II), mucopolysaccharide storage disorders and trisomy 4pS.

Figure 9.11 Untreated Severe Graves Disease in a Pregnant Mother. The small-for-dates boy was born to a mother with severe Graves disease. The baby was hyperthyroid at birth and required iodine therapy to control his symptoms. Transplacental thyroid stimulation caused these problems.

Figures 9.12 Hyperthyroidism in an Adolescent. Hyperthyroidism is shown here in a 13-year-old girl who presented with emotional lability, tremor, weight loss, increased sweating, heat intolerance and accelerated growth. **Figure 9.12** shows a diffuse, firm goitre.

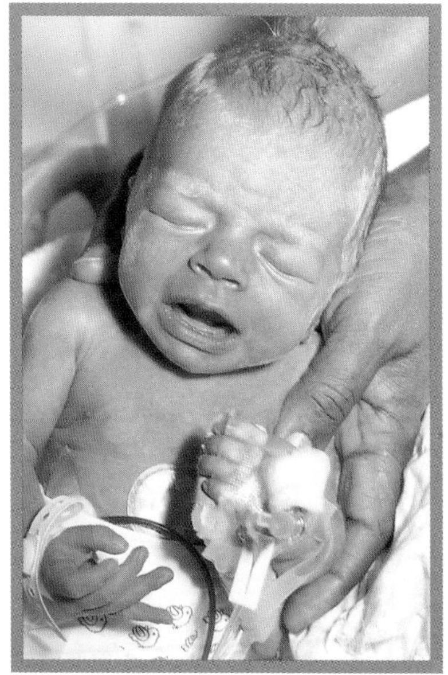

↑**9.11**

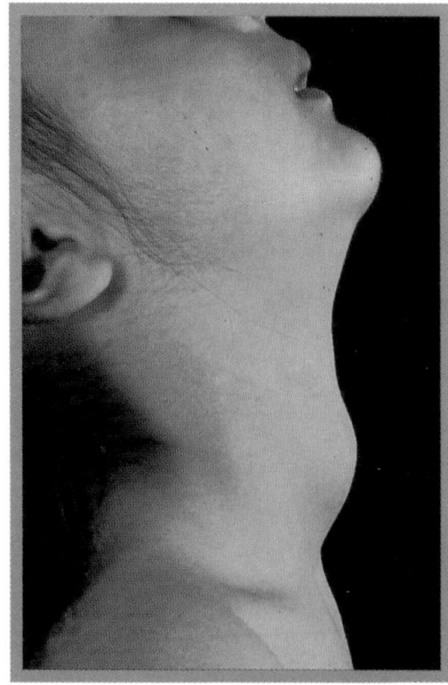

↑**9.12**

Figure 9.13 Exophthalmos. In the same girl there was also tachycardia and systolic hypertension present. Investigations revealed that T4 and T3 were raised, with TSH levels being reduced. Hyperthyroidism in childhood is usually autoimmune, occurring more frequently in girls, and is often familial.

Treatment consists of administration of propranolol acutely and antithyroid drugs, *e.g.*, carbimazole. Approximately 50% of cases remit spontaneously and many will become hypothyroid.

Figure 9.14 Myxedema in a 9-year-old Girl with Acquired Juvenile Hypothyroidism. The girl shown here presented with a reduced growth velocity and an increasing weight-for-height. She has myxedematous skin changes. She complained of constipation, and had been injured in her self-defence class as her reflexes had slowed. She had a history of acute anterior neck pain starting some 8 weeks previously. On examination, she had a diffusely enlarged, firm, painless thyroid with no audible bruit. There was associated dry skin and hair with delayed relaxation of her deep tendon reflexes. Thyroid function showed a grossly elevated thyroid stimulating hormone (TSH) level. Thyroid microsomal autoantibodies were positive and she responded well to daily thyroxine.

Figures 9.15 and 9.16 Cushingoid Facies. In pediatric practice cushingoid facies are most commonly due to exogenous steroids. Shown here are the 'full moon facies', plethora, hirsutism and obesity. Striae over the abdomen, an interscapular fat pad (the 'buffalo hump'), easy bruising, growth retardation and hypertension were also present.

Differential diagnosis includes simple obesity, in which case the striae are pink as distinct from the purplish striae of Cushing syndrome. The patient is not usually hypertensive and has normal growth.

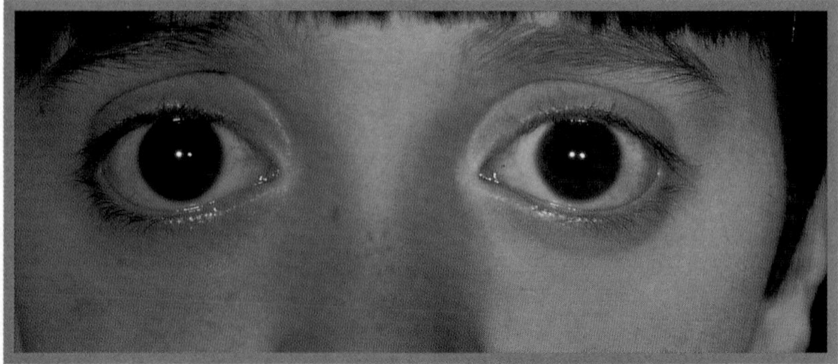

↑9.13

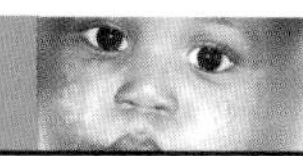

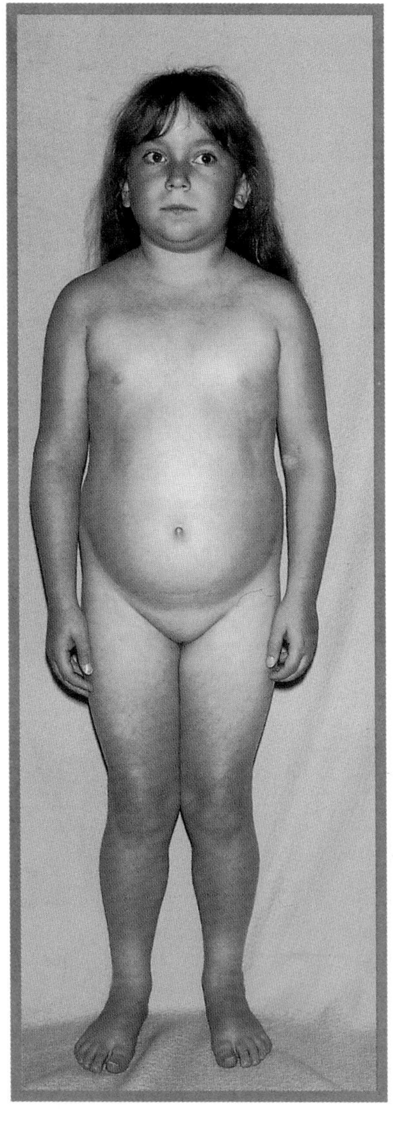

↑9.14

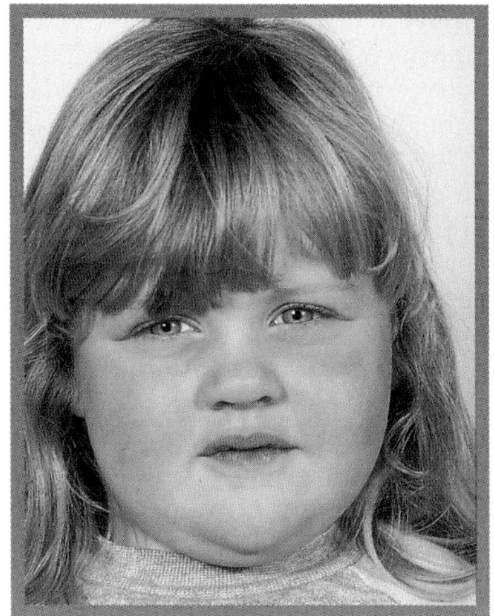

↑9.15

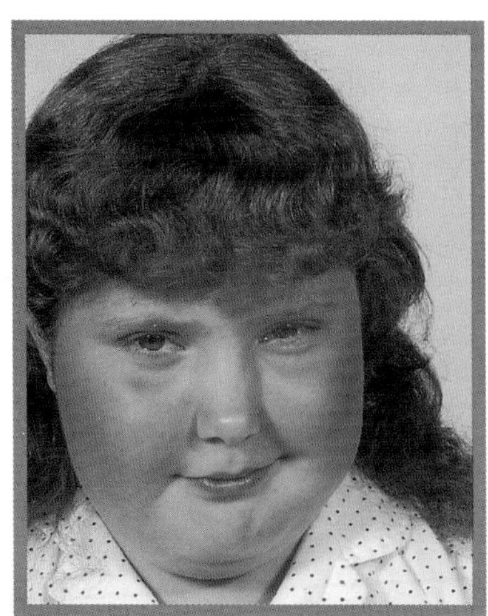

↑9.16

Figure 9.17 Obesity. The 4-year-old Afro-Caribbean girl shown here weighs 44 kg, which is well over the 99th centile. Her height is 120 cm, which is over the 97th centile. She has no striae, and is of normal development. Her mother and father are similarly overweight. The differential diagnoses of Cushing syndrome, Prader–Willi syndrome, Laurence–Moon–Biedl syndrome, hypothyroidism and Turner syndrome would all be associated with short stature.

Figure 9.18 Addison Disease. Increased pigmentation of the tongue is shown. The child presented with progressive lassitude, muscle weakness, constipation, abdominal pain and an increased pigmentation in the buccal mucosa and palmar creases due to ACTH melanocyte stimulation.

Laboratory investigations revealed hyponatremia, hyperkalemia, anemia, and fasting hypoglycemia. ACTH levels were raised and adrenal autoantibodies were present. The most common cause of Addison disease is autoimmunity, although tuberculosis is still a significant cause.

A patient presenting as an acute Addisonian crisis (with hypotension and collapse) necessitates urgent treatment. This should take the form of

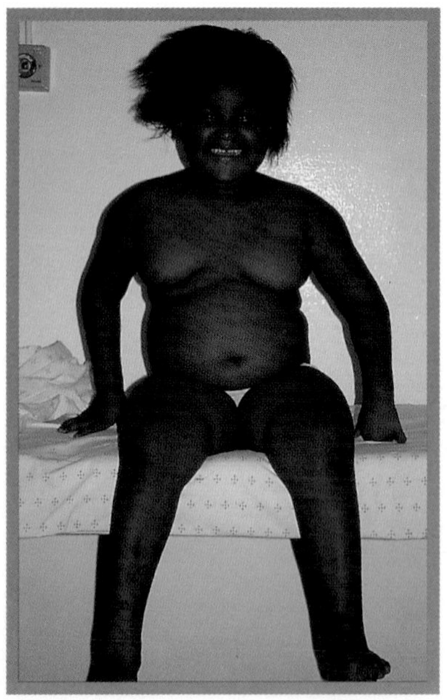

↑9.17

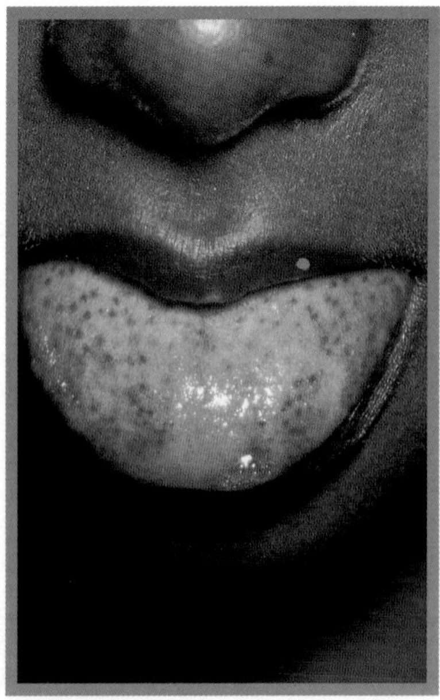

↑9.18

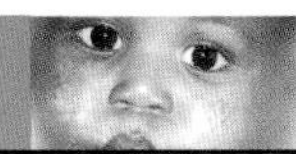

resuscitation with plasma, hormone replacement and correction of the electrolyte disturbance and hypoglycemia. Long-term treatment consists of life-long oral hydrocortisone and mineralocorticoid administration.

Figure 9.19 Achondroplasia. The baby shown here has achondroplasia. Note the macrocephaly with prominent forehead, hypotonia, low nasal bridge, proximal shortening of all four limbs (rhizomelia), small thoracic cage, and small hands. Also shown is mild midfacial hypoplasia. The child's hands were tridentate in nature when open. This autosomal dominant condition may be complicated by hydrocephalus secondary to the narrow foramen magnum, spinal cord or root compression secondary to kyphosis, spinal cord stenosis or herniated discs. X-rays demonstrated short tubular bones with thick broadened and cupped ends.

Figures 9.20 Russell–Silver Dwarfism without Asymmetry. A 14-month-old girl with her normal sized 9-year-old brother and 10-year-old sister is shown. Note the child's short stature, which was on the third centile at the age of 6 months. She was small-for-dates.

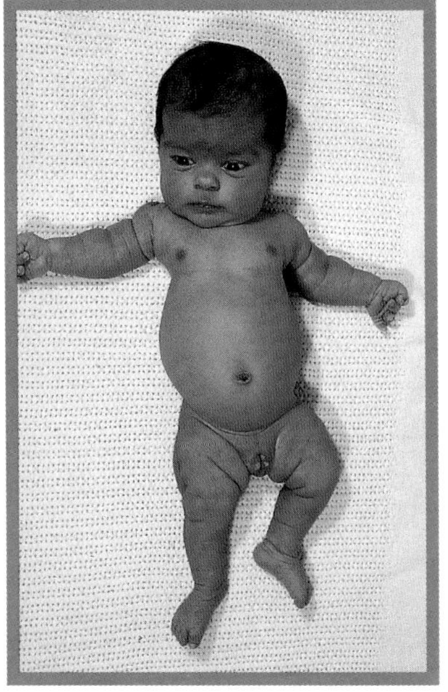

↑9.19

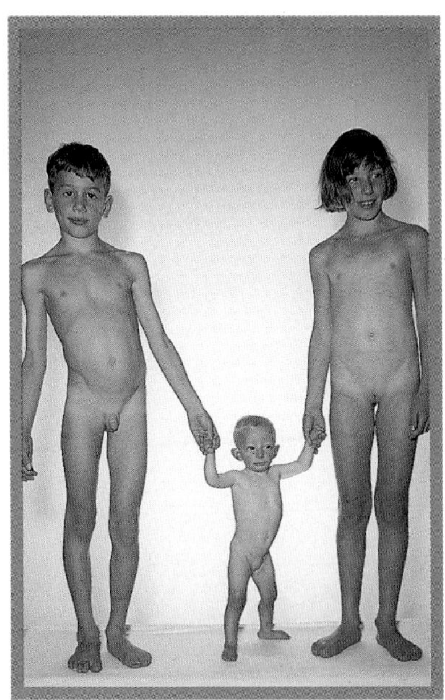

↑9.20

Figure 9.21 Russell–Silver Dwarfism. The girl shown here has the characteristic facial features of Russell–Silver dwarfism. The face is small and triangular with frontal bossing, thin lips, protruding ears and micrognathia. The head circumference is normal. The girl had normal intellegence and clinodactyly of the fifth finger. Some children additionally show asymmetry of the limbs and café-au-lait patches.

Figures 9.22 and 9.23 Familial Short Proximal Upper Limb in Father and Child. Note that on flexion of the elbow there is overshooting of the thumb

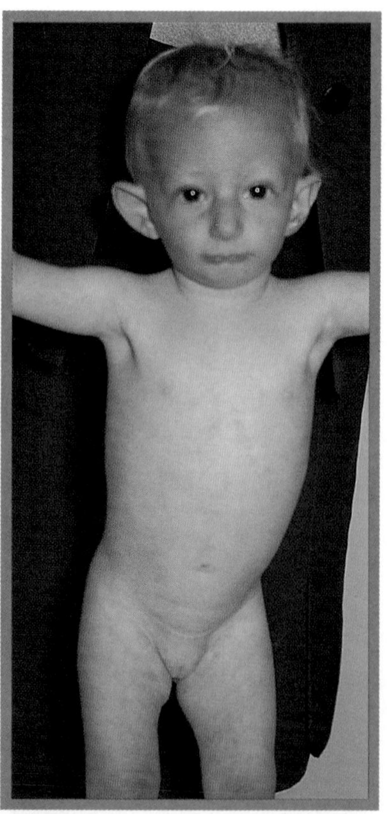

↑9.21

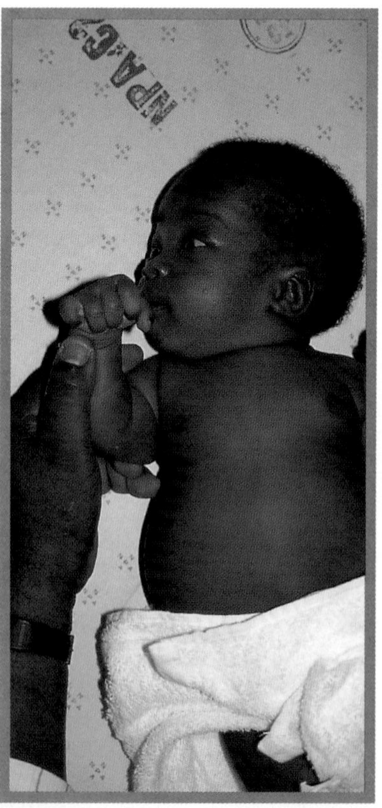

↑9.22

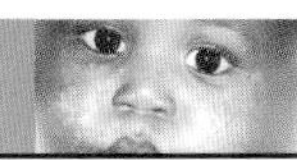

above the shoulder line. This is an indication of shortening of the proximal upper limb. Note that there is also brachydactyly, as the fingers should be of a length at least equal to that of the palm.

Figures 9.24–9.27 Turner Syndrome.

Figure 9.24 Note the wide elbow-carrying angle (cubitus valgus), the widely spaced nipples, short stature, and prominent ears.

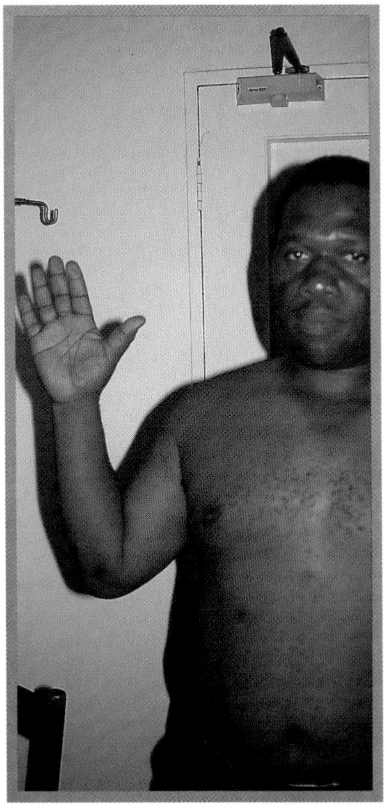

↑9.23

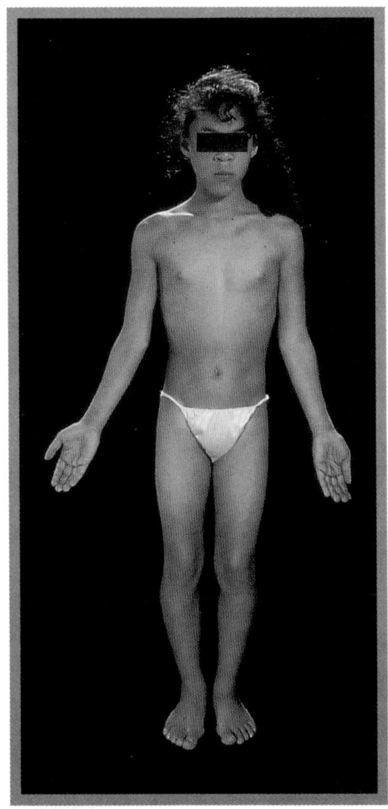

↑9.24

Figure 9.25 Note the webbed neck and low posterior hair line.
Figure 9.26 The nails are narrow, dysplastic and spoon-shaped.
Figure 9.27 There is shortening of the fourth and fifth metacarpals (which also occurs in pseudo and pseudo-pseudohypoparathyroidism).

Cases also have a tendency to congenital heart disease, particularly coarctation of the aorta, and renal tract abnormalities, *e.g.*, horseshoe kidney, duplex ureters, and streaked ovaries with failure of development at puberty. Most cases have an XO karyotype in all cells, but some are mosaic.

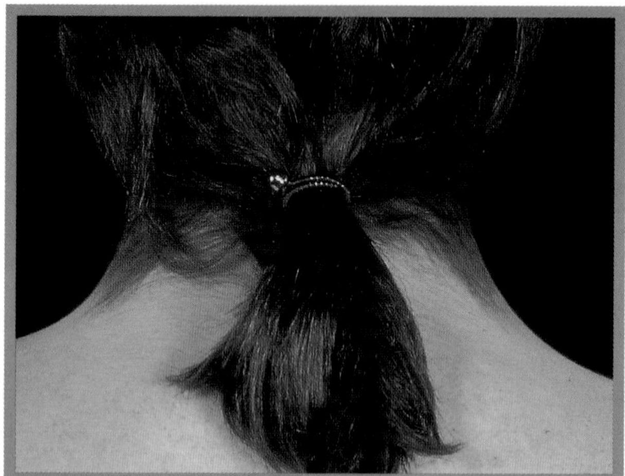

←9.25

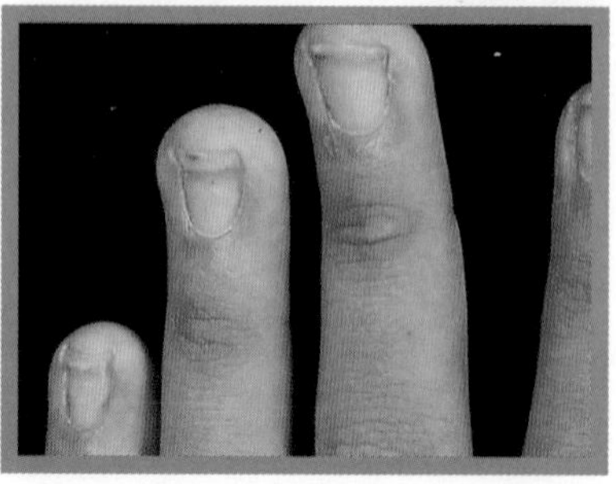

↑9.26

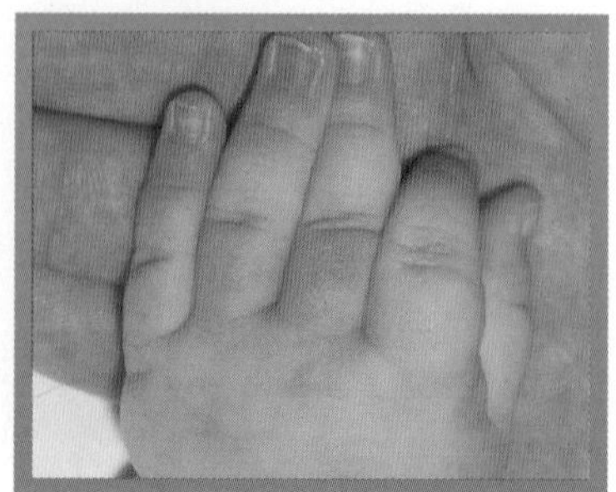

↑9.27

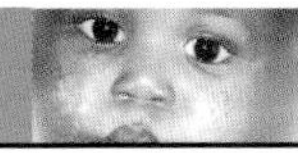

Figures 9.28 and 9.29 Noonan Syndrome. The girl shown here with Noonan syndrome has short stature, a short neck with webbing, and widely spaced nipples. She also has the characteristic facial features of hypertelorism, downward-slanting eyes with ptosis, a well-grooved philtrum, a broad nose tip, and wavy hair. This condition is autosomal dominant and is often associated with congenital heart disease, particularly pulmonary stenosis. In addition a characteristic feature in boys are undescended testes.

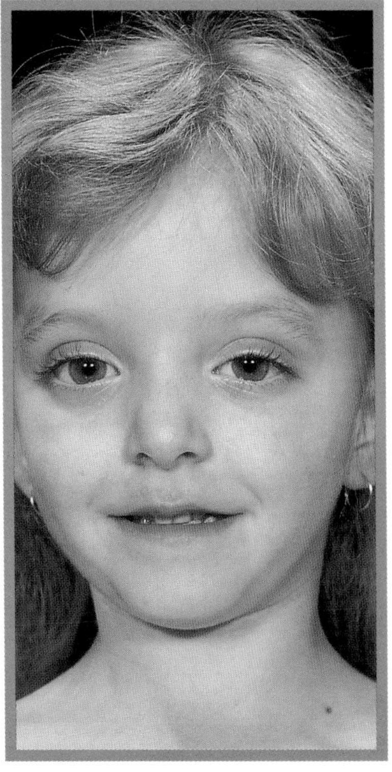

↑ **9.28**

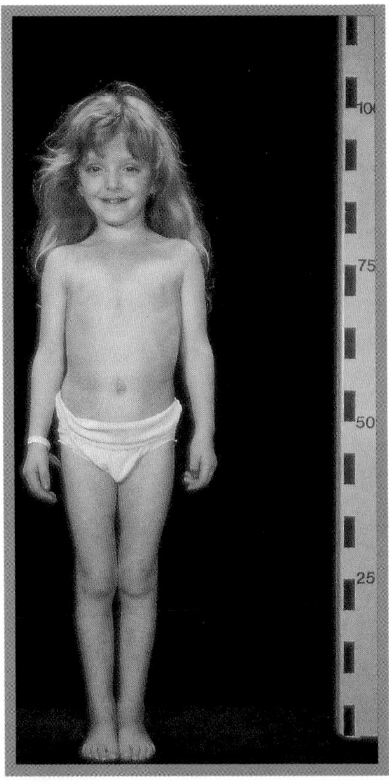

↑ **9.29**

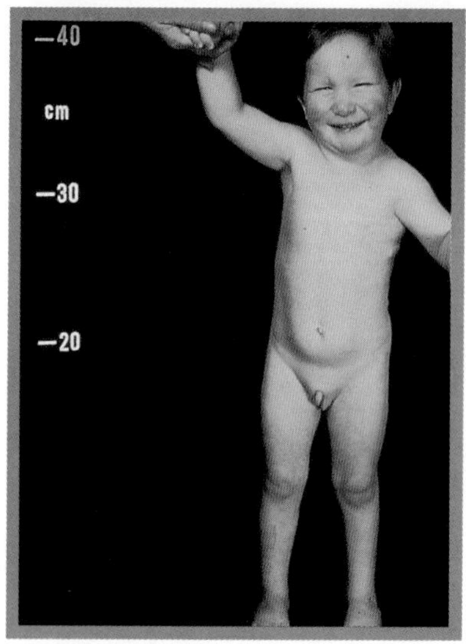

—40
cm
—30
—20

↑9.30

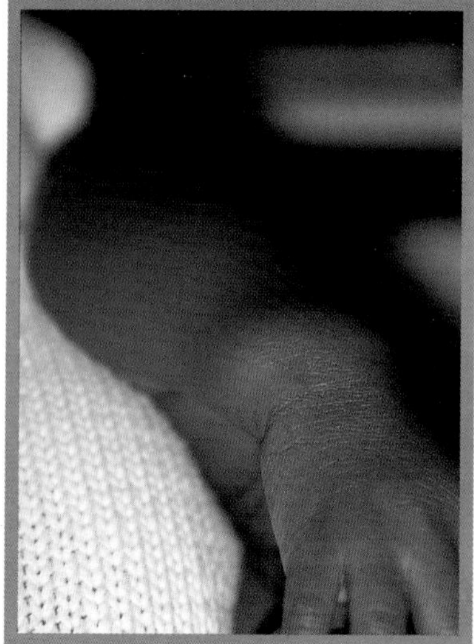

↑9.31

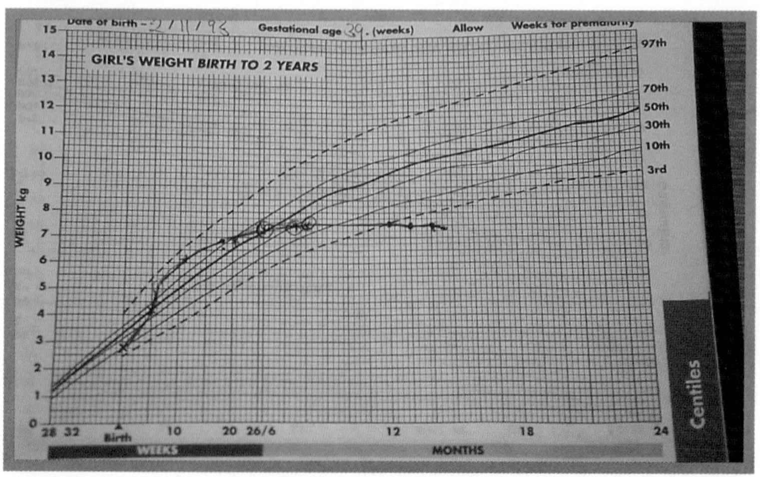

Date of birth –
Gestational age
. (weeks)
Allow
Weeks for
GIRL'S WEIGHT BIRTH TO 2 YEARS
WEIGHT kg
15
14
13
12
11
10
9
8
7
6
5
4
3
2
1
0
97th
70th
50th
30th
10th
3rd
28
32
Birth
10
20
26/6
12
18
24
WEEKS
MONTHS
Centiles

↑9.32

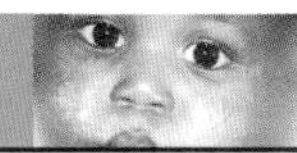

Figure 9.30 Congenital Hypopituitarism. The 1-year-old boy shown here presented in the newborn period with hypoglycemia and jaundice. He failed to grow in height due to growth hormone deficiency. He is normally proportioned with truncal obesity. The testes are typically undescended and a micropenis is present. Treatment consists of growth hormone injection,and oral cortisone and thyroxine administration. Sex hormone replacement will be required at puberty.

Figures 9.31–9.34 Rickets shows vitamin-D-deficiency rickets in a 15-month-old girl.

Figure 9.31 shows swelling of the wrist.

Figure 9.32. The growth chart demonstrates a fall from the 70th centile to below the third centile.

Figure 9.33 and 9.34. A Rachitic rosary, *i.e.* beading of the costochondral junction of the ribs is shown.

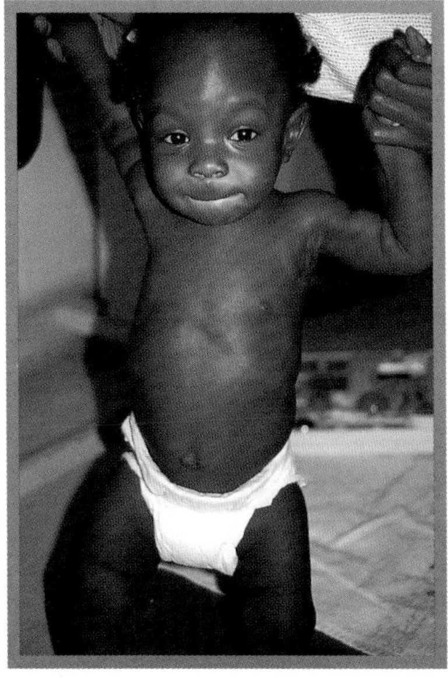

↑9.33

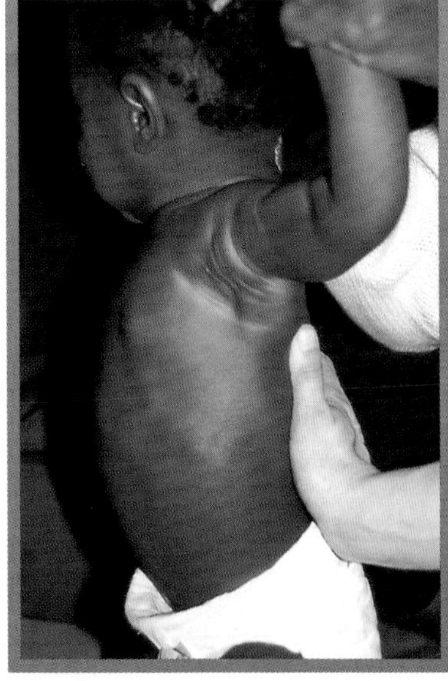

↑9.34

Figure 9.35 Genu varum (tibial bowing) due to rickets is shown, although this is very often normal up to the age of 2 years. In this child there was reduced serum 25 hydroxycholecalciferol present, a reduced serum phosphate level, increased alkaline phosphatase and raised parathyroid hormone levels.

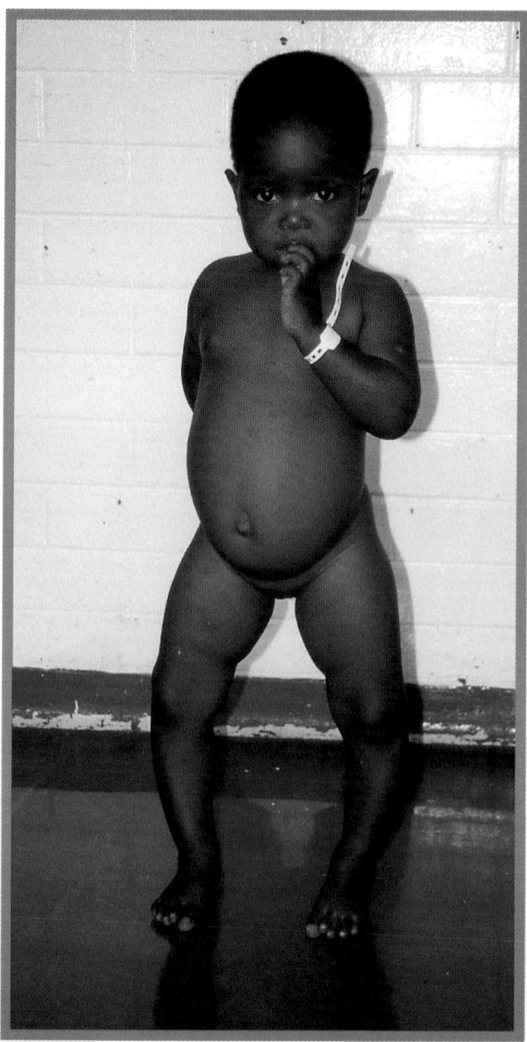

←9.35

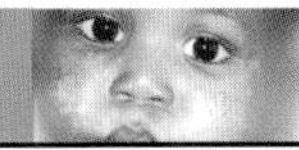

Figure 9.36 Genu valgum (knock knees) is seen here in a 7-year-old.
Figure 9.37 This 1-year-old girl with rickets has marked occipital and frontal bossing, giving the head a box-like appearance of 'caput quadratum'.

→ 9.36

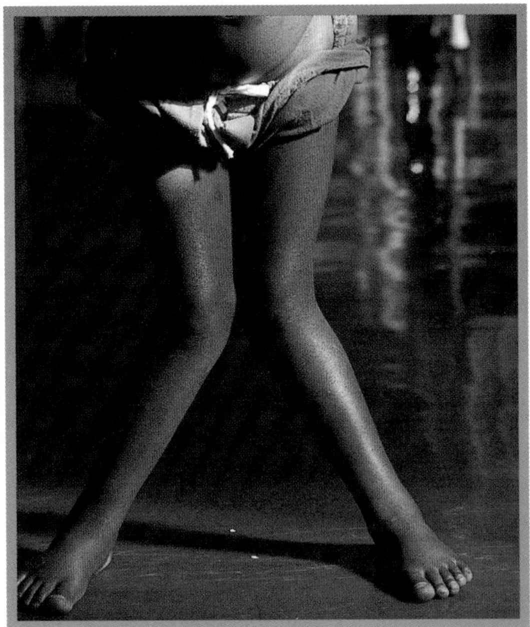

→ 9.37

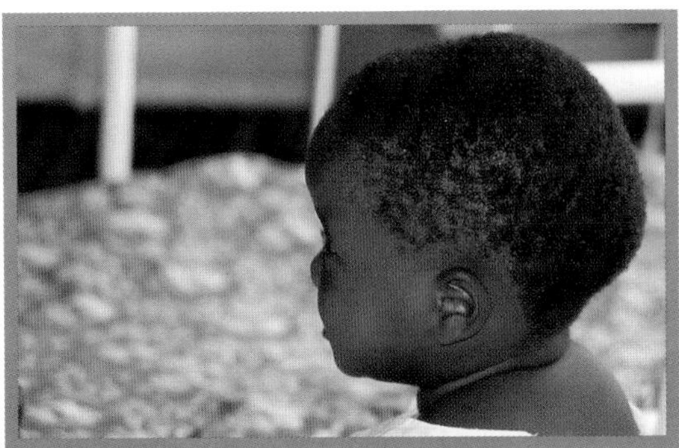

Figure 9.38 The wind-swept appearance of the legs seen here in a 4-year-old child results from nutritional rickets.

Figure 9.39 X-ray of child with rickets. (a) Splaying and irregularities of the metaphyses are shown with predominantly cartilagenous epiphyses and delayed ossification.

Figure 9.39(**b**) The same case is shown following treatment. Accelerated ossification is seen in the sclerosed epiphyseal plate, as is an enlargement of the ossified epiphyses toward the normal configuration.

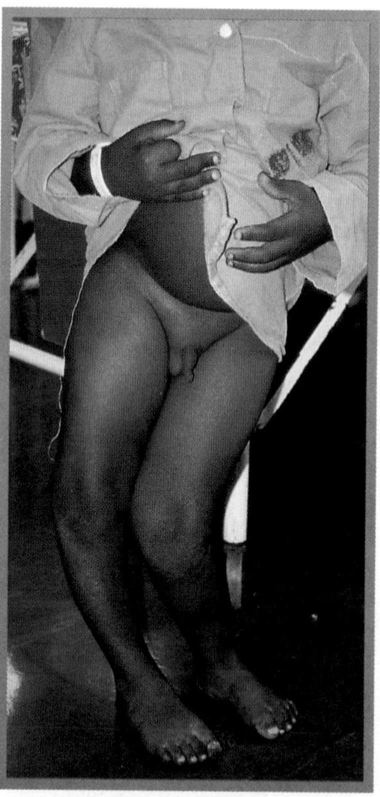

↑9.38

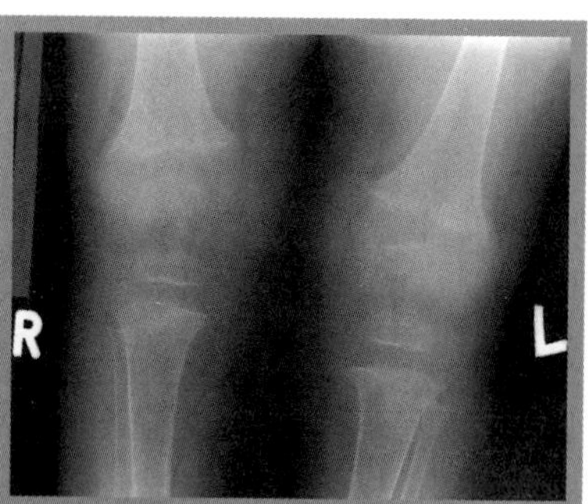

↑9.39a

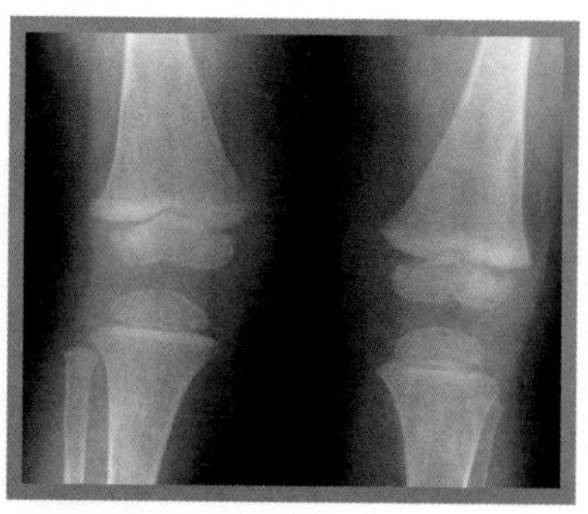

↑9.39b

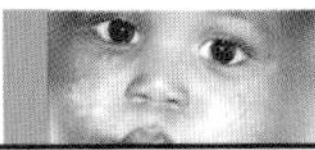

Figure 9.40 Physiological Bowing (Genu Valgum). This is seen here in a 3-year-old normal boy. It can be observed up to the age of 8 years.
Figure 9.41 Striae in Adolescence. The 15-year-old boy displayed here has pink striae on his back as a result of his pubertal growth spurt. Striae may be mistaken for marks associated with skin trauma due to child abuse.

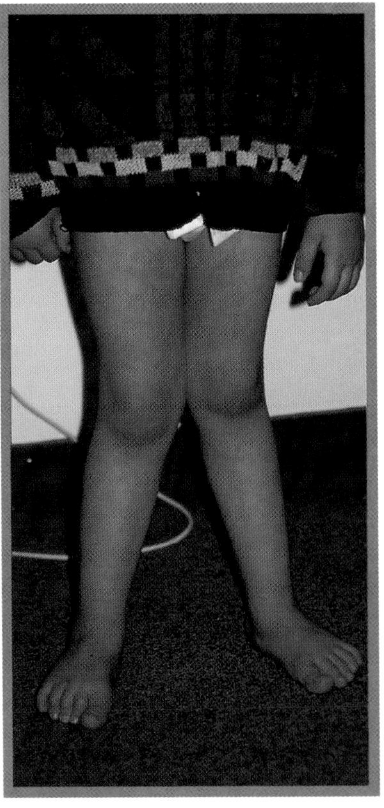

↑9.40

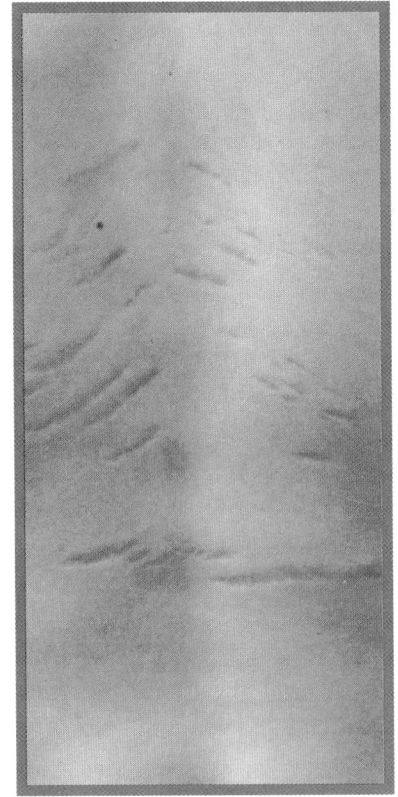

↑9.41

Figure 9.42 McCune–Albright Syndrome (Polyostotic Fibrous Dysplasia). In this case there was precocious puberty associated with skeletal abnormalities and irregular café-au-lait patches. These have a characteristic irregular outline – the 'coast of Maine' – as shown in this child. The pigmented lesions tend to be most severe on the side with the most pronounced bone involvement. The endocrinopathy is usually much more severe in girls.

McCune–Albright syndrome is also characterized by multiple areas of fibrous dysplasia in the bones, which often results in deformed or thickened bones with associated pathological fractures.

The differential diagnoses for the café-au-lait nevi are neurofibromatosis, Russell–Silver dwarfism, ataxia telangiectasia, Bloom syndrome, Fanconi syndrome and multiple lentigines (Leopard) syndrome.

Figure 9.43 Ambiguous Genitalia in a Neonate. This finding constitutes a medical emergency. This was a case of congenital adrenal hyperplasia in a genotypical girl. She presented in the newborn nursery with clitoral hyperplasia, fusion of the labioscrotal folds (forming a penile urethra), and thickening of the labia majora to resemble a scrotum. She was not

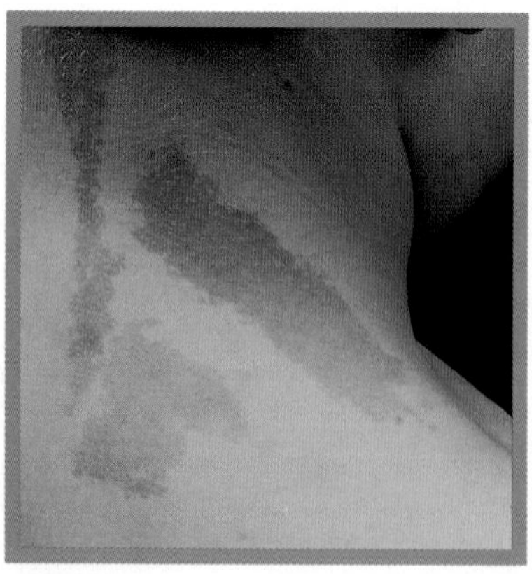

9.42

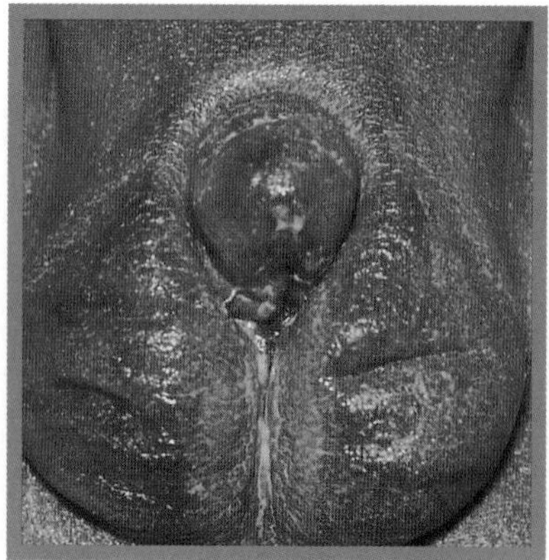

9.43

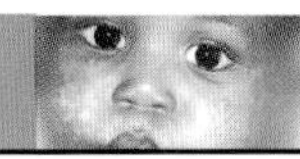

hypertensive and there was no associated salt loss. Biochemical studies revealed a grossly elevated 17-hydroxyprogesterone level consistent with the diagnosis. Salt loss occurs in 66% of cases, and in male infants usually results in collapse at about 10–14 days of age due to hyponatremic dehydration. Investigations must include genotypic and ultrasound tests to ascertain the presence of gonads, and DNA studies on the parents in order to make an antenatal diagnosis in subsequent pregnancies. Antenatal treatment with dexamethasone will prevent masculinization of a female fetus.

Other causes of ambiguous genitalia are testicular feminization due to end-organ insensitivity to male sex hormones.

Figure 9.44 Hypogonadotrophic Hypogonadism. The 6-year-old boy had hypogonadism from primary gonadotrophin deficiency. Note the cryptorchidism and micropenis. Syndromes associated with gonadotrophin deficiency and obesity include Laurence–Moon–Biedl syndrome (with polydactyly and retinitis pigmentosa) and Prader–Willi syndrome. Hypogonadism in association with anosmia occurs in Kallmann syndrome.

→9.44

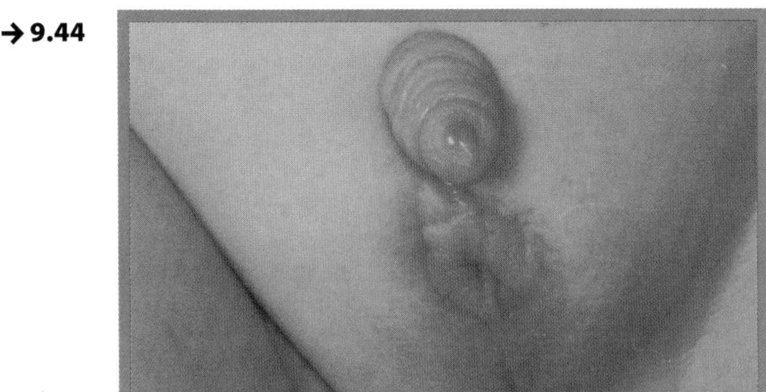

Figure 9.45–9.47 Prader–Willi Syndrome. The 6-year-old boy has Prader–Willi syndrome. He was hypotonic at birth and required nasogastric feeding. He subsequently required strict control of his eating habits as he showed a tendency to overeat.
Figure 9.45 shows the feature of almond-shaped eyes.

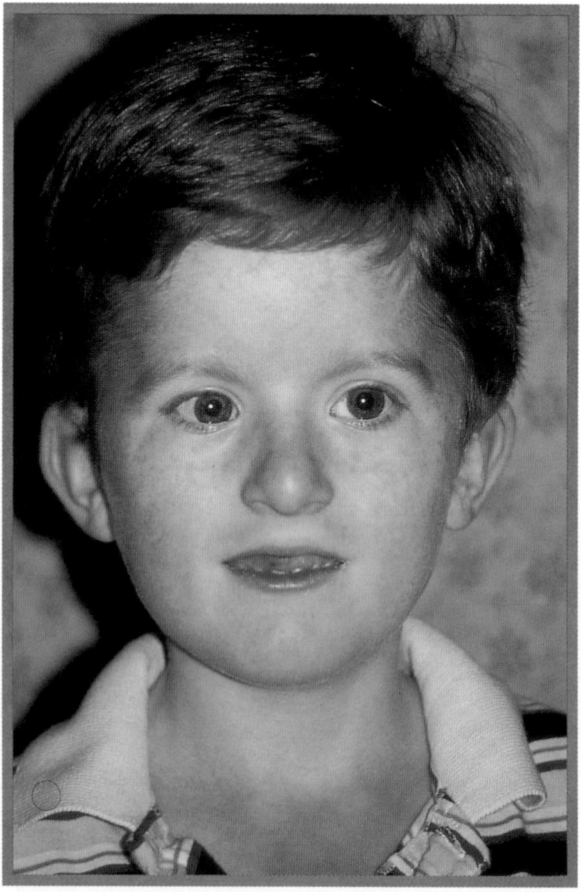

←9.45

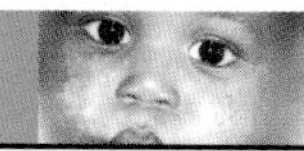

Figure 9.46 shows the feature of small hands.
Figure 9.47 shows hypogonadism, scrotal hypoplasia, a micropenis and repaired cryptorchidism.

The child had short stature and developmental delay. Approximately 70% of patients have been shown to have a paternally derived deletion of the long arm of chromosome 15; others have a maternal disomy for part of chromosome 15.

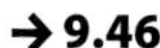

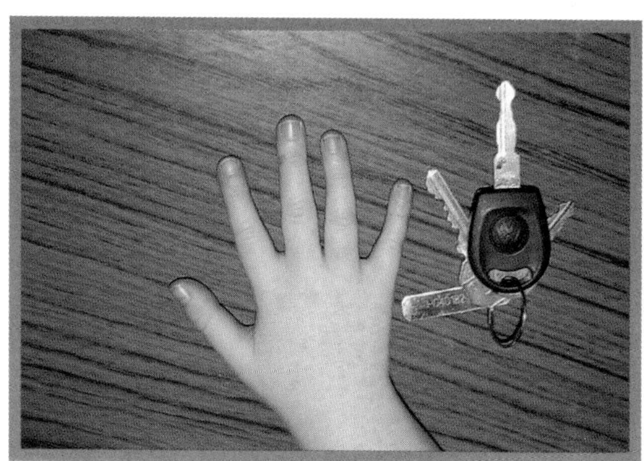

→9.47

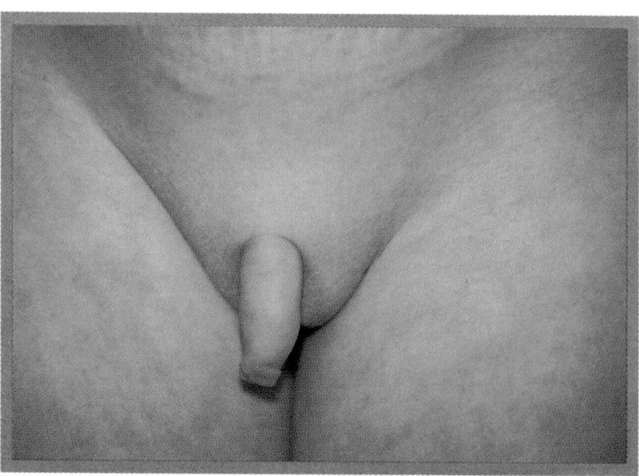

Figure 9.48 Precocious Puberty. The 4-year-old boy shown here has precocious puberty caused by an adrenocortical tumor. The sexual development is consistent with a boy of 12 years. Note the accelerated growth, pubic and axillary hair and large penis (**9.48a**). The lateral view (**9.48b**) shows abdominal distension due to the tumor.

Figure 9.49 Hurler Syndrome. Hurler syndrome is an autosomal recessive mucopolysaccharidosis in females. Note the coarse facial features, the thick lips, coarse hair, hypertrichoses, corneal opacification and macroglossia. The child also had hepatosplenomegaly an umbilical hernia, mental retardation, upper airway obstruction, short stature, kyphosis and immobility. Levels of heparin sulfate and dermatan sulfate were increased in the urine, and the

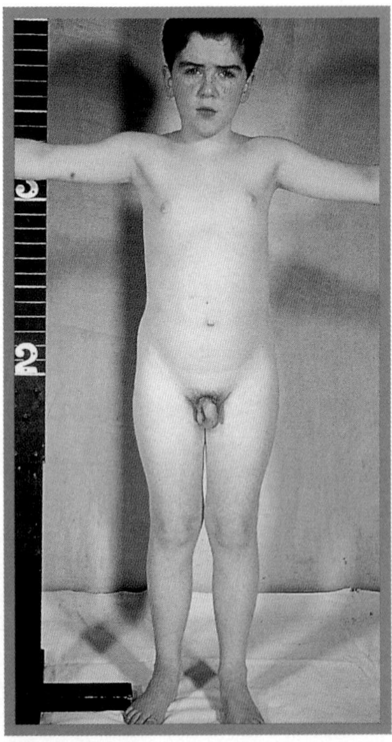

↑ **9.48a**

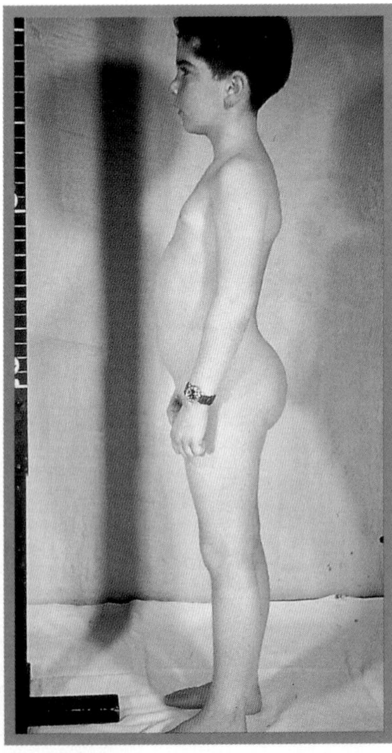

↑ **9.48b**

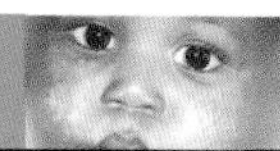

child's leukocytes showed decreased activity of α-L-iduronidase. The differential diagnosis includes other mucopolysaccharidoses and hypothyroidism.

Figure 9.50 Morquio Disease (Mucopolysaccharidosis Type IV). This figure shows Morquio disease in a 1-year-old child. Note the large head, protruding chin, coarse facial features, short neck and trunk, and pigeon chest. There is a marked lordosis and the short, deformed limbs are fixed in semi-flexion.

Corneal clouding, aortic regurgitation, mental impairment and odontoid hypoplasia lead to atlantoaxial instability. This disorder is autosomal recessive.

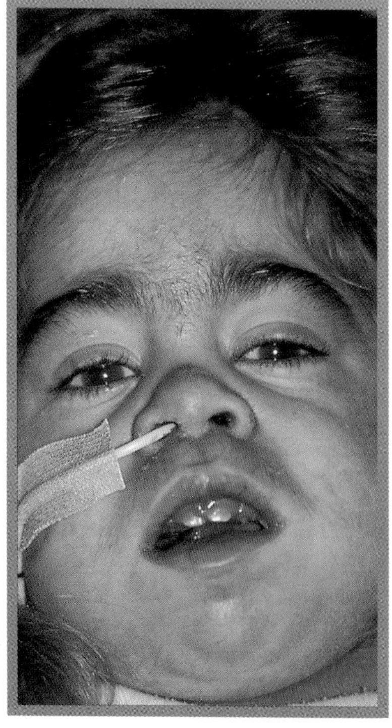

↑9.49

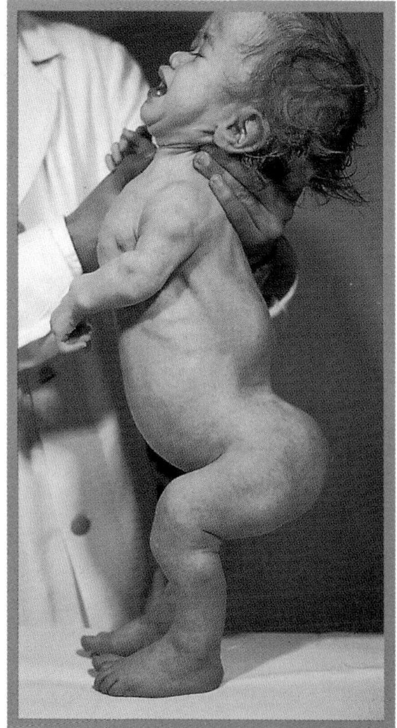

↑9.50

Figure 9.51 Fragile X Syndrome. A 13-year-old boy with fragile X syndrome is shown. Note the long face, large ears and coarse features. He also had behavioral problems, specifically with hyperactivity and speech delay. On examination, his testicular size was increased. Autistic behavior occurs in up to 10% of children affected. Molecular analysis shows an unstable p(CCG)n trinucleotide repeat sequence in the responsible (fMR-1) gene on the X-chromosome.

Figure 9.52 Soto Syndrome (Cerebral Gigantism). The 15-year-old boy shown here presented at birth with both weight and head circumference above the 97th centile. Presently he is tall, with large hands and feet and behaves in a clumsy manner. Note the macrocephaly, downward-slanting palpebral fissures, high prominent forehead and pointed chin. Most cases are sporadic.

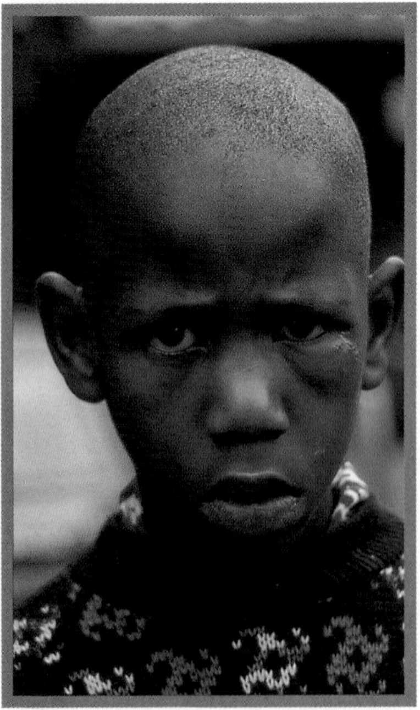

↑9.51

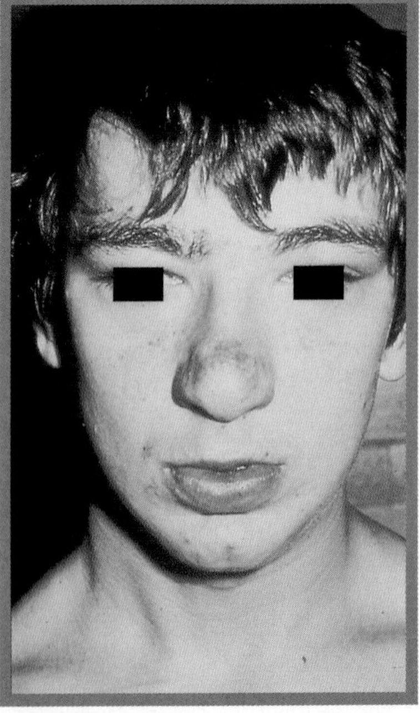

↑9.52

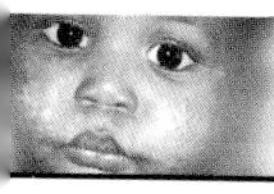

10 Rheumatological and musculoskeletal disorders

Figure 10.1 Prader–Willi Syndrome. The child presented as a floppy infant. Note the small hands and feet and the frog-like posture. Prader–Willi syndrome usually presents in the neonatal period as hypotonia and poor feeding, which commonly causes failure to thrive. Other features include small, almond-shaped eyes, a tent-like mouth, and a narrow forehead. Diagnosis in up to 50% of cases is confirmed upon cytogenetic tests as a small deletion at 15q 12 – an example of uniparental disomy. Other characteristics are short stature, hypogonadism, cryptorchidism, and obesity after the first year due to an increased appetite and low resting metabolic requirements. The IQ is affected to a variable degree. There is an increased incidence of diabetes mellitus.

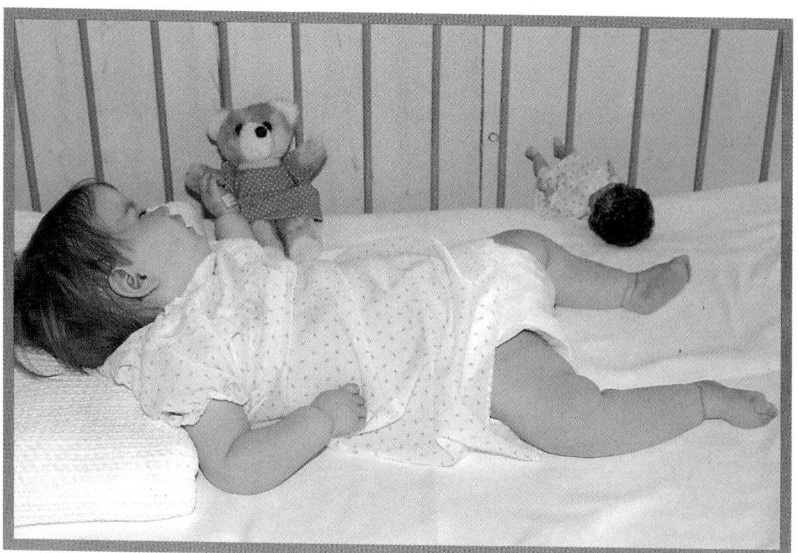

↑ 10.1

Figure 10.2 Floppy Infant. Note the straight arms and marked head lag. The infant shown has dystrophia myotonica. The differential diagnosis is very wide. Cases are classed as floppy and weak, or floppy only. Floppy and weak cases are usually caused by neouromuscular diseases (*e.g.*, myopathy, myasthenia, and spinal muscular atrophies), whereas floppy only cases are usually caused by CNS abnormalities or chromosomal conditions with CNS effects (*e.g.*, trisomy 21).
Figure 10.3 Floppy Infant. Plaster of Paris ankle casts are used to correct talipes.

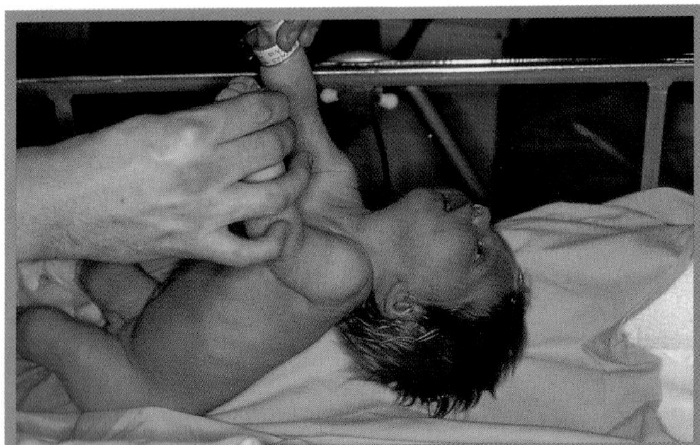

←**10.2**

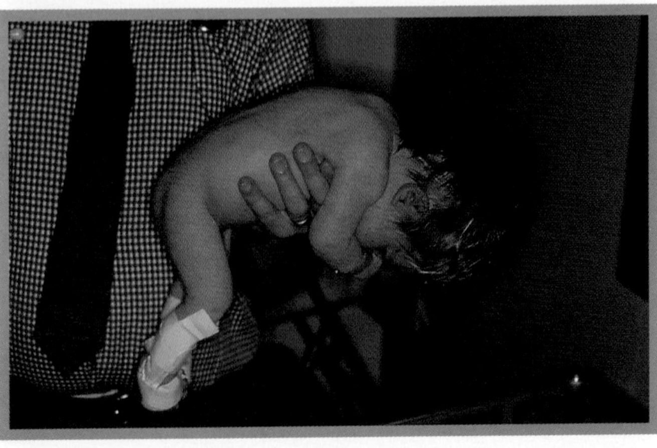

←**10.3**

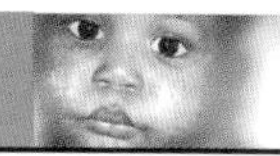

Figure 10.4 Ligamentous Laxity. Note the opposition of the thumb on to the flexor surface of the forearm. This condition is usually familial. It may present as delayed motor milestones, and musculoskeletal pain may occur during growth spurts. A diagnostic criterion is the demonstration of the laxity in five specific areas:

1. Passive abduction of the thumb, as shown here.
2. Passive hyperextention of the fingers so they are parallel to the extensor surface of the forearm.
3. Hyperextension of the elbow.
4. Hyperextension of the knee (genu recurvatum).
5. The ability to place the palms on the floor when the knees are extended.

Normal investigations. The condition improves with age. It can be associated with intrauterine moulding. Differential diagnosis includes connective tissue disorders, *e.g.*, Ehlers–Danlos syndrome and Marfan syndrome, and chromosomal conditions, e.*g.*, trisomy 21.

→ **10.4**

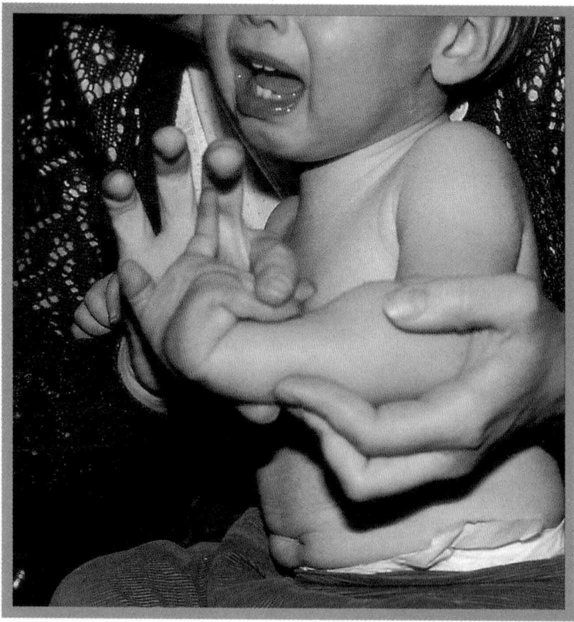

Figures 10.5 and 10.6 Ehlers–Danlos Syndrome in Two Infants. Figure 10.5 demonstrates that the skin folds can be pulled away from the body easily. **Figure 10.6** shows hyperflexibility of the shoulder joint. Extreme fragility of the skin also occurs. Ehlers–Danlos syndrome is a connective tissue disorder with hyperelastosis and a reduction of collagen.

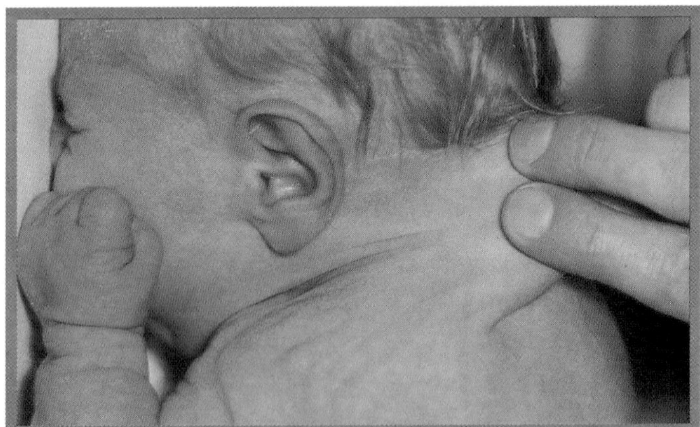

← 10.5

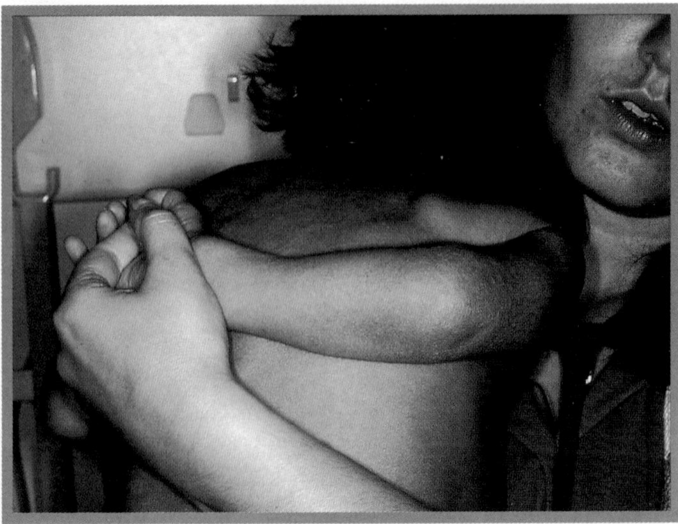

← 10.6

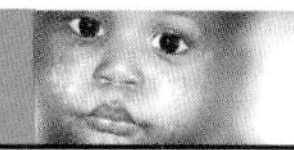

Figures 10.7–10.9 Congenital Myopathy. Shown here are the typical facies and chest of a child with a myopathy. The reflexes are reduced or absent. The facial muscles are involved, as are respiratory muscles.

Kyphosis is progressive, but can be controlled by spinal bracing. Myopathies can be classed as central-core disease, myotubular myopathy, metabolic myopathy and mitochondrial myopathy.

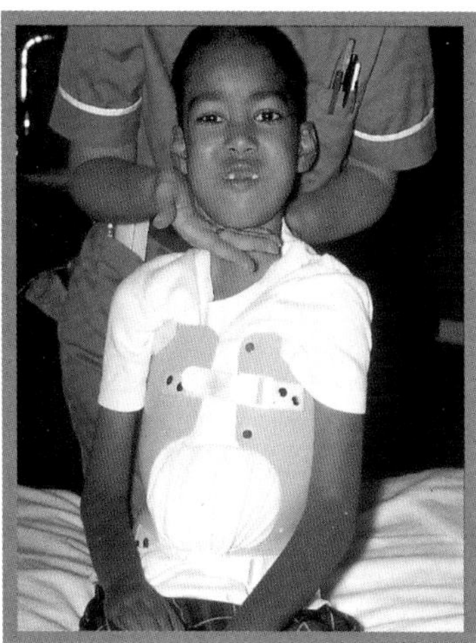

↑ **10.7**

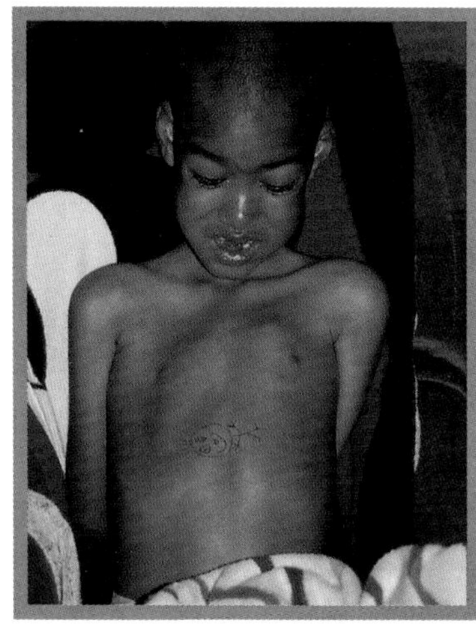

↑ **10.8**

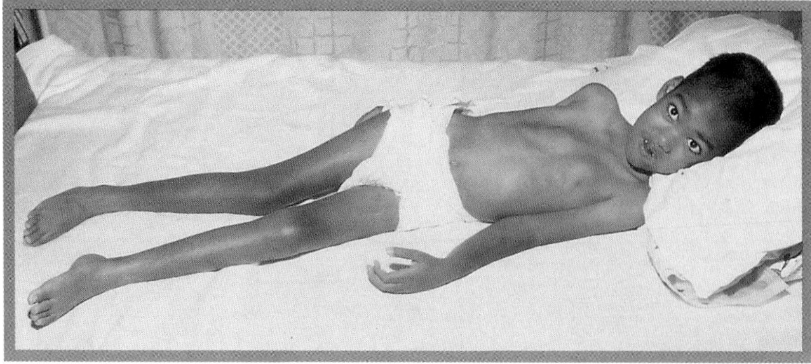

↑ **10.9**

Figure 10.10 Negative Pressure Ventilator (Iron Lung). The child shown here required nocturnal ventilation due to the effect of the myopathy on the respiratory muscles. Nocturnal ventilation using a cuirass device is also available for those children with alveolar hypoventilation.
Figure 10.11 Dystrophia Myotonica. Droopy myopathic facies are shown. This is an autosomal dominant condition, with the locus being on the long arm of chromosome 19. Babies born to mothers with the disease show a much more profound weakness, and will frequently have respiratory problems in the neonatal period. Feeding difficulties often occur for the first few weeks of life. The hypotonia persists, but most of the children will eventually walk unaided. There is generally some degree of learning difficulty.

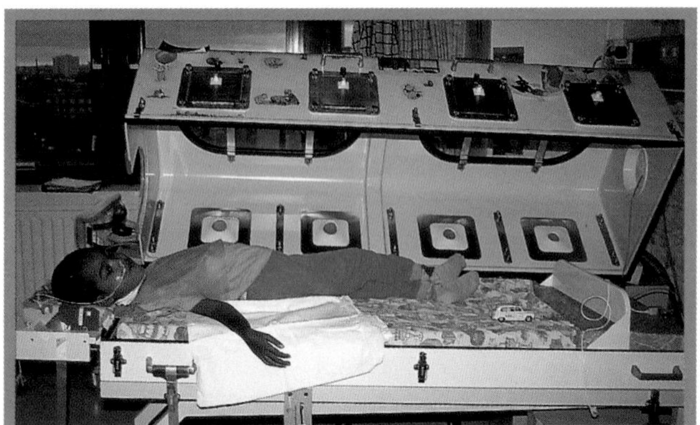

← 10.10

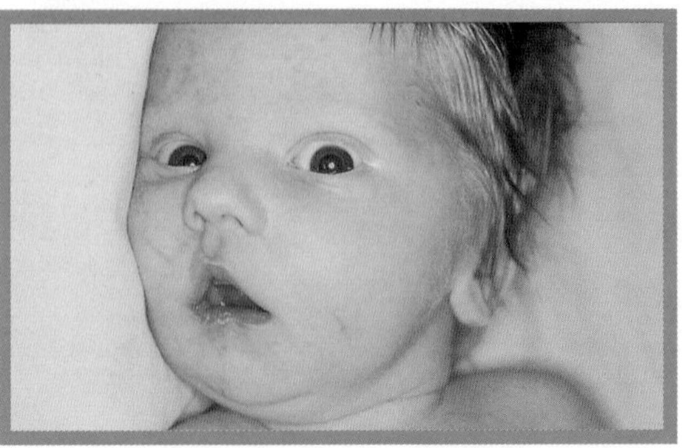

← 10.11

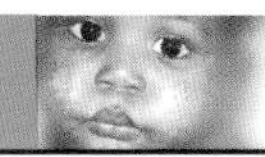

Figure 10.12 Dystrophia Myotonica. This figure shows talipes due to reduced intrauterine movement. The condition is associated with polyhydramnios due to swallowing difficulties and ventricular dilatation. Treatment consists of intensive physiotherapy.

Figure 10.13 Dystrophia Myotonica. Dystrophia myotonica is shown in the mother of a baby with the same condition. Note the droopy myopathic facies, particularly the inability to bury her eyelids. Other findings are a masculine hair line, cataracts, muscular stiffness and a myotonic grasp, especially on a cold day. Investigation should be undertaken along with electromyography (EMG) of the small muscles of the hand.

→10.12

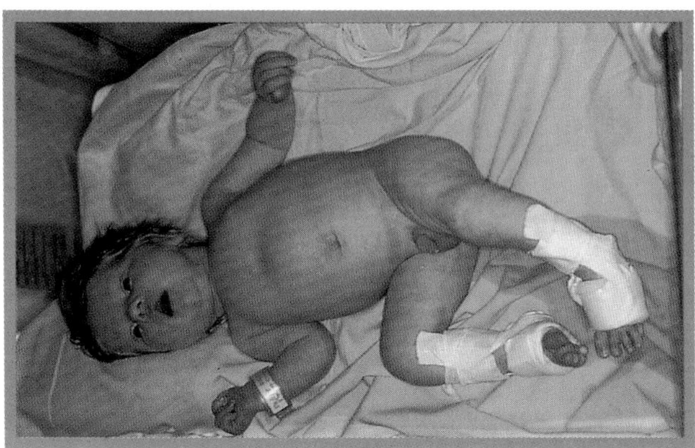

→10.13

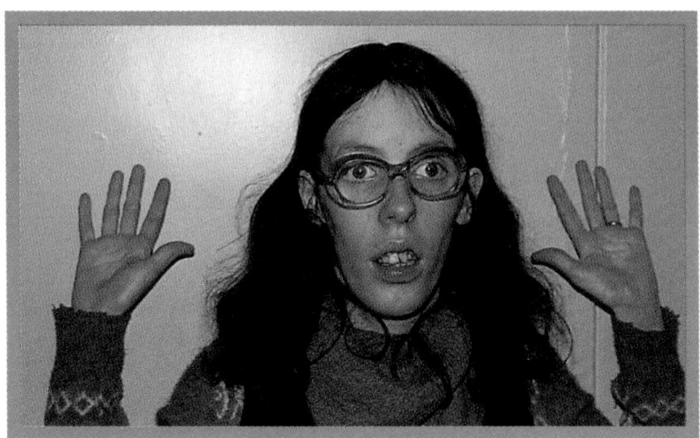

Figures 10.14 and 10.15 Ptosis. This case was caused by congenital myasthenia gravis, which is an autosomal recessive condition. There is oculomotor involvement only in this child. The ptosis was demonstrated clearly when the child tried to look up (**Figure 10.15**). In this form of the disease, and as in this case, the mother is rarely affected. Symptoms are often subtle and not easily detected, and affected children may present as floppy. This condition is not caused by receptor antibodies and responds poorly to therapy.

Neonatal myasthenia gravis is another form of this condition. It is transient, and occurs in 12% of babies born to affected mothers. It is caused by the transfer of maternal acetylcholine receptor antibodies across the placenta.

The third form of the condition is the juvenile myasthenia gravis associated with thymoma. This is treated with anticholinergics and, in severe cases, by thymectomy and the use of plasmaphoresis. Differential diagnosis includes botulism, ocular myopathy, congenital ptosis, Möbius syndrome, Guillain–Barré syndrome and poliomyelitis.

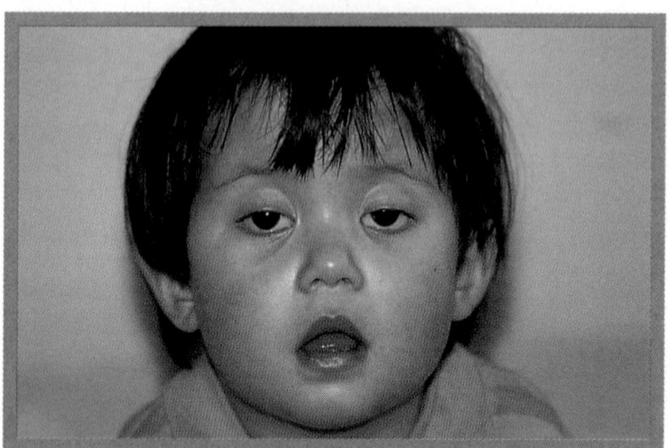

←10.14

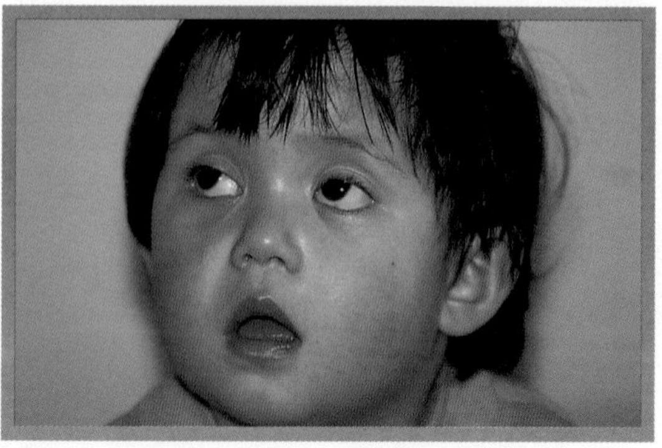

←10.15

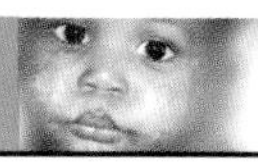

Figures 10.16–10.18 Dermatomyositis. The 7-year-old girl shown in **Figure 10.16** has a typical facial heliotrope (violaceous) red rash in a malar distribution. The rash does not spare the nasolabial folds, unlike systemic lupus erythematosis.
Figure 10.17 The 10-year-old boy shown here has edematous hands with periorbital edema. There is calcification in the soft tissues (**Figure 10.18**) following inflammation of the muscle and skin. The predominant symptom is proximal muscle weakness affecting the neck, the abdominal muscles, and the pelvic and shoulder girdles.
Figure 10.18 shows the rash after its progression to a scaly atrophic appearance.

→ 10.16

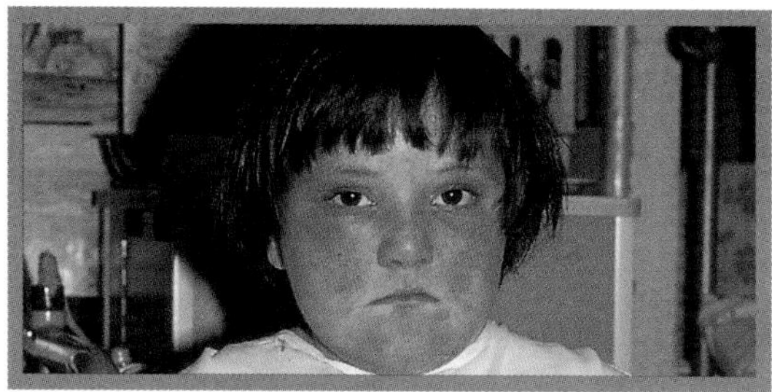

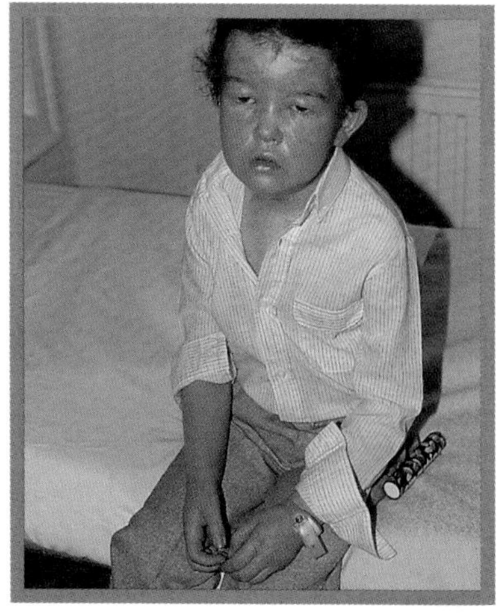

↑ 10.17

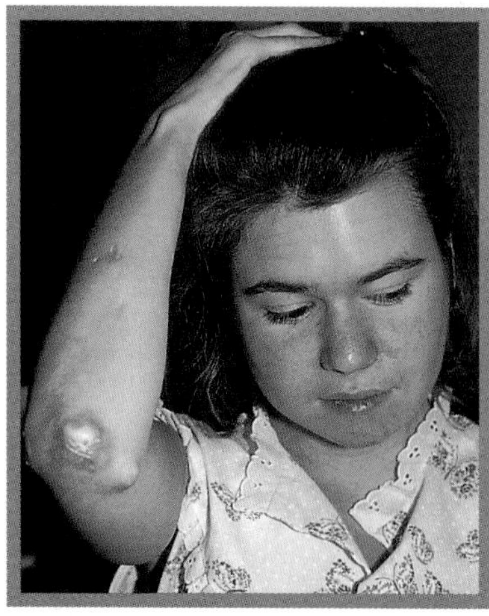

↑ 10.18

Diagnosis is based on the clinical features, the muscle enzyme levels (particularly creatine phosphokinase), and MRI scanning of muscle. Confirmation requires the biopsy of an area with an abnormally high signal, which usually demonstrates the degeneration of muscle fiber with some cellular infiltrate. Treatment consists of administration of high-dose steroids and the use of chemotherapy. As in most vasculitides, psychological disturbance may occur before weakness and rashes. Dermatomyositis, being a generalized vasculitis, may progress to infarction of the bowel and fits.

Figures 10.19 and 10.20 Duchenne Muscular Dystrophy. Affected boys aged 8 and 9 years show pseudohypertrophy of the calf muscles. Both boys presented with delayed motor skills. Findings included a waddling gait, and difficulty in climbing stairs and in getting up from the lying position (Gower's sign). EMG investigation shows a decreased amplitude and duration of bursts. Ultrasound investigation of muscle is also used, and blood CPK is raised. The family history is very important. The disease is X-linked recessive, with the gene being in band Xp21. A gene probe is available both for diagnosis and genetic counselling of relatives.

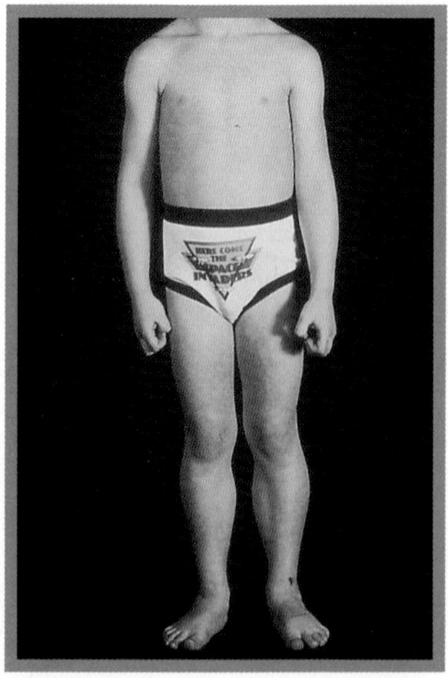

↑ 10.19

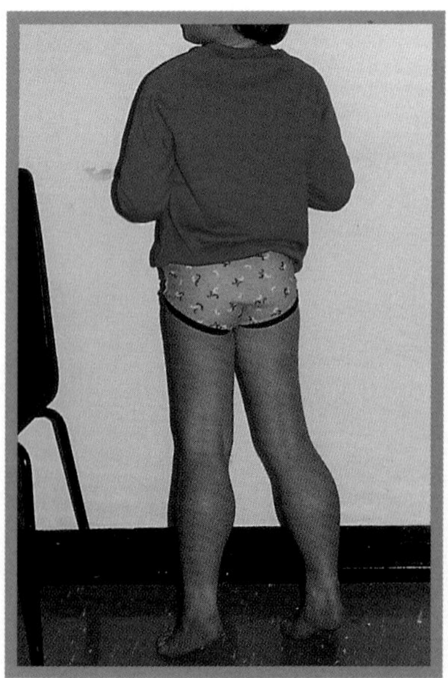

↑ 10.20

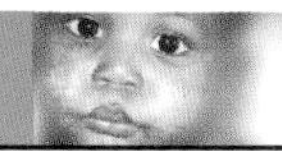

Figures 10.21 and 10.22 Henoch–Schönlein Purpura. This is a vasculitic rash associated with an arthropathy and synovitis. It is usually triggered by hemolytic streptococcal or viral illness. The rash is urticarial, evolving into purpuric macules that are usually found on the legs, feet and buttocks. Localized areas of soft-tissue edema affect the hands and feet, and can spread over the genitalia. Arthritis is usually transient and affects the large joints.

Henoch–Schönlein purpura can give severe abdominal pain mimicking appendicitis. Renal involvement occurs in approximately 50% of cases, with 5% going into end-stage renal failure. Hematuria occurs in up to 70% of children, usually within the first month of the illness. The condition generally resolves spontaneously, but can be very chronic and may rarely cause chronic renal failure.

The ESR is high, and there is a normal full blood count. Serum IgA is often raised, and complement C4 and C3 levels are low. Symptomatic treatment only is given, unless there is renal impairment or gastrointestinal hemorrhage, in which case immunosuppressants are used to good effect.

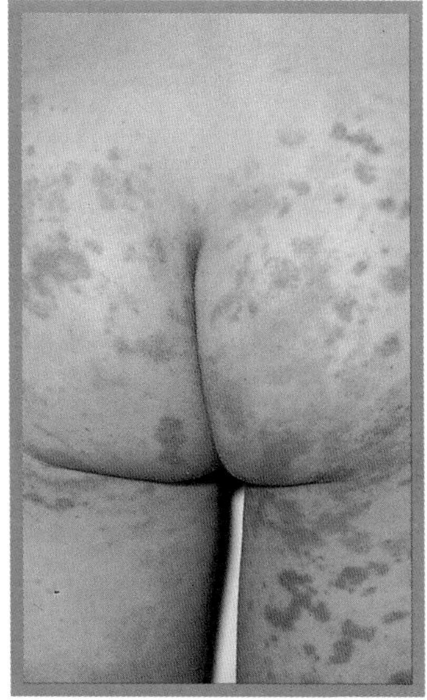

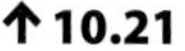
10.21

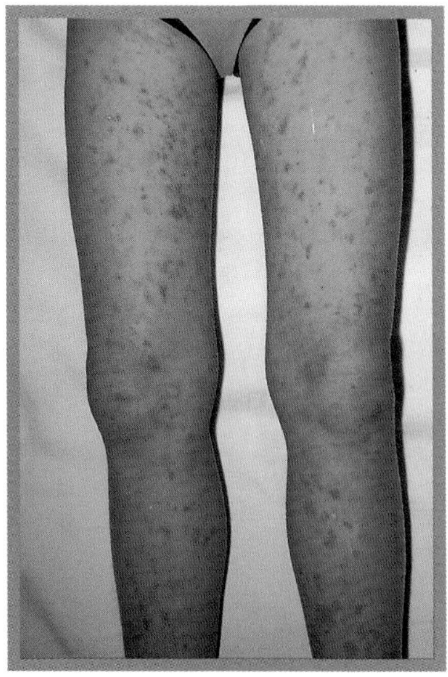

↑ 10.22

Figures 10.23–10.26 Systemic Lupus Erythematosis. This is most commonly found in Afro-Caribbean girls. The 5-year-old girl shown here presented with a butterfly rash and a systemic upset. She had arthralgia, a generalized vasculitic rash of erythema multiforme, and conjunctivitis. The condition was precipitated by oral herpes (**Figure 10.23**). Onset usually occurs after 5 years of age, with a female:male prepubertal ratio of 4:1, and a postpubertal ratio (up to age 18) of 5:1.

There may be associated complement deficiencies. The clinical features are manifest and variable. There is weight loss and malaise, with arthralgia or arthritis. Skin rashes can be papular, vesicular, or purpuric, and tend to be vasculitic. Oral ulceration and a photosensitive rash also occur. Renal involvement is common, and may be the presenting symptom. Any of the connective tissues may be involved, and neurological involvement may give rise to seizures.

Laboratory diagnosis can be based on a positive anti-DNA and on low complement C4 tests. Other antineutrophil antibodies may also be positive. Hematological abnormalities including anemia, thrombocytopenia and lymphopenia may occur. The course of the disease is highly variable and the severity relates closely to the degree of systemic involvement. Sepsis is a common and severe complication. Meticulous monitoring is essential. Treatment involves the use of steroids, cytotoxics and anticoagulants in the case of phospholipid syndrome.

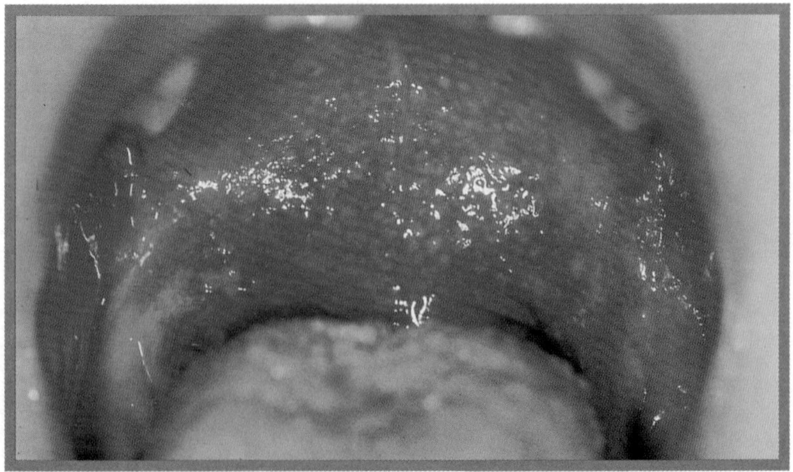

↑ 10.23

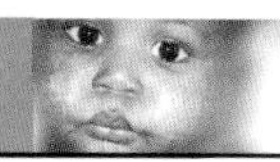

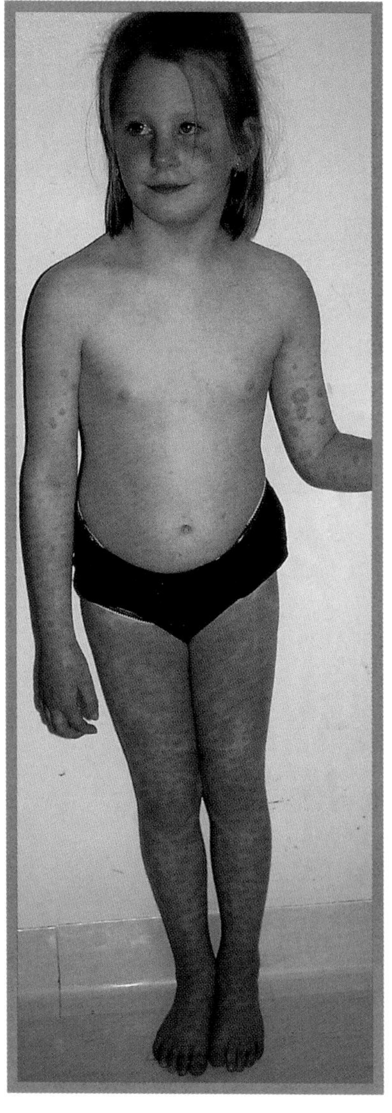

↑ 10.24

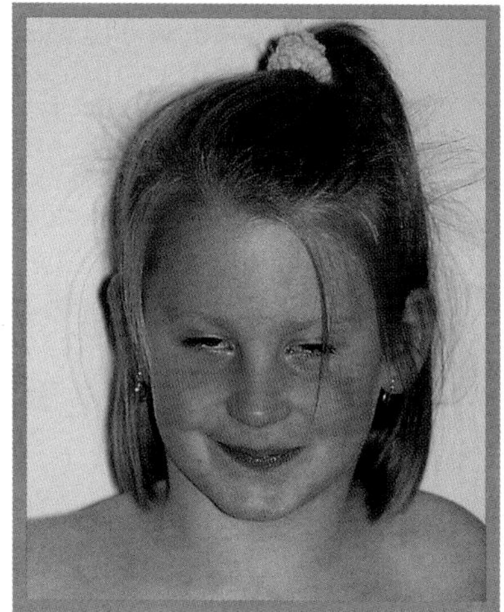

↑ 10.25

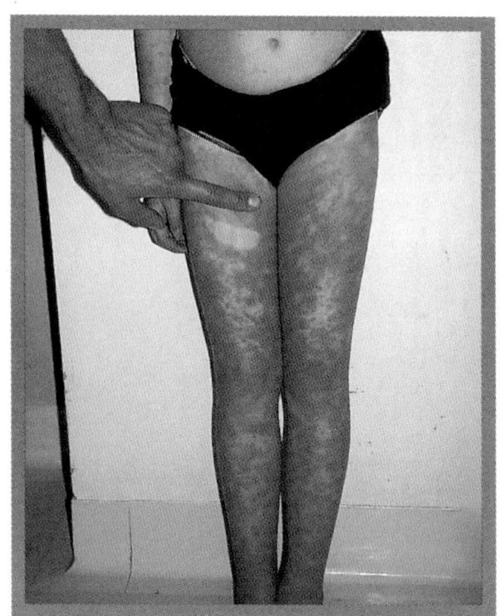

↑ 10.26

Figures 10.27–10.34 Juvenile Spondyloarthropathy. The 14-year-old boy shown here presented with pyrexia of unknown origin. He subsequently developed an arthropathy affecting the cervical and lumbar spine (**Figures 10.28 and 10.29**), with reduced flexion of the right knee (**Figures 10.31–10.32 , page 270**) and reduced mobility of the right wrist (**Figures 10.33 and 10.34, page 271**). He also had severe chronic anemia requiring pulsed methylprednisolone therapy.

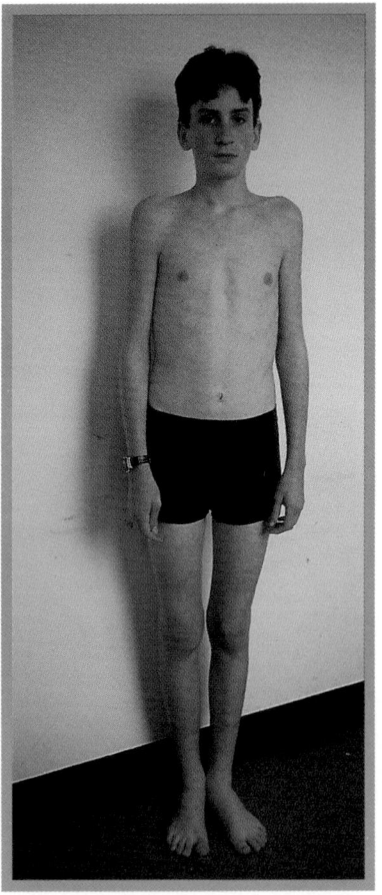

↑ **10.27**

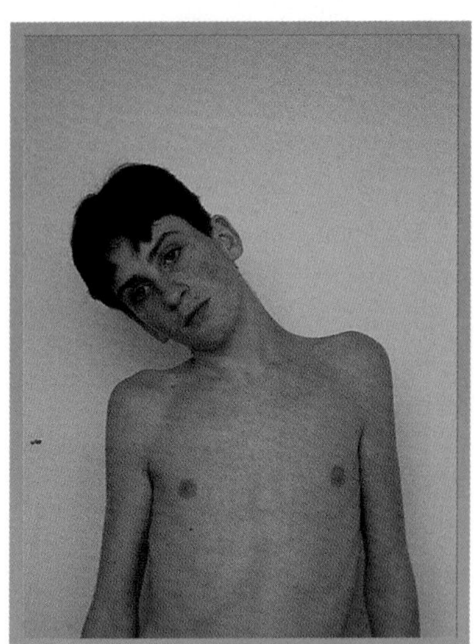

↑ **10.28**

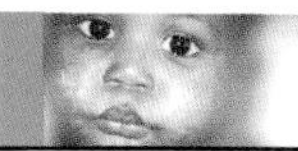

This disorder tends to affect males and is more common in those over 9 years old. He has predominantly peripheral arthritis with associated inflammation of tendons, *e.g.*, the achilles and patella.

The IgM rheumatoid factor was negative, and HLA-B27 was present. Treatment includes non-steroidal, anti-inflammatory treatment and the use of sulfasalazine. Physiotherapy is important in preserving function. There is a good outcome in two thirds of cases over time, but the remainder can develop cervical and other spinal involvement as well as features of spondylitis.

Arthropathy can be the presenting feature of inflammatory bowel disease, Reiter's syndrome, psoriasis, and postinfective diarrheal reactive arthritis.

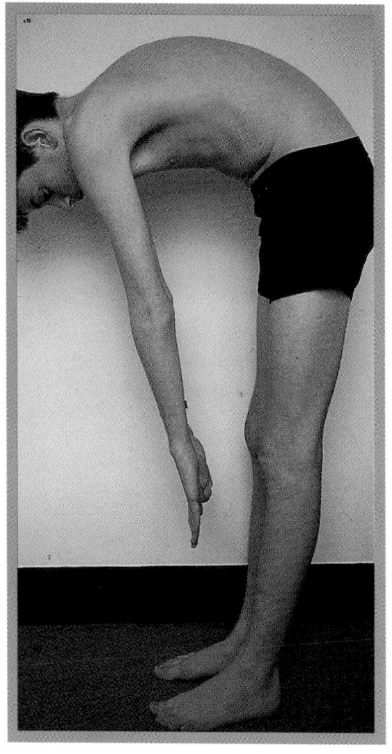

↑ **10.29**

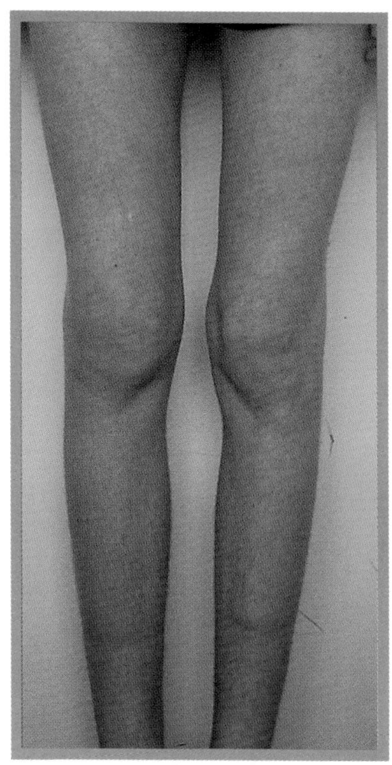

↑ **10.30**

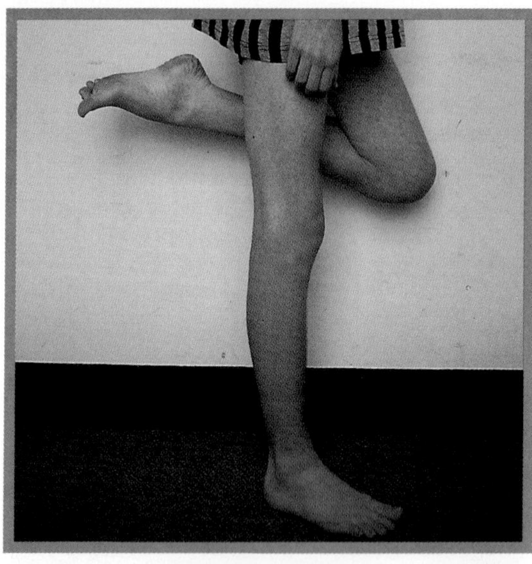

← 10.31

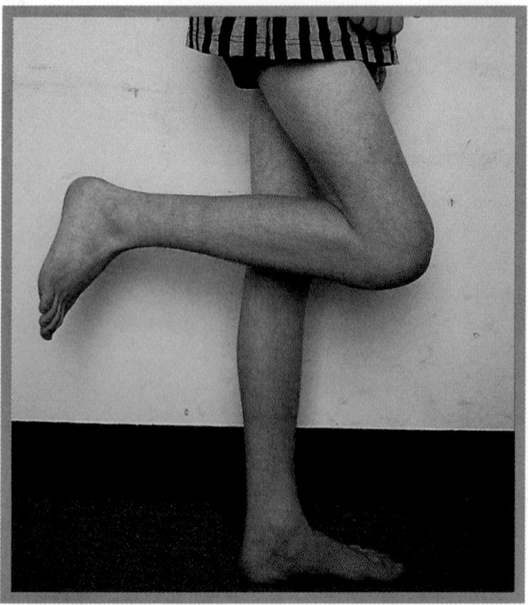

← 10.32

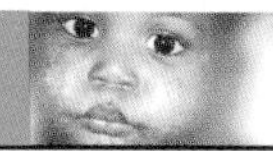

→ 10.33

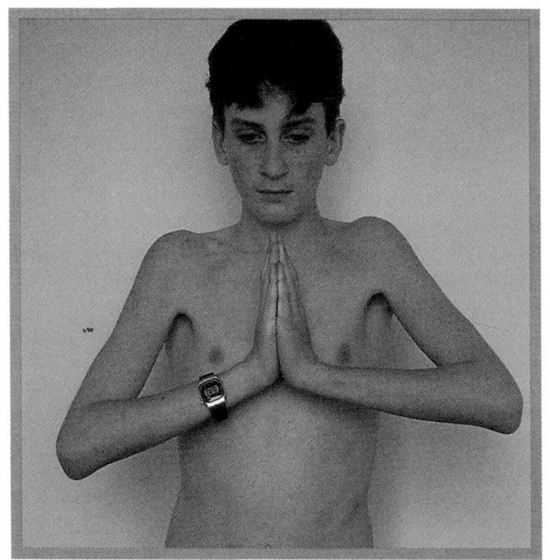

→ 10.34

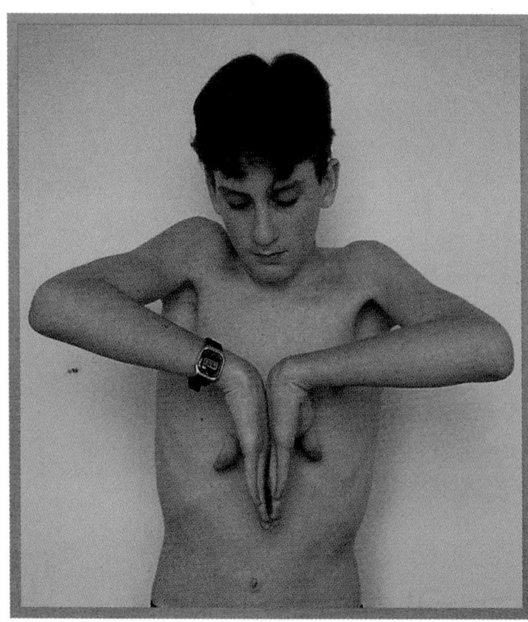

Figure 10.35 Juvenile Spondyloarthropathy – Effusion of the Right Knee. This is an example of pauciarticular-onset (four or fewer joints involved) juvenile chronic arthritis (JCA) in a 12-year-old boy. He had a 1-year history of flitting arthralgia and arthropathy. Only the right knee was involved. The effusion was tapped, and showed an inflammatory exudate. All investigations – ESR, rheumatoid factors, antinuclear antibodies, antineutrophil cytoplasmic antibody (ANCA) – were negative. The child was histocompatible leukocyte antigen (HLA) type B27 positive.

Figures 10.36 and 10.37 Wrist and Foot of Pauciarticular-onset Juvenile Chronic Arthritis (JCA). Figure 10.36 shows effusion of the right wrist with limited flexion. In this case of pauciarticular JCA in a 5-year-old girl, all investigations had negative results. The condition improved upon non-steroidal, anti-inflammatory treatment.

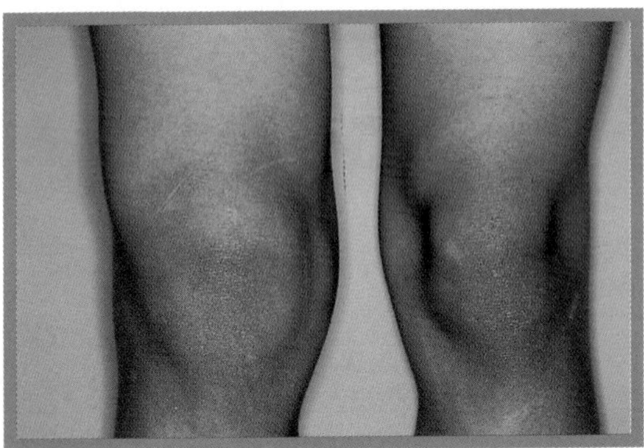

← 10.35

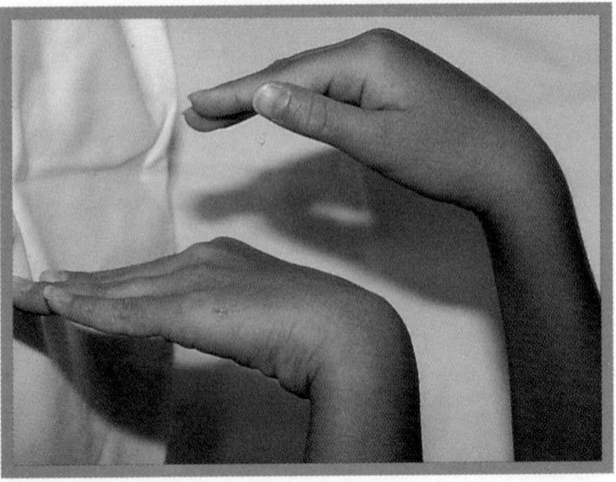

← 10.36

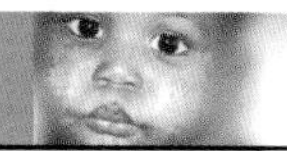

Figure 10.37 shows left ankle valgus deformity due to pauciarticular JCA. If antinuclear antibody tests are positive then there is an increased risk of chronic iridocyclitis as a complication, and regular ophthalmological follow-up is indicated. Treatment consists of administration of non-steroidal, anti-inflammatory drugs, intra-articular steroid injections and physiotherapy. The overall prognosis is good, as the disease remits in approximately 70% of treated patients.

Figure 10.38 Polyarticular Juvenile Chronic Arthritis. The 3-year-old girl discussed here has polyarthritic onset JCA. There is involvement of both wrists, the proximal interphalangeal joints, and mainly the right thumb and metacarpophalangeal joints of the right hand. Investigations revealed the IgM rheumatoid factor to be negative.

→10.37

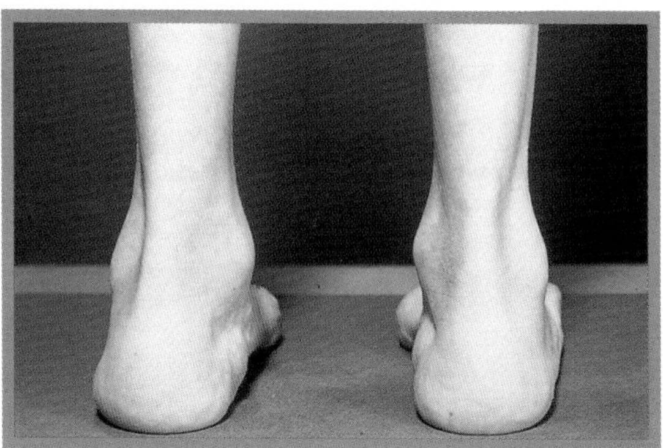

→10.38

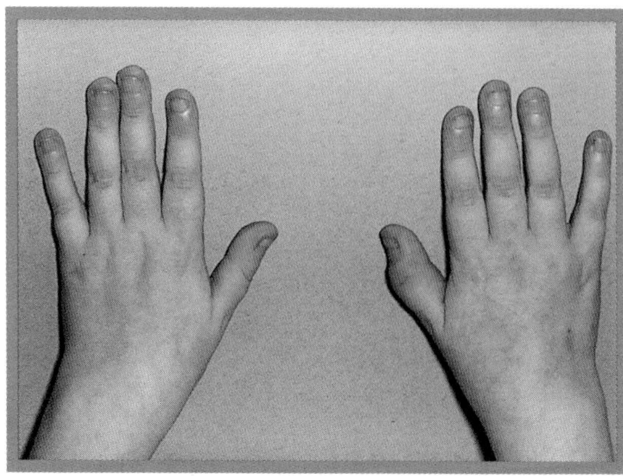

Figure 10.39 Juvenile Rheumatoid Arthritis. The 9-year-old girl shown here has IgM rheumatoid-factor-positive arthritis. Micrognathia is demonstrated, resulting from chronic involvement of the temperomandibular joint. She was also HLA-DR4 positive.

Figure 10.40 Septic Arthritis of the Ankle. This 5-year-old shown here presented with severe ankle pain, swelling, and loss of function. The joint space was drained, and the patient responded well to intravenous antistaphylococcal treatment. This is a pediatric emergency, as the child will be systemically unwell until the infection is controlled, and the joint may be destroyed.

Figure 10.41 Reactive Arthropathy Secondary to Disseminated Atypical TB in an Immunocompromised Host. The child discussed here had two siblings with the same disorder. Reactive arthritis usually occurs after an intercurrent infection without evidence of the causative organism in the joint. It affects any age group, and particularly males. ANA tests are negative, with a high incidence of HLA-B27 tests being positive. The presence of arthritis, urethritis, balanitis, cystitis, conjunctivitis, mouth ulceration, fever and rashes may suggest Reiter's syndrome.

Treatment is targeted against the causative organism if found, along with physiotherapy to maintain function, and administration of non-steroidal, anti-inflammatory drugs, sulfasalazine being used if the symptoms persist. It should be remembered that reactive arthropathy can affect any joint.

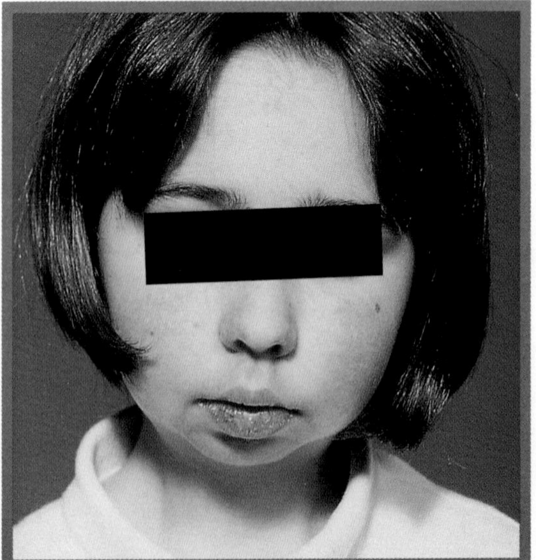

← **10.39**

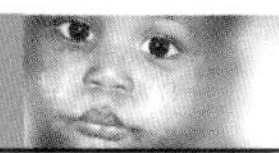

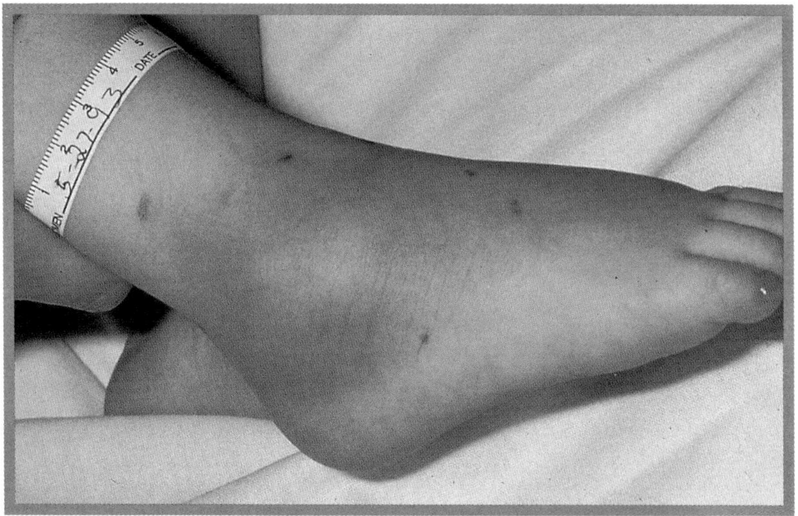

↑ 10.40

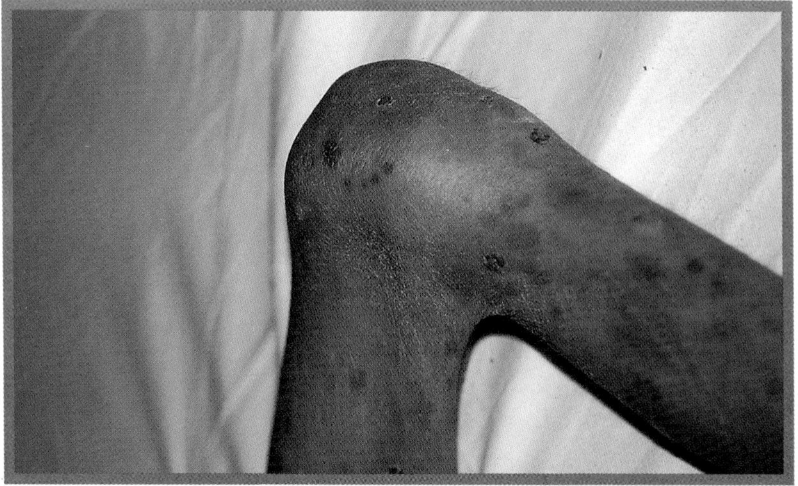

↑ 10.41

Figure 10.42 Langerhan's Cell Histiocytosis. The skin lesions involved are often mistaken for eczema. They are now recognized as Langerhan's cell tumors. Langerhan's cell histiocytosis may also present as musculoskeletal pain (see **Figure 14.15**).

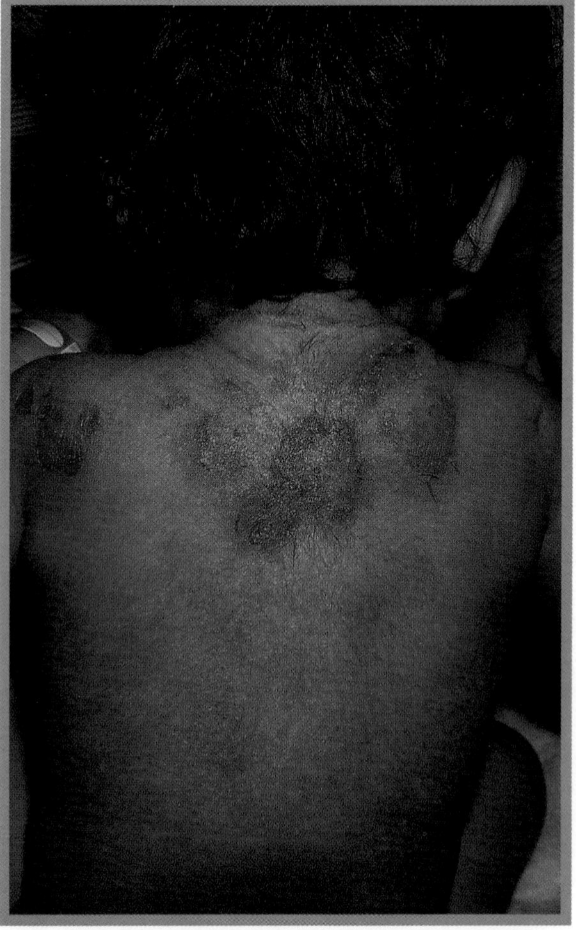

←10.42

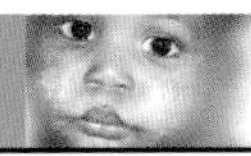

Figure 10.43 Arachnodactyly. The elongated fingers of Marfan syndrome in a newborn are shown. Other features include hypermobility of the joints, a tall stature, and an arm span that exceeds the height. Facial features include a high arched palate, long narrow facies, heterochromia of the iris, blue sclerae, myopia and lens subluxation. Cardiac involvement includes aortic and mitral regurgitation due to dilatation, and aneurysmal dilatation of the aorta. Thoracic features include pectus carinatum (pigeon chest), pectus excavatum, kyphoscoliosis and cystic lung disease. Diagnosis is made by clinical assessment, checking that the arm span is greater than the height, by radiological assessment, and by the identification of gene mutation and the fibrillin gene.

An important differential diagnosis is homocystinuria, as the phenotypical features are identical. The two diseases may be differentiated by the presence of homocysteine in the urine in homocysteinuria.

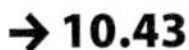

→ 10.43

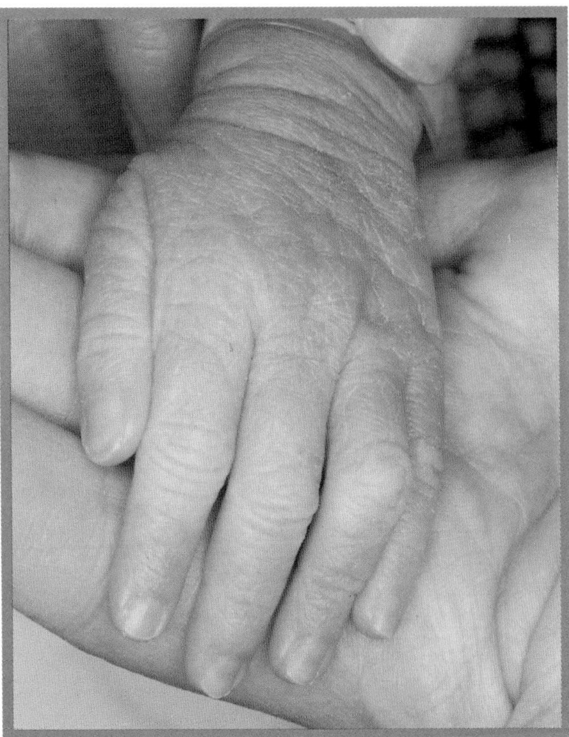

Figures 10.44 and 10.45 Arthrogryposis Multiplex in a Newborn. Congenital joint contractures were noted on routine ultrasound examination at 21 weeks, gestation. There is involvement of both the large and small joints. Other findings include hip subluxation and talipes equinovarus. Treatment is principally aimed at maintaining function, with cosmetic appearance being a secondary consideration. Physiotherapy is used, with orthotic splinting and orthopedic correction. Causes are usually neuromuscular disorders, e.g. congenital muscular dystropy.

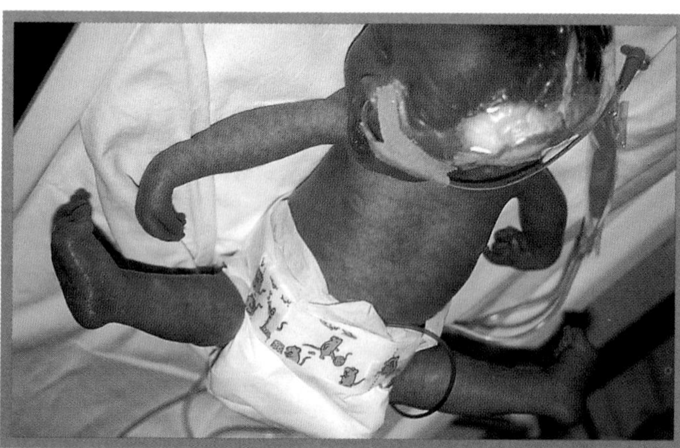

← **10.44**

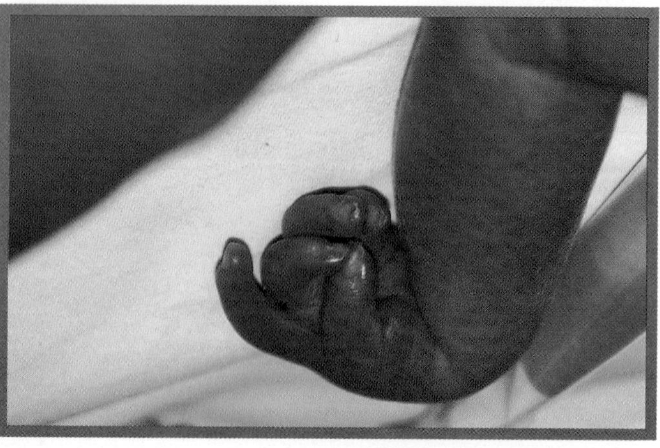

← **10.45**

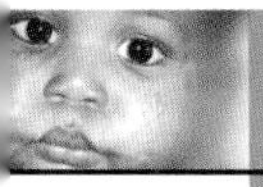
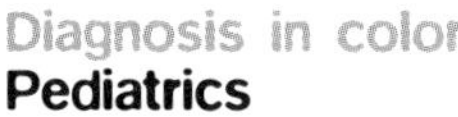

11 Dermatology

Figure 11.1 Mongolian Blue Spots. These usually present as several, ill-defined, blue-grey pigmented areas of varying size, usually over the lumbosacral area. They are more common in dark skins, and tend to fade with age. It is important to document them in view of the differential diagnosis of bruising.

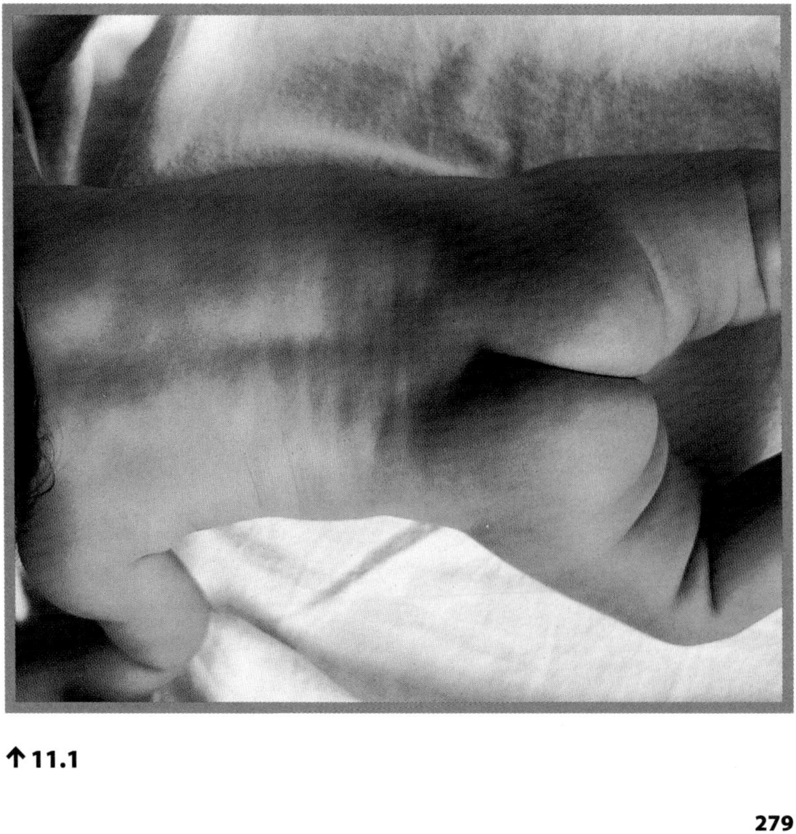

↑11.1

Figure 11.2 Congenital Melanocytic Nevus. A nevus on the thoracolumbar region is shown, but it can occur at any site. This is associated with a Mongolian blue spot. The occurrence of malignant change has probably been exaggerated in the past, and is in fact exceedingly low.

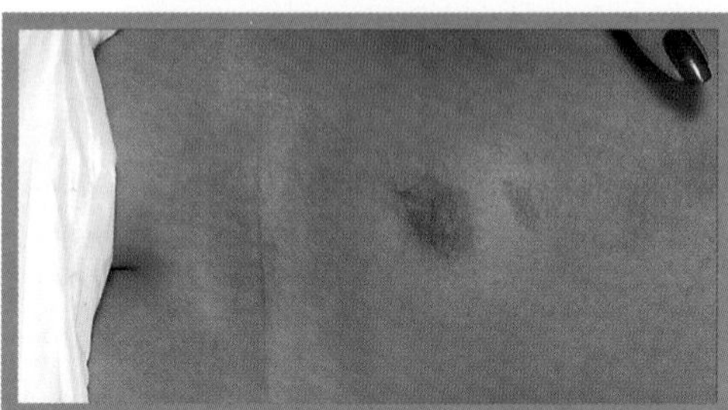

←11.2

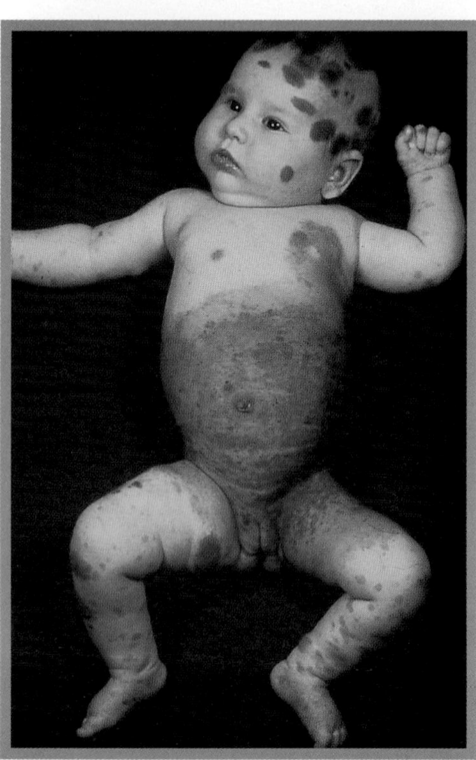

←11.3

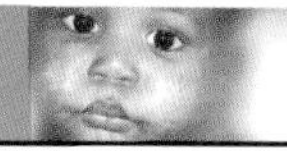

Figure 11.3 Giant Congenital Melanocytic Nevi. These are extensive pigmented lesions of varied shades of brown-to-black, and are raised in parts. Note the presence of multiple smaller nevi over the rest of the body.

There is an increased risk of malignant melanoma of about 1%. Management is by referral to a nevus clinic and plastic surgery. The use of tissue expanders allows even large nevi to be successfully removed over a period. Underlying neurological conditions are frequent.

Figure 11.4 Infantile Hemangioma. These lesions are often removed on esthetic grounds by surgery.

Figure 11.5 Collodion Baby. Congenital ichthyosis is rare. The baby shown here was born encased in a shiny membrane resembling collodion. The skin is thickened and fissured, and the hair is sparse. Movements of the joints are limited, and ectropion (everted eyelashes and lids) is present. Heat and water loss is a problem in these infants. Management is by the use of emollients. There is a tendency for significant improvement over a period of time, although some cases may end up with severe ichthyosis.

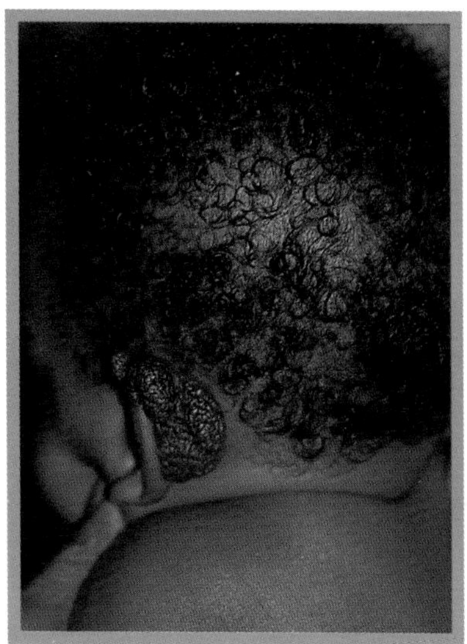

↑**11.4**

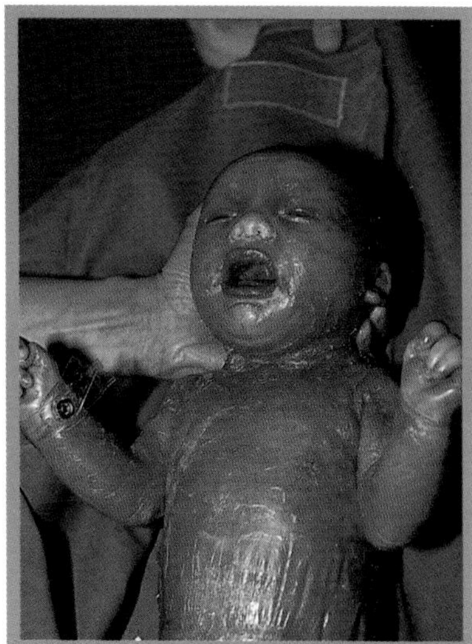

↑**11.5**

Figures 11.6 and 11.7 Lamellar Ichthyosis. Plate-like scales are seen over the trunk and face. Successive episodes of desquamation occurred. This case was treated with keratolytics and emollients.

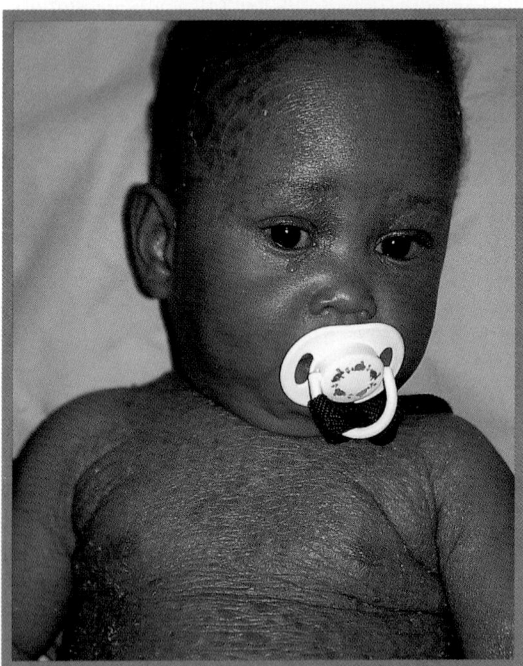

←11.6

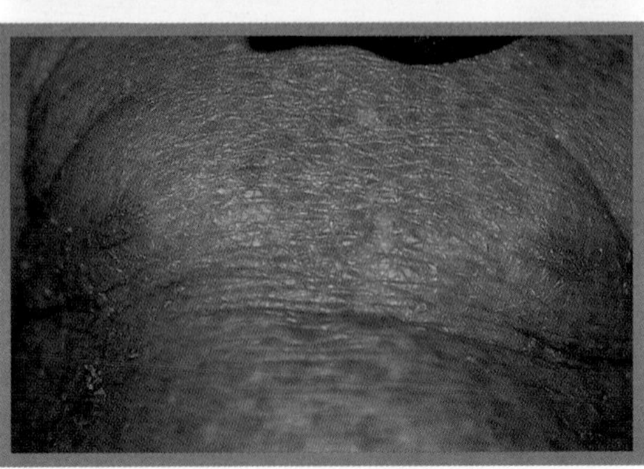

←11.7

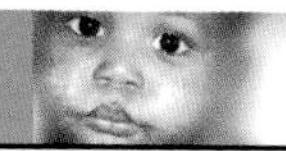

Figures 11.8–11.10 Sebaceous Nevi. Sebaceous nevi are shown affecting a number of tissues.
Figure 11.8 shows nevi on the face and scalp of an infant from the Middle East. They are hairless, linear plaques that are reddish-brown in color.
Figure 11.9 shows ocular involvement causing corneal opacification.

→11.8

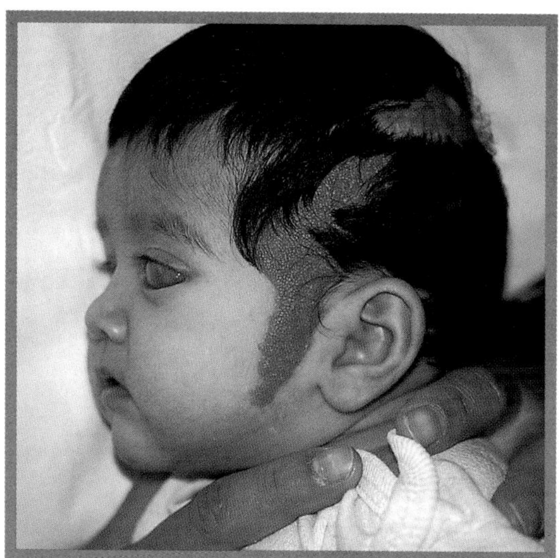

→11.9

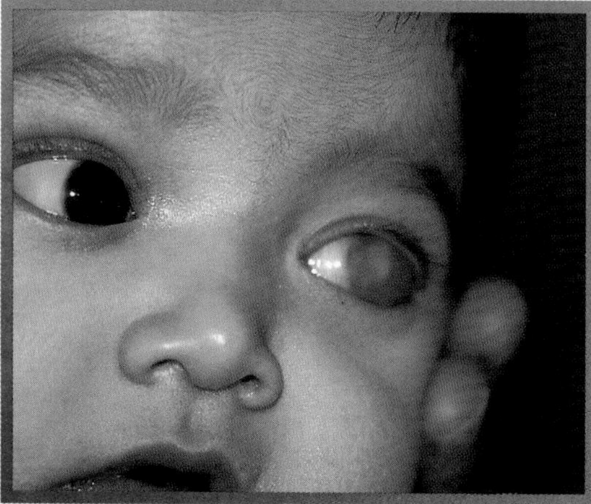

Figure 11.10 shows more lesions on the trunk. These are browner and more warty.

Epidermal nevus syndrome constitutes the association of these nevi with neurological, ocular, and skeletal abnormalities. Treatment is difficult, and is by the use of retinoic acid, diathermy, cryothermy and surgical excision. Complications include malignant change in later life.

Figure 11.11 Port Wine Stain (Nevus Flammeus). A reddish-purple macular nevus is shown over the left aspect of the trunk. It has an irregular shape and clear margins, and was present from birth. Such nevi are usually found unilaterally on the face and limbs, and can be quite extensive. They may be associated with arteriovenous malformations, limb hypertrophy (Klippel–Trenaunay syndrome) or, when over the ophthalmic division of the trigeminal nerve, with Sturge–Weber syndrome.

Treatment is by early referral to a dermatologist or plastic surgeon and consideration of laser therapy.

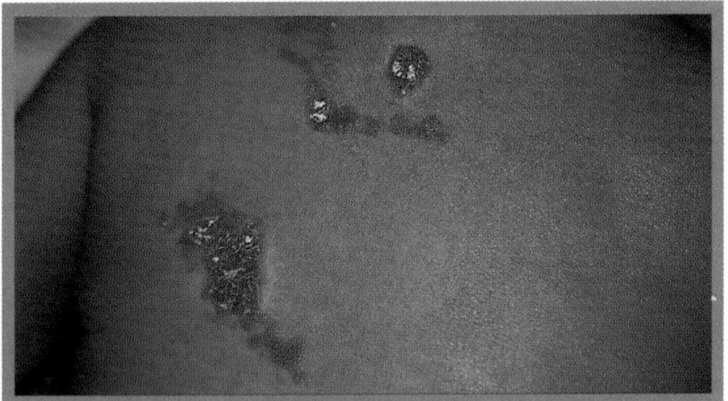

←11.10

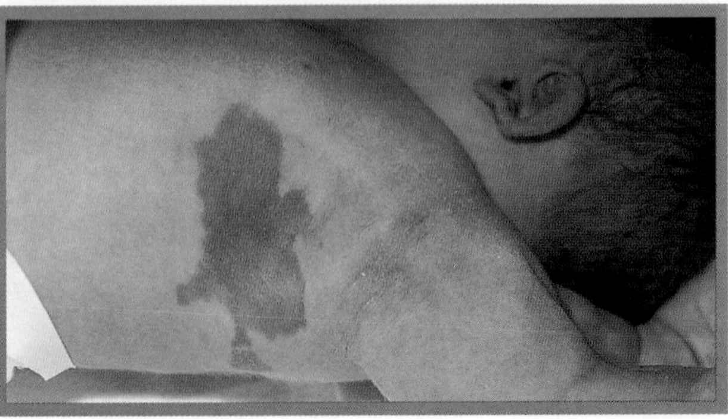

←11.11

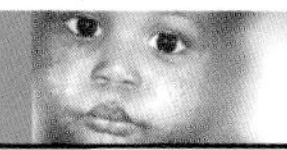

Figure 11.12 Klippel–Trenaunay–Weber Syndrome. The port wine stain seen here was associated with a deeper vascular malformation causing overgrowth of the affected limb. To avoid scoliosis a built up shoe is required as well as orthopedic treatment to fuse the epiphysis and prevent massive asymmetry.
Figures 11.13–11.20 Infantile Hemangioma. Figures 11.13 and 11.14 show strawberry nevi. It is a well-demarcated, compressible, red or blue lesion shown here in the axilla (**Figure 11.13**) and lateral to the eye (**Figure 11.14**).

→11.12

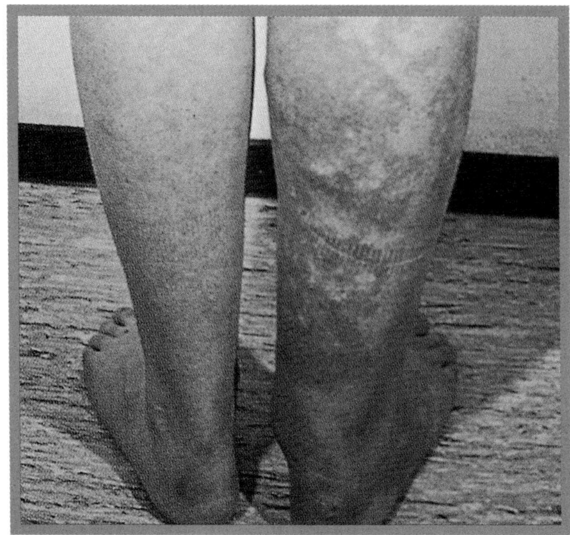

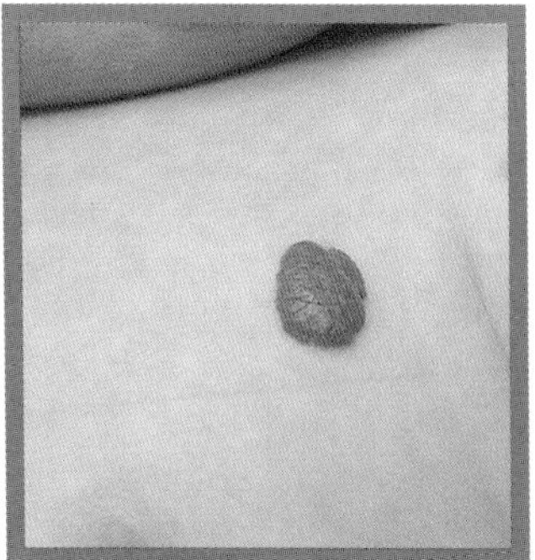

↑11.13

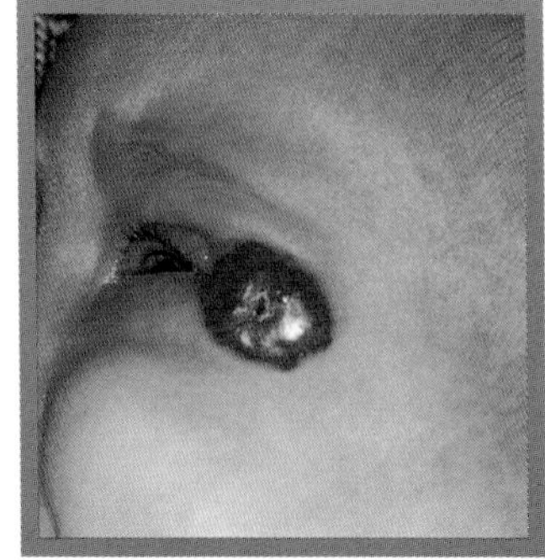

↑11.14

These lesions can be very superficial or are in the deeper tissues where they tend to take on a bluish hue. The surface may ulcerate and hemorrhage. The size tends to increase in the first 6 months and then regress over the next 2–4 years.

Figures 11.15 and 11.16 Superficial Hemangioma. This 1-year-old had a superficial hemagioma on the right hand that subsequently resolved completely (**Figure 11.16**).

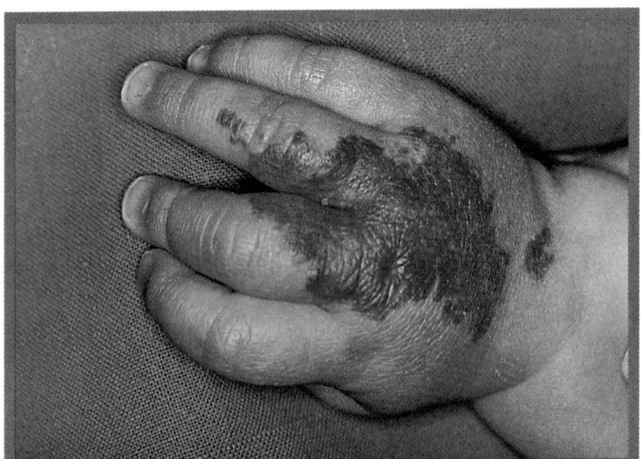

←11.15

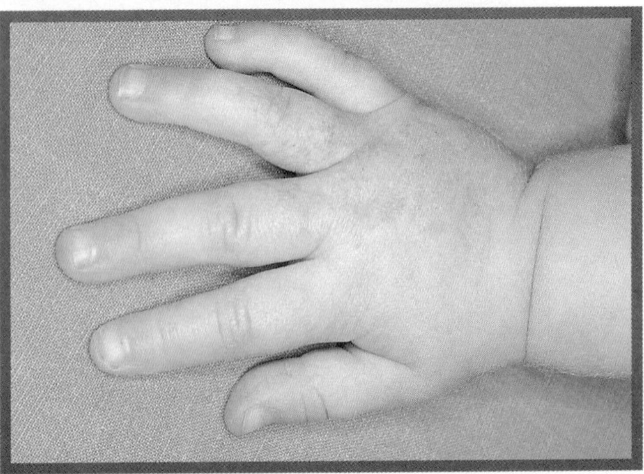

←11.16

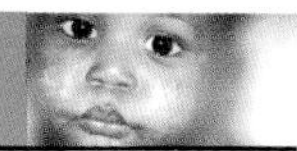

Figures 11.17–11.20 Cavernous Hemangioma. These figures show the massive nature and temporal progress of this mixed cavernous hemangioma. It was associated with the destruction of the cartilage of the ear and nose. Resolution is mostly spontaneous, but both laser and interferon therapy were used in this case. A mass effect on the eye can cause impaired vision.

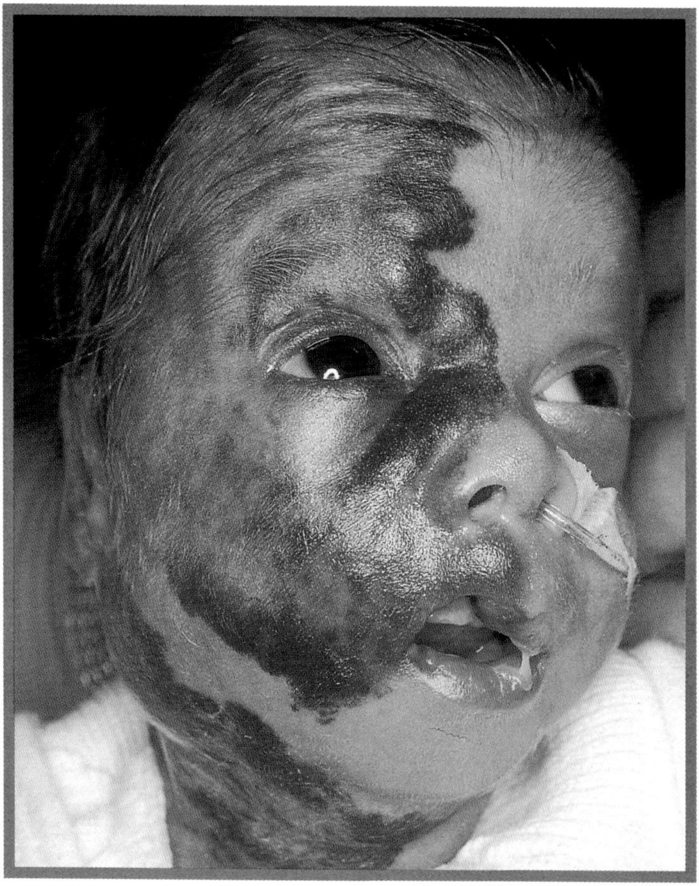

↑11.17

Cavernous hemangiomas generally grow in the first 6–9 months and then remain static for about 12 months. Fifty percent resolve by 5 years, and 70% by 7 years. Complications caused by local pressure effects may occur during the growth phase, and these may be an indication for intervention. Other indications for intervention are thrombocytopenia (Kasabach–Merritt syndrome, see **Figure 11.20**), cardiac failure from high output, restriction of movement, and ulceration or bleeding. Various treatment options are available in such instances, *e.g.*, pressure bandages, prednisolone, laser treatment, embolization, interferon and surgery.

Figures 11.21 and 11.22 Infantile Atopic Dermatitis (Eczema). Figure 11.21 shows pruritic, red, scaly excoriated lesions with crusting seen on the cheeks. An infraorbital line (Morgan's fold) is commonly seen in atopic infants. Serum IgE levels may be raised but are non-specific. This child developed asthma and had a family history of atopy.

Figure 11.22 shows flexural eczema in a 2-year-old child. The skin is generally dry with lichenification and excoriation. Involvement of most of the legs has occurred with a preponderance over the flexural aspects of the limbs.

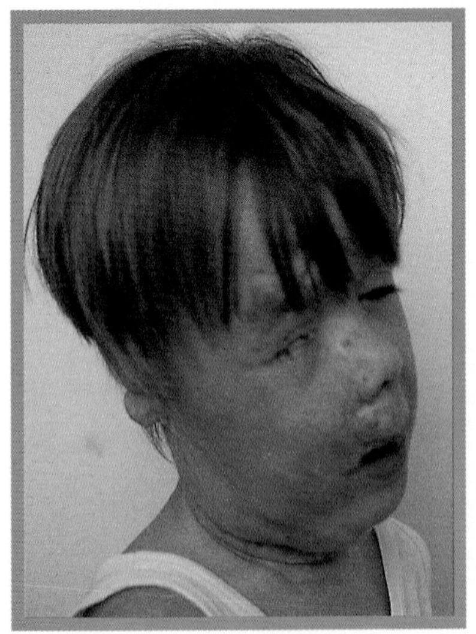

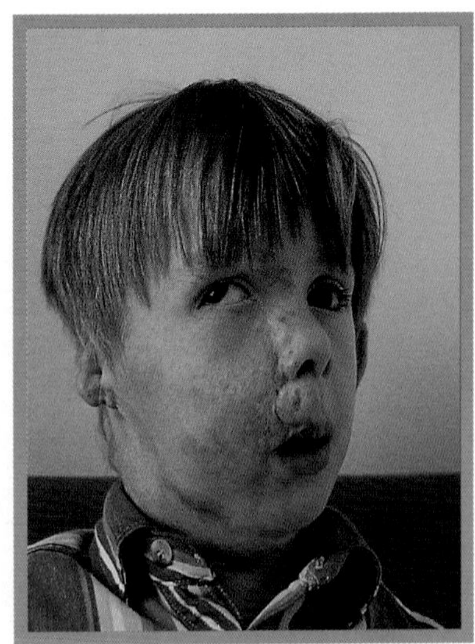

↑11.18

↑11.19

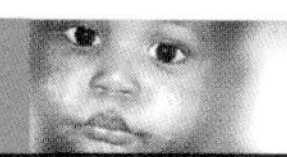

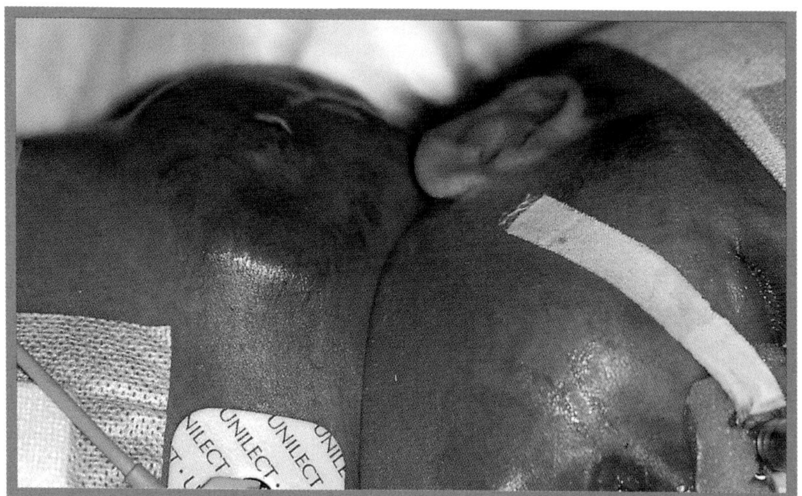

↑ 11.20

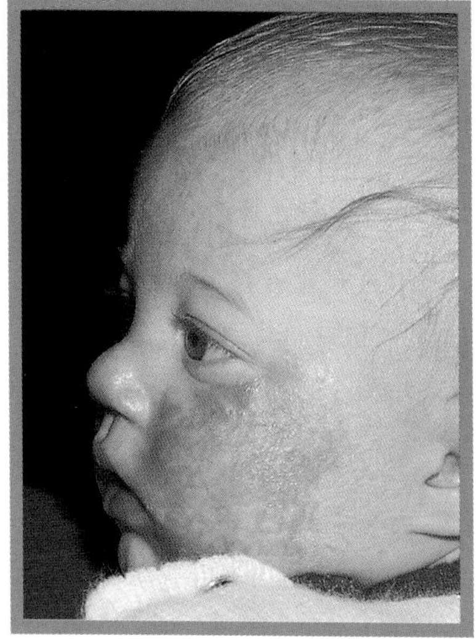

↑ 11.21

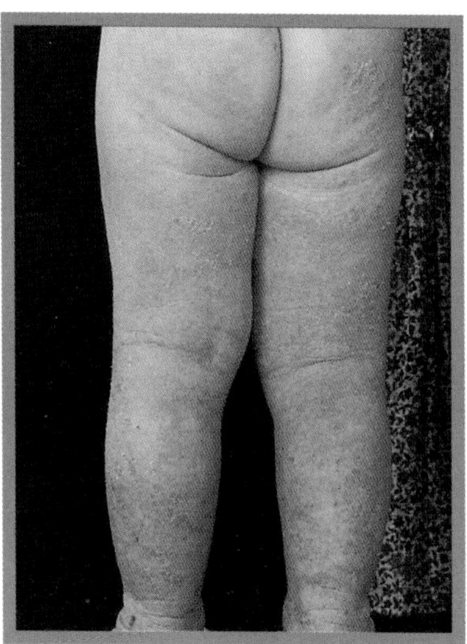

↑ 11.22

Figure 11.23 Discoid Pattern of Atopic Eczema. The well-defined patch of eczema shown here was seen in a symmetric distribution over the flexural areas (in older children such eczema may occur over the extensor surfaces). Note the post-inflammatory pigment changes, which are more noticeable on pigmented skin. In Asian and Oriental children, it is not uncommon for lesions to take the form of disks. The differential diagnosis is of tinea and psoriasis.

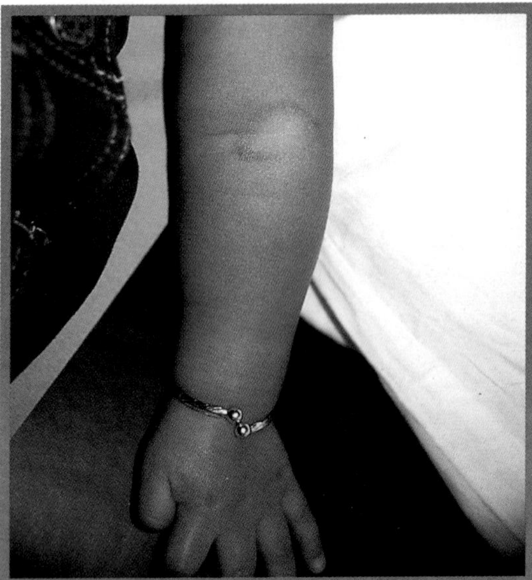

←**11.23**

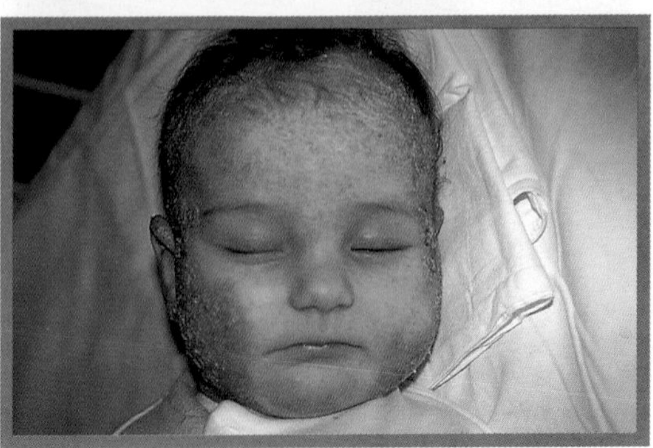

←**11.24**

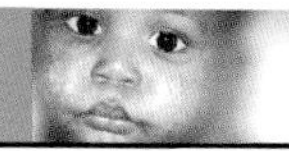

Figures 11.24–11.26 Complications of Eczema. Figure 11.24 shows secondary bacterial infection in eczema. Yellow crusting is shown, with impetiginization on the face and scalp of an infant. The usual infective organism is *Staphylococcus.*

Figure 11.25 Eczema Herpeticum. This shows a severe, secondary, herpes simplex infection in an infant with eczema. The pustular lesions are 2–4 mm in diameter and may coalesce.

Figure 11.26 Eczema Herpeticum Lesions. Viral warts are shown in the left axilla. Molluscum contagiosum also tends to flourish in eczematous areas. Treatment consists of administration of oral antibiotics and acyclovir.

The following may be used in the treatment of eczema:

1. Suitable clothing: wool should be avoided; cotton is ideal; perfumed products should be avoided.
2. Aqueous creams and bath oils.
3. Emollients applied regularly to hydrate the skin.
4. Topical steroids at the lowest effective concentration.
5. Occlusive wet dressings.
6. Antibiotics for infected eczema.
7. Antihistamines to reduce itching.
8. Pets and dietary avoidance in selected cases.

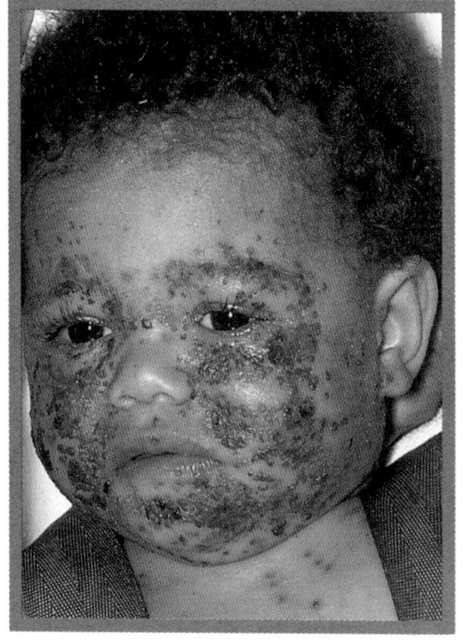

↑ 11.25

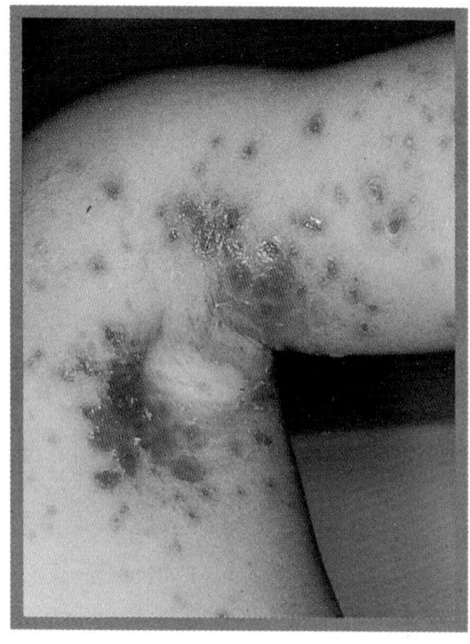

↑ 11.26

Figures 11.27 and 11.28 Seborrheic Dermatitis 'Cradle Cap'. Seborrheic dermatitis is shown in a 3-month-old child (top) and in a 12-year-old (bottom). There are generally greasy, yellow scales on the scalp, with round, red lesions over the trunk. The condition is non-pruritic in nature. The groin, neck and limb flexures may also be involved. Secondary candidal infection is common. Treatment consists of administration of weak topical steroids, antifungals if appropriate, and sulfur and salicylic acid preparations (keratolytics).

The differential diagnosis consists of drug reactions, atopic dermatitis, ammoniacal dermatitis (diaper or nappy rash), and psoriasis.

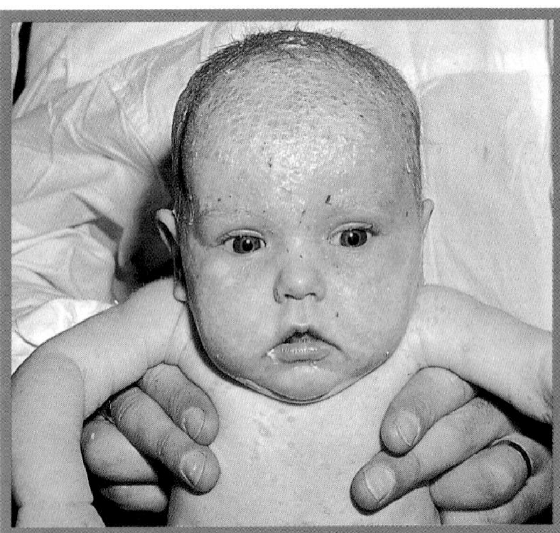

←11.27

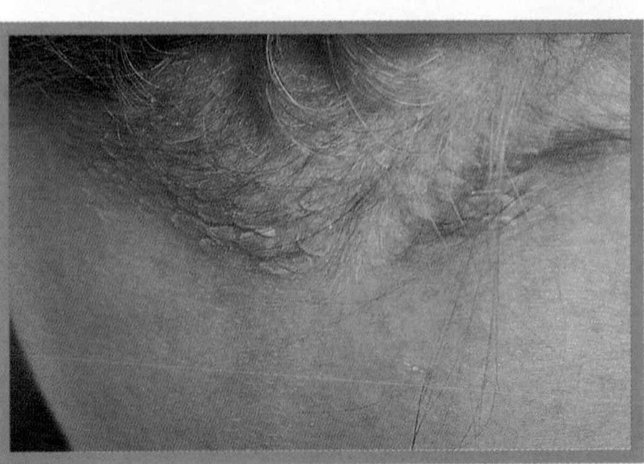

←11.28

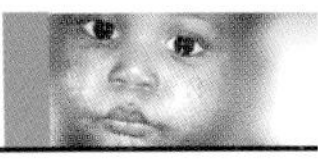

Figures 11.29–11.35 Erythema Multiforme. Figures 11.29 and 11.30 show erythema multiforme in a 5-year-old girl with systemic lupus erythematosis and herpes simplex infection. There are circular lesions with peripheral erythema and blue, discolored centers. The rash is confluent in places, is non-pruritic, and is distributed over the face, trunk and limbs, although it is characteristically distributed over the periphery. Note the blancing on pressure.

→ 11.29

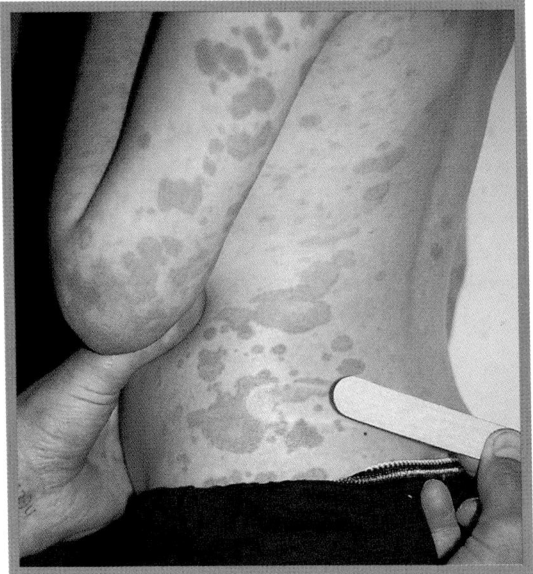

→ 11.30

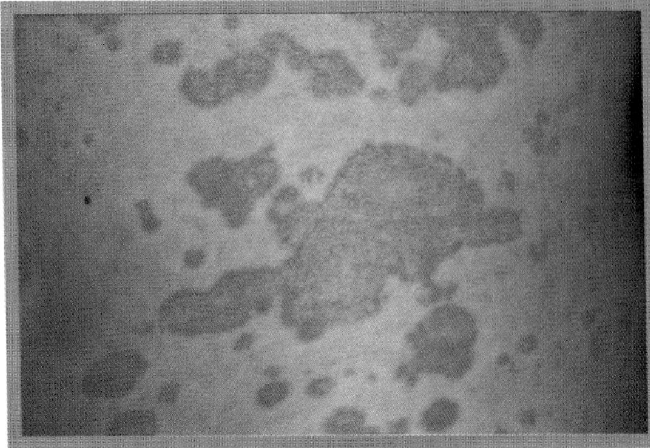

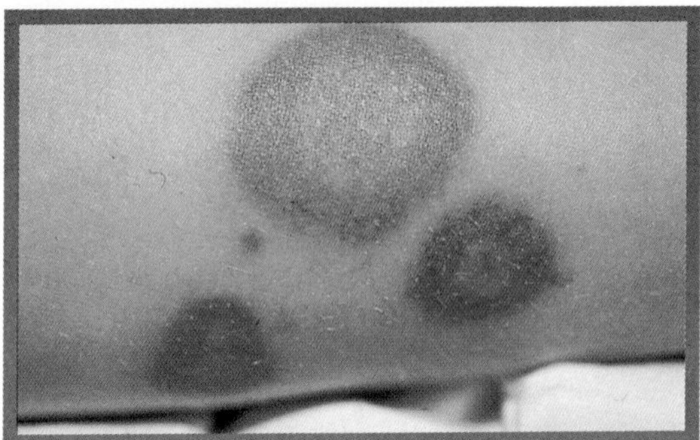

←11.31

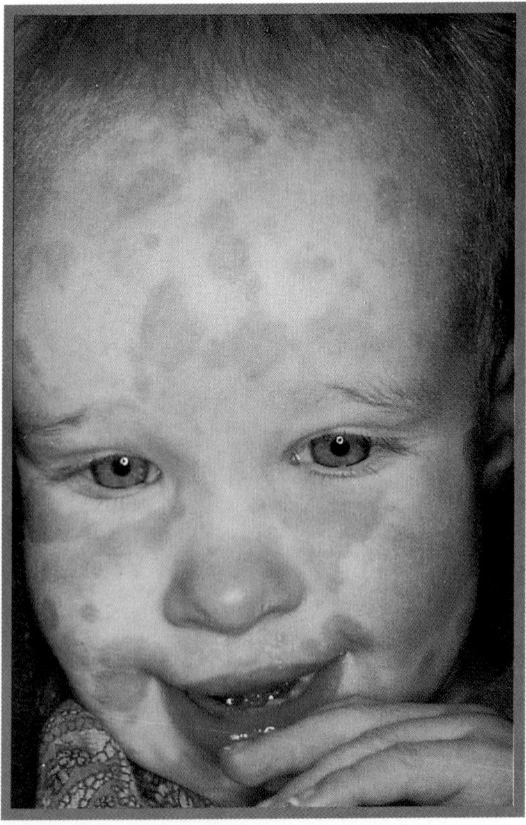

←11.32

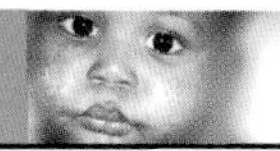

Figure 11.31 shows a **'target' lesion**, with a pale center and bright red borders.
Figure 11.32 shows erythema multiforme involving the face.
Fifty percent of cases are idiopathic, but known causes include:

1. Infection, *e.g.*, by herpes simplex, mycoplasma, Orf, streptococci, yersinia, and tuberculosis. .
2. Connective tissue diseases or neoplasia.
3. Drugs, *e.g.*, sulfonamides, sulfonylurea, penicillin, and salicylates.

Figures 11.33–11.35 Bullous Erythema Multiforme (Stevens–Johnson Syndrome). The figures show a severe, bullous form of erythema multiforme in a 13-year-old girl. There is a rash over her limbs, hands, eyes and ears, with involvement of the mucous membranes. It was associated with pyrexia and malaise. The condition was triggered by penicillin. Intravenous fluids were required due to the severe stomatitis. There is a significant morbidity and mortality. Treatment is by administration of steroids, and particular care should be paid to the eyes since corneal ulceration may cause blindness.

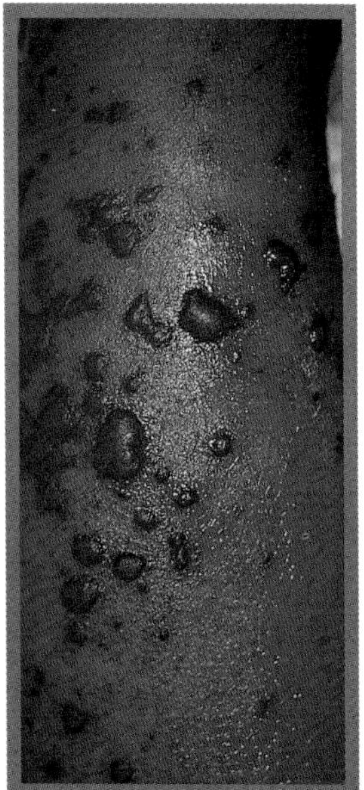

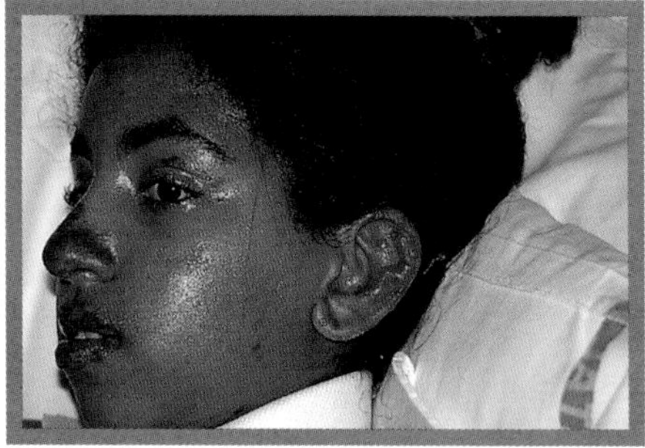

↑11.34

↑11.33 **→11.35**

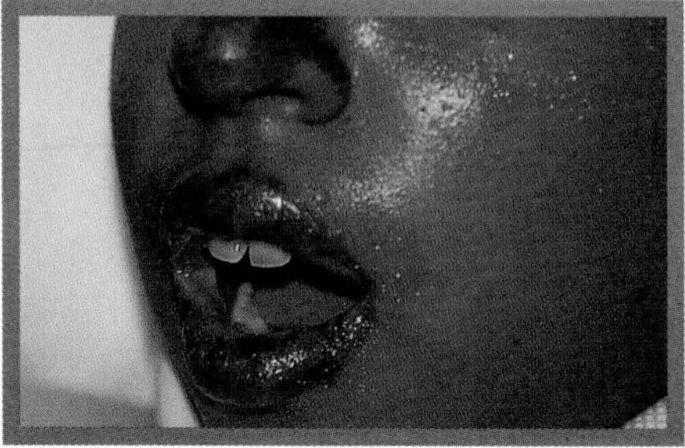

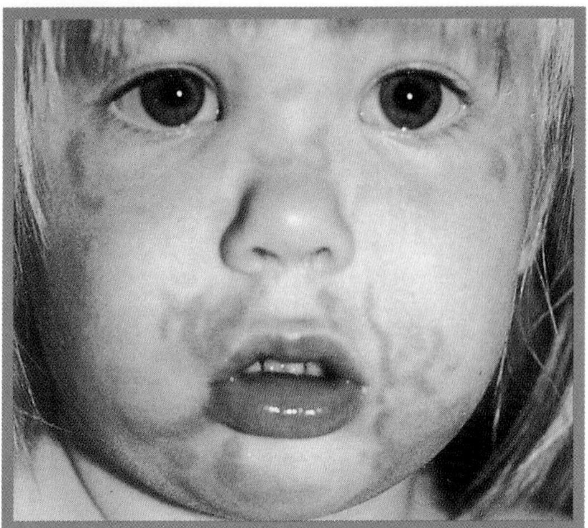

←11.36

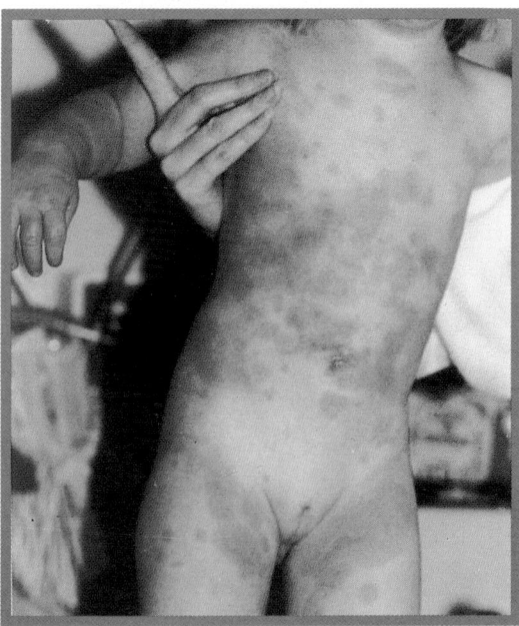

←11.37

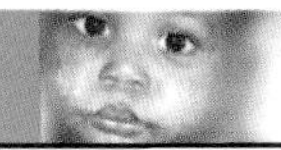

Figures 11.36 and 11.37 Urticaria. Generalized urticaria is seen here in a child with an allergy to milk. Note the wheal and flare. Both confluent and discrete lesions are seen. There is angioedema of the eyes and lips, and of the subglottic area. The rash is usually only transient, but may be recurrent.
The causes are:

1. Cold.
2. Heat, sunlight and cold water.
3. Foods, especially milk and peanuts.
4. Viral infections.
5. Exercise.
6. Hot baths.
7. Spicy foods and emotional stress.

Figures 11.38 and 11.39 Erythema Marginatum. A macular erythematous rash is seen here on the right forearm and face. The rash has a circular nature with pale centers of normal skin. Erythema marginatum is a major feature of rheumatic fever, and only occasionally occurs. The lesions vary in shape and site from hour to hour.

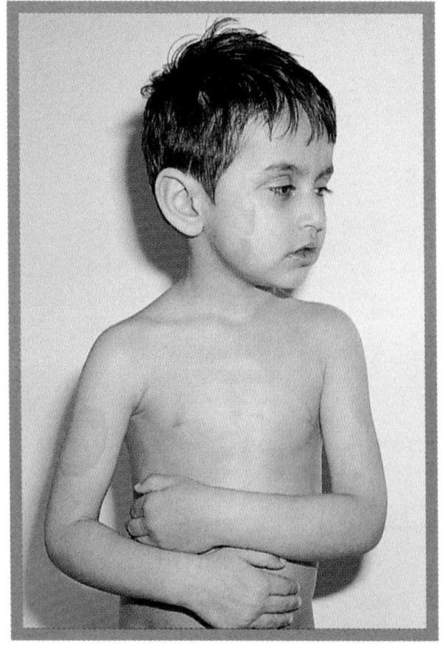

↑ **11.38**

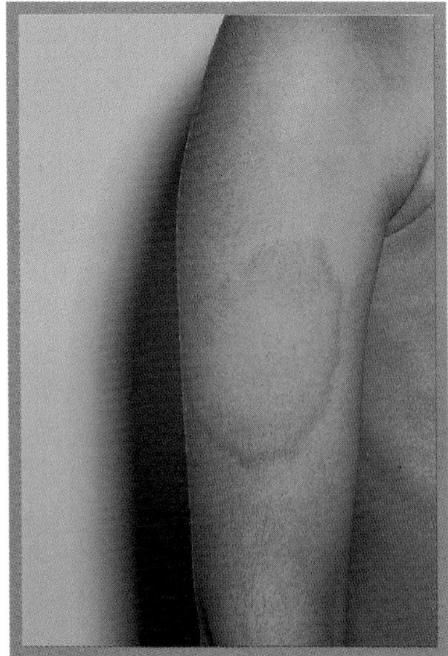

↑ **11.39**

Figures 11.40 and 11.41 Erythema Nodosum. Erythema nodosum is shown on the anterior lower legs of this 10-year-old girl. The painful red nodules of varying size are hot to the touch. In this case, they were post-streptococcal and faded to leave a pigmented area.

Erythema nodosum may occur in association with tuberculosis, inflammatory bowel disease, oral contraceptives, sensitivity to BCG, SLE and sarcoidosis. No cause is identified in 50% of cases.

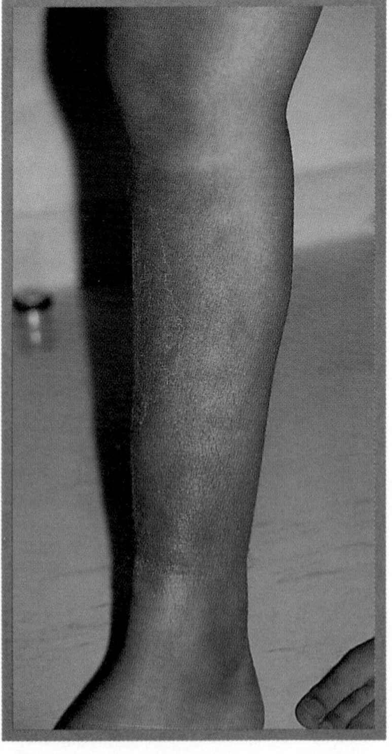

↑ 11.40

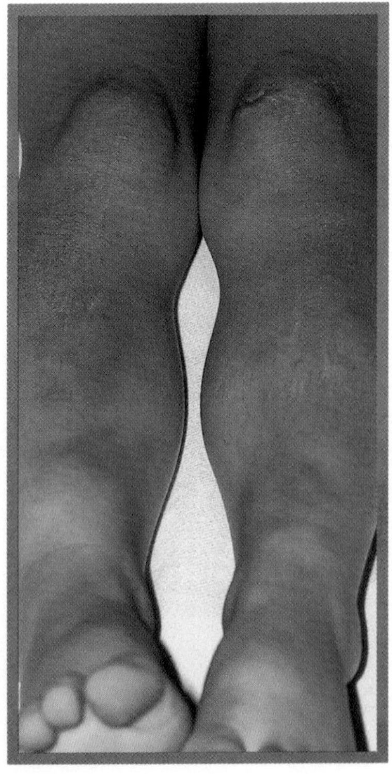

↑ 11.41

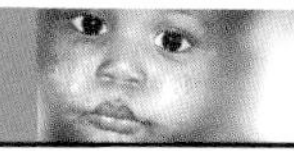

Figure 11.42 Acne. Infantile acne commencing over the first few days of life is shown. The pustules, seen over the cheeks, are due to stimulation of the sebaceous glands by maternal androgens. The condition usually resolves by 10 weeks of age.

Figure 11.43 Molluscum Contagiosum. Molluscum contagiosum is seen over the groin of a 3-year-old girl. There are pearly-white, spherical lesions present with umbilicated centers. Common sites are the anogenital region, axillae and trunk. Caseous material can be expressed from the lesions. In this case, the lesions were allowed to resolve spontaneously. Molluscum contagiosum is caused by the pox virus. Treatment is rarely indicated. The differential diagnosis is of warts, skin tags, and dermatofibromas.

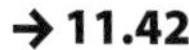

→ 11.42

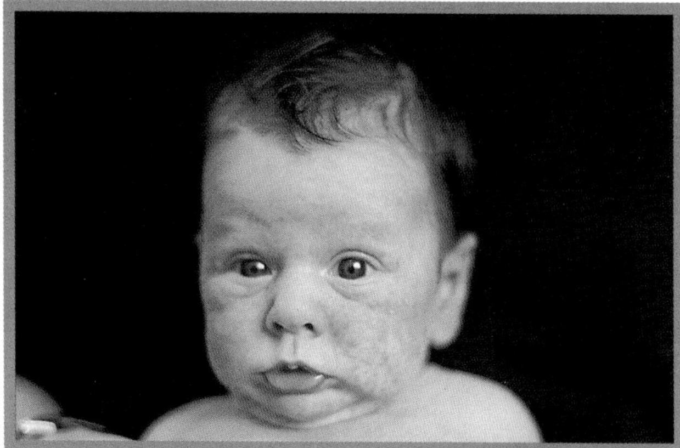

→ 11.43

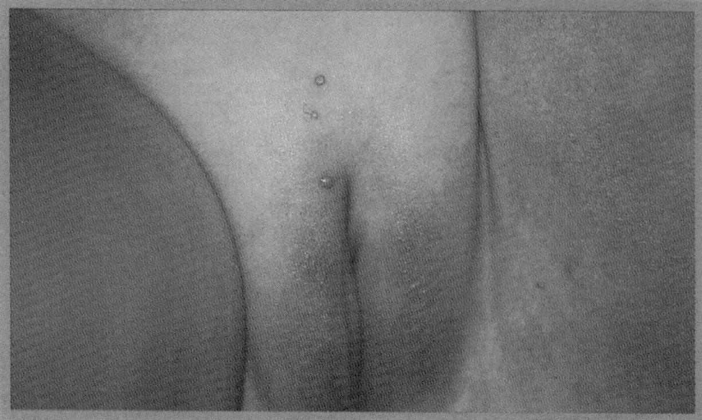

Figures 11.44–11.46 Tinea Corporis. Tinea corporis is shown on both black and white skin. The lesions are scaly and itchy. Treatment is with topical antifungals on the localized areas. Oral antifungals are used for chronic lesions in the skin and for all nail and hair infections.

Figures 11.47 and 11.48 Tinea Capitis. Circular patches of hair loss with scaling are shown. Both patients complained of pruritus. There are three main patterns of scalp infection, and these patterns determine the rate of hair breakage and clinical appearance.

The differential diagnosis is of alopecia areata, traumatic alopecia (hair twisting) and, in diffuse hair loss, hypothyroidism, hypopituitarism, iron deficiencies, and the effects of chemotherapy.

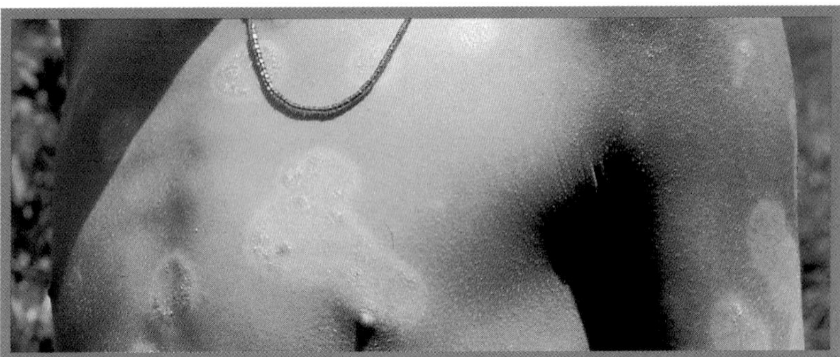

↑ 11.44

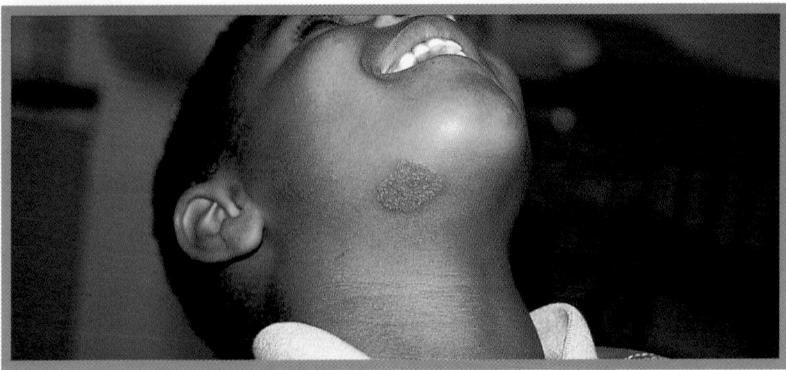

↑ 11.45

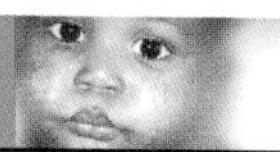

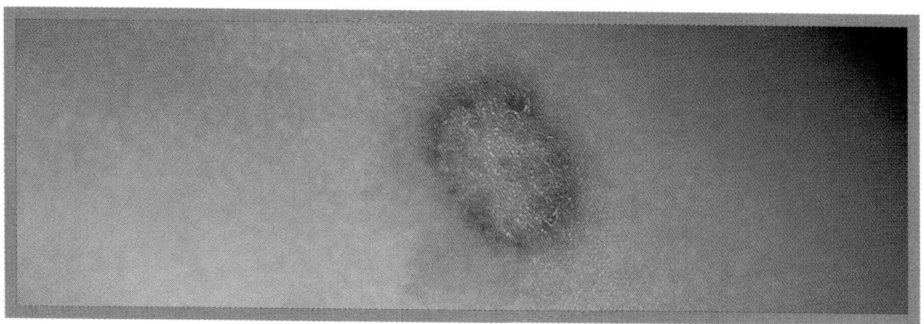

↑ 11.46

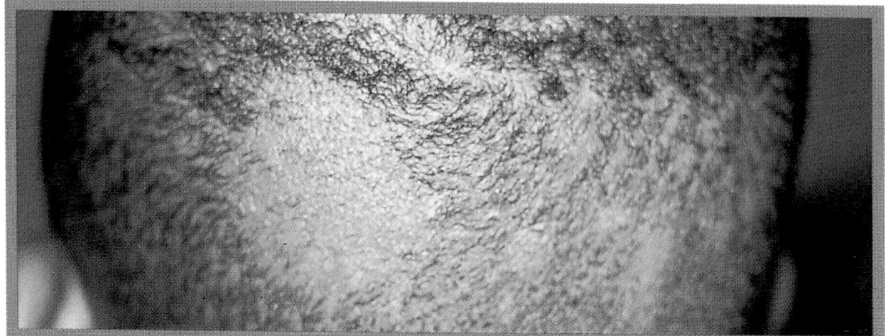

↑ 11.47

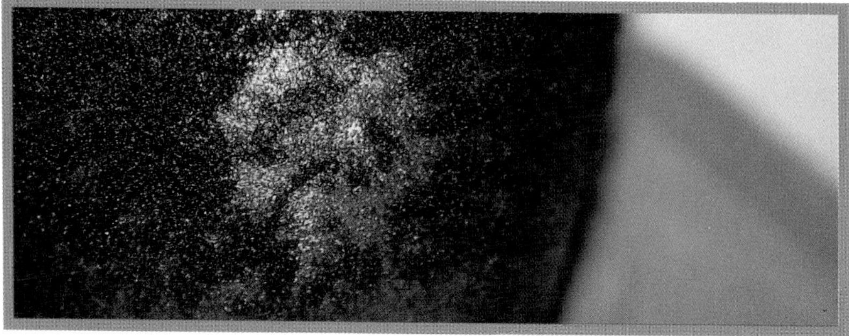

↑ 11.48

Figures 11.49 and 11.50 Lupus Vulgaris. The Nepalese child shown in **Figure 11.49** has a father (**Figure 11.50**) with cutaneous tuberculosis. The lesions may remain as discrete pustules or may coalesce. The differential diagnosis is of lupus erythematosus, sarcoidosis, syphilis, and leprosy. Treatment is with anti-TB therapy.
Figure 11.51 Vitiligo. Vitiligo usually affects the eyelids, perioral skin, and

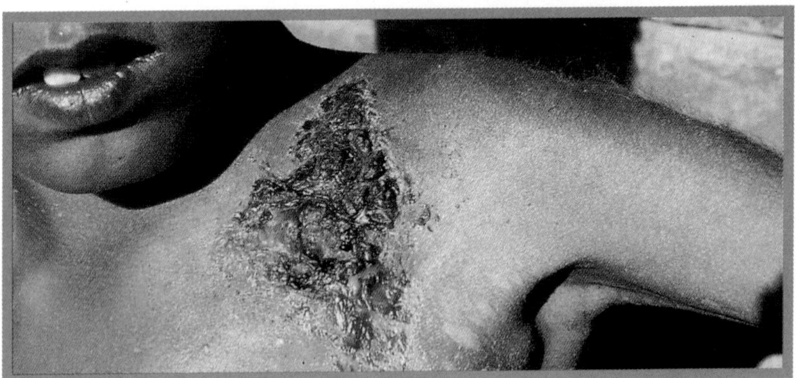

↑ 11.49

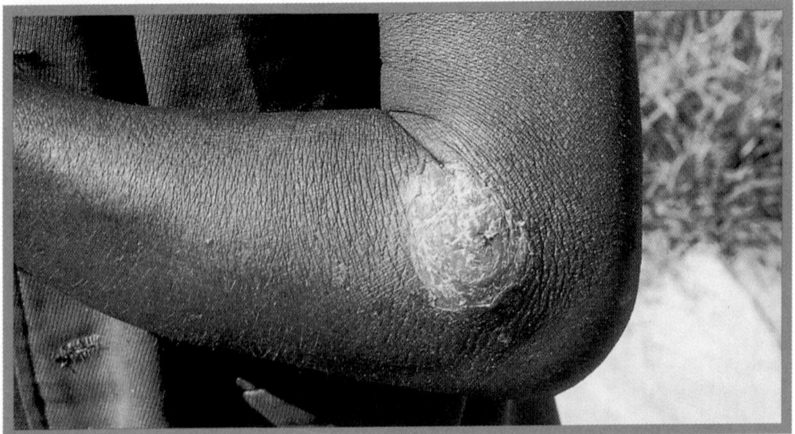

↑ 11.50

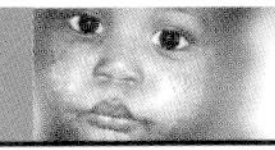

hands. It may be precipitated by trauma. It is occasionally associated with autoimmune disorders, *e.g.*, thyroiditis, Addison disease, and diabetes. Treatment is with application of camouflage makeup, administration of steroids rarely, and photochemotherapy.

Figure 11.52 Oral Candidiasis. The 2-month-old shown here has oral thrush. There are white patches that can be scraped off to reveal a red mucosa. Treatment consists in administration of an oral antifungal agent.

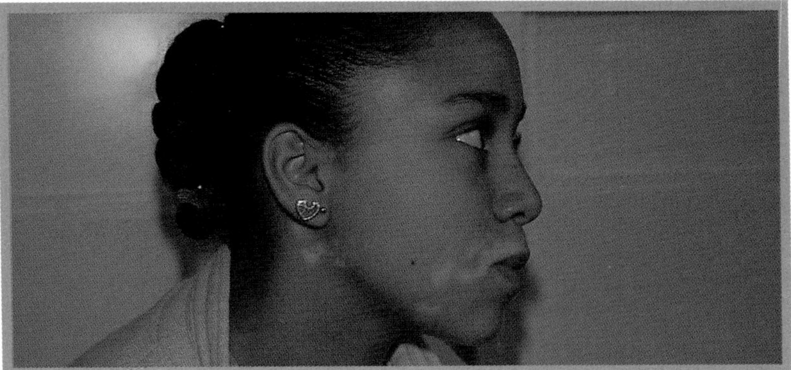

↑11.51

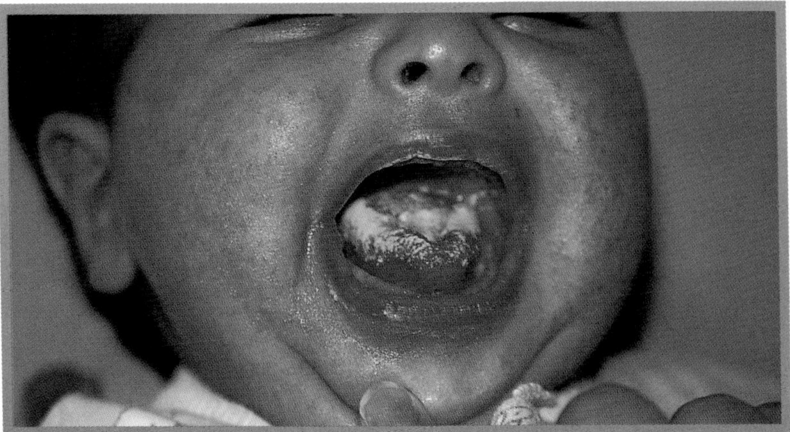

↑11.52

Figure 11.53 Erysipelis. A tender, red, edematous area can be seen over the left leg. The area has a well-demarcated edge. The patient was systemically unwell, with malaise and fever. This case was associated with hemorrhagic blistering and tender lymphadenopathy, and was caused by streptococcal group A infection. Treatment was with antibiotics.

Figure 11.54 Onychomycosis. This fungal nail infection occurred in a child with HIV infection. This is caused by a range of fungi.

Figure 11.55 Leukonychia. Diffuse whitening of all the nails is seen. This may be congenital or acquired.

Acquired causes are:

1. Liver disease.
2. Stress and nail trauma.
3. Cardiac disease.
4. Renal disease.
5. Neoplasia.
6. Psoriasis.
7. Dermatophyte infection.

This was a congenital case with other family members being affected.

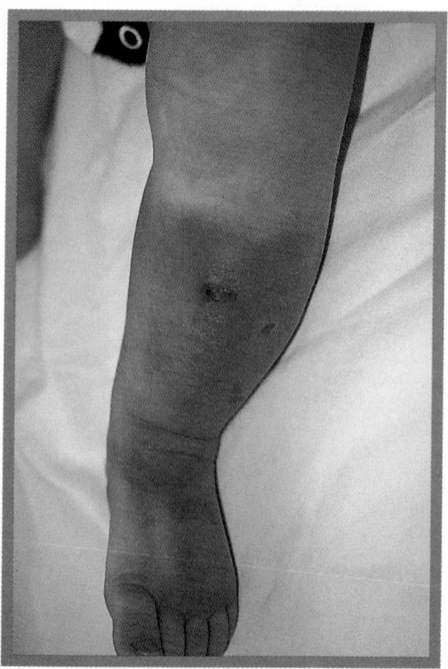

←11.53

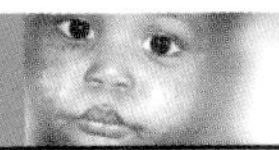

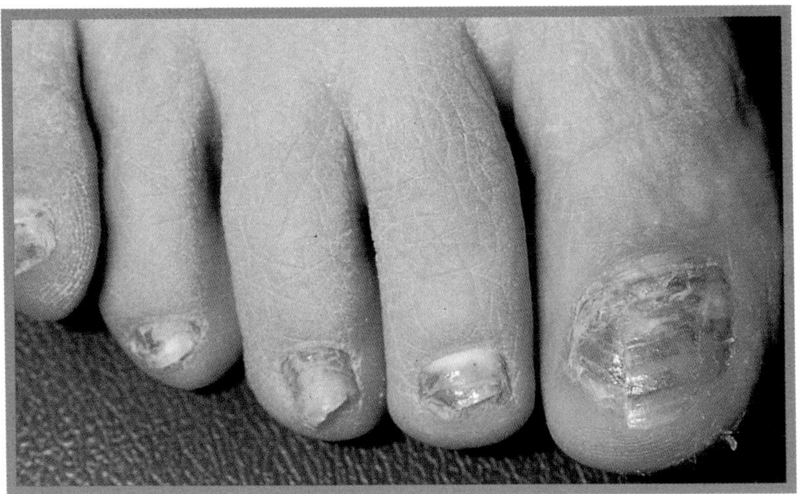

↑ 11.54

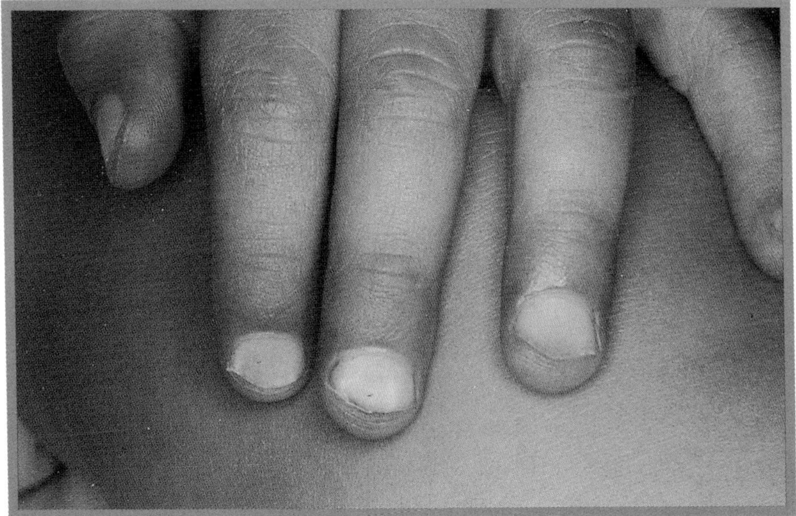

↑ 11.55

Figure 11.56 Tetracycline Staining of the Teeth. Tetracycline taken in pregnancy or early childhood can cause disfiguring brown staining of the teeth. Tetracyclines should not be given to children under 12 years of age.

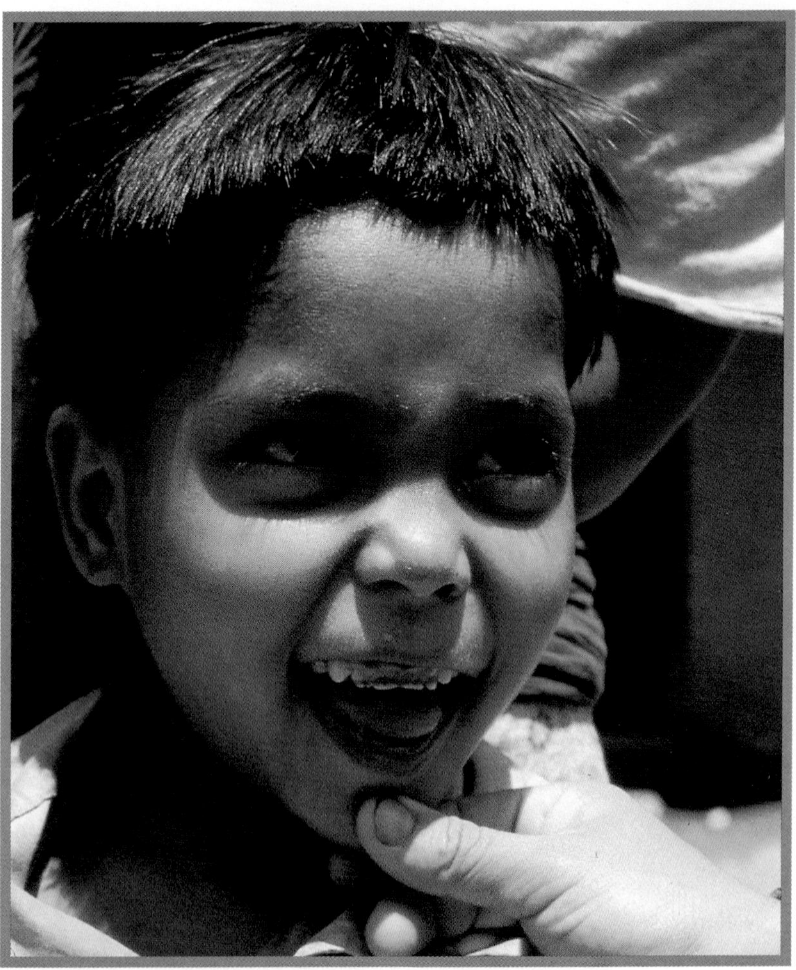

↑11.56

12 Infection and immunity

Figure 12.1 Roseola Infantum in an Infant. The child shown here presented with an abrupt onset of high fever that reached 40°C and lasted for 3 days. The fever was followed by a widely distributed, nonconfluent, maculopapular rash that started on the trunk. The rash persisted for 1 day and then disappeared. Complications include febrile convulsions and, in rare cases, encephalitis. Roseola is caused by human herpes virus 6 (HHV-6)

→ 12.1

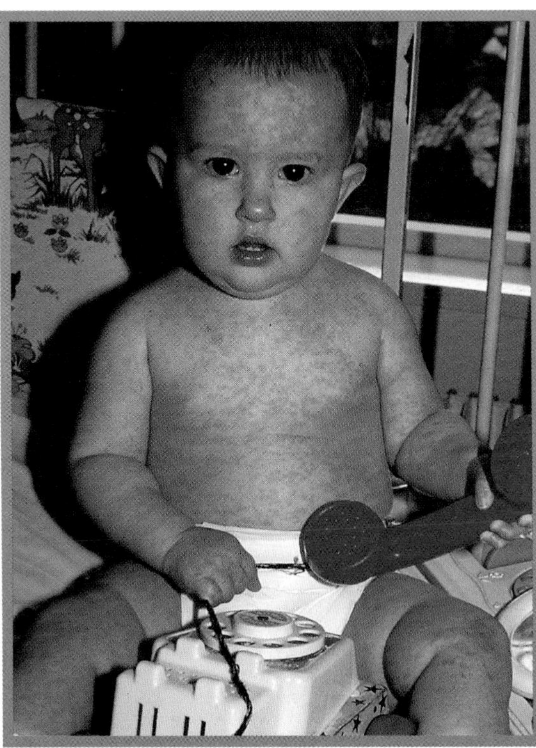

Figure 12.2 Infectious Mononucleosis. The adolescent shown here presented with malaise, fever, sore throat, lymphadenopathy, splenomegaly and an erythematous rash. Blood film tests revealed atypical lymphocytosis. A Paul–Bunnell test gave a positive result.

Infectious mononucleosis is caused by the Epstein–Barr virus. Complications of infection are:

1. Hematological: autoimmune hemolytic anemia, thrombocytopenia, and neutropenia.
2. Tonsillar hypertrophy leading to airway obstruction.
3. Neurological: aseptic meningitis. transverse myelitis, Bell palsy, and Guillain–Barré syndrome.
4. Cardiac: myocarditis and arrhythmias.
5. Pneumonia.
6. Gastrointestinal disorders.
7. Hepatitis.
8. Splenic rupture if traumatized.
9. Renal dysfunction.

The disease may follow a protracted course, sometimes lasting many months.

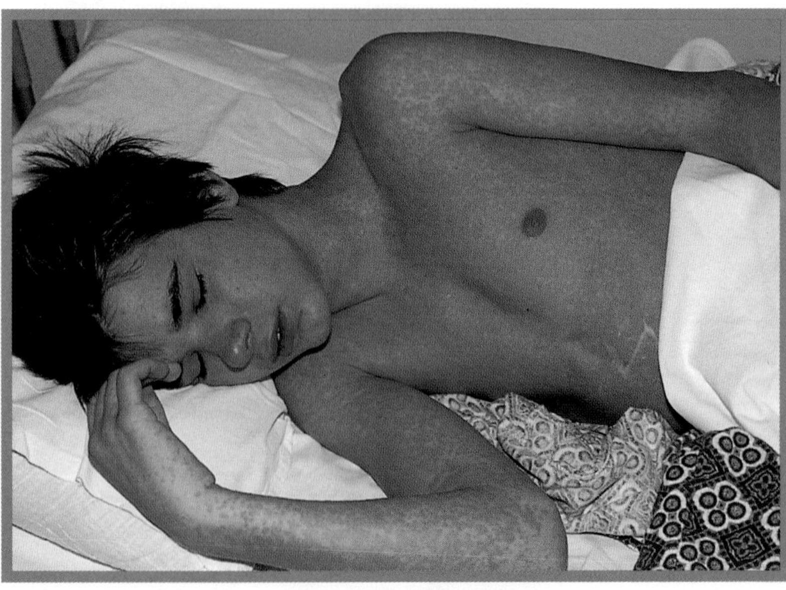

↑ 12.2

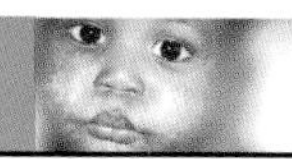

Figures 12.3–12.5 Measles. Measles is shown in an infant and child respectively. Note the erythematous, maculopapular rash, which is confluent in parts and is distributed on the face up to the hair line and on the trunk. Also note the eyelid edema and conjunctivitis particularly on the second child. In both cases the rash began on the head and spread to the torso. It faded in the same sequence.

Measles is caused by an RNA virus. Its incidence has decreased since the introduction of measles, mumps,and rubella (MMR) vaccine, but it is still a significant cause of morbidity and mortality, particularly in developing countries.

The incubation period is 10–14 days. Koplick spots (white papules) occur 1–2 days prior to and after the onset of the rash.

Early complications are otitis media, bronchopneumonia, encephalitis, corneal ulcers, stomatitis and appendicitis. A late complication is subacute sclerosing panencephalitis.

Treatment with vitamin A in deficient individuals has been shown to reduce the complications of measles. Immunoglobulin should be given to immunocompromised children who have had contact with measles, as in these children, disseminated measles carries a high mortality.

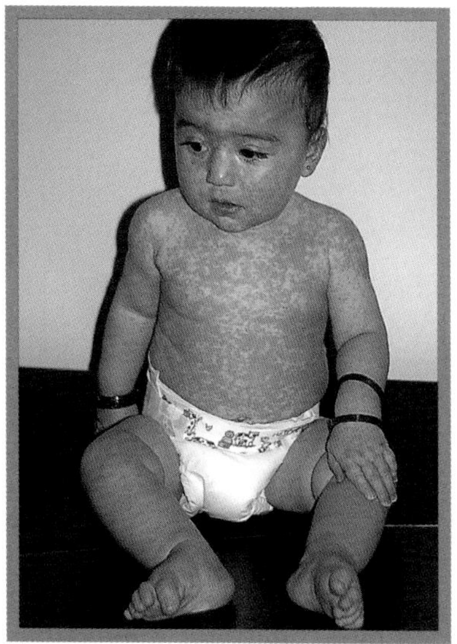

↑12.3

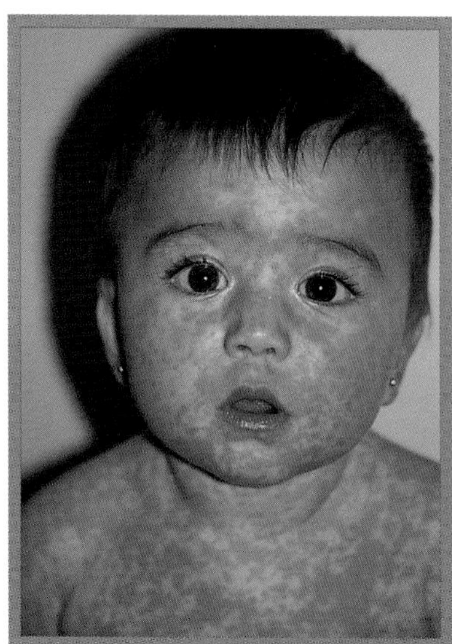

↑12.4

Figures 12.6–12.8 Scarlet Fever. Scarlet fever is shown following infection of a foot burn by an erythrogenic-toxin-producing strain of group A β-hemolytic streptococci. The child shown presented with fever, headache, sore throat and anorexia.

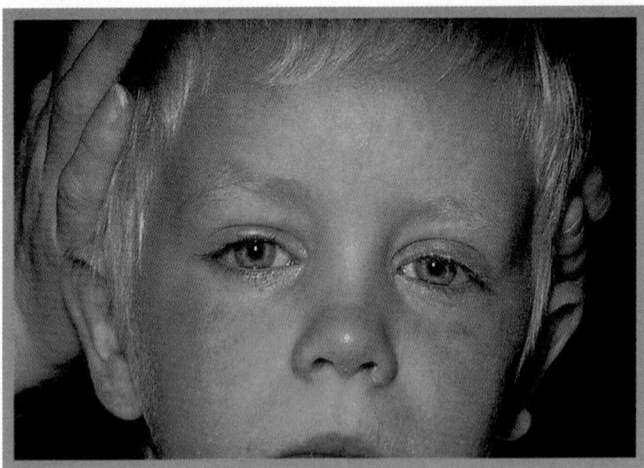

← 12.5

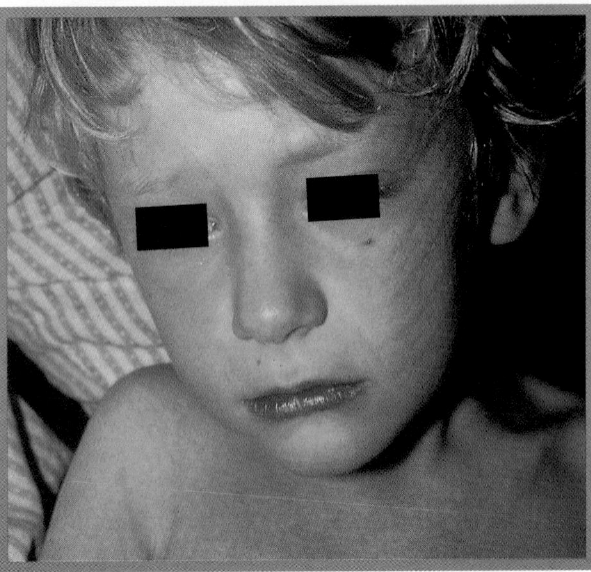

← 12.6

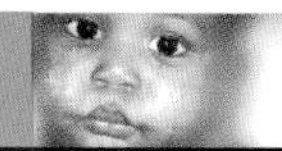

A diffuse erythematous rash covering all surfaces of the body is seen. The rash blanches on pressure (**Figure 12.8**) and has a rough surface. The face is flushed with a mild circumoral pallor. The tongue is swollen and has a yellowish-white coating and prominent papillae ('strawberry tongue'). Desquamation occurred later in the disease process, and started on the face. There was a significant rise in the serum antistreptolysin O (ASO) titre.

Scarlet fever is typically caused by a mucocutaneously acquired infection with streptococci. The rash is due to absorption of toxin. However, there has been an increased incidence of invasive group A streptococcal disease in many countries, which has been associated with the focal infection of bones, joints, soft tissues, lungs and brain. Invasive disease is associated with a high mortality and occasionally toxic-shock syndrome.

Later immunological manifestations of the disease include: rheumatic fever, acute glomerulonephritis, and erythema nodosum. Early treatment with antibiotics will help to prevent complications.

Differential diagnoses are toxin-producing strains of *Staphylococcus aureus* (which can produce a similar rash), measles, Kawasaki syndrome, and drug reactions.

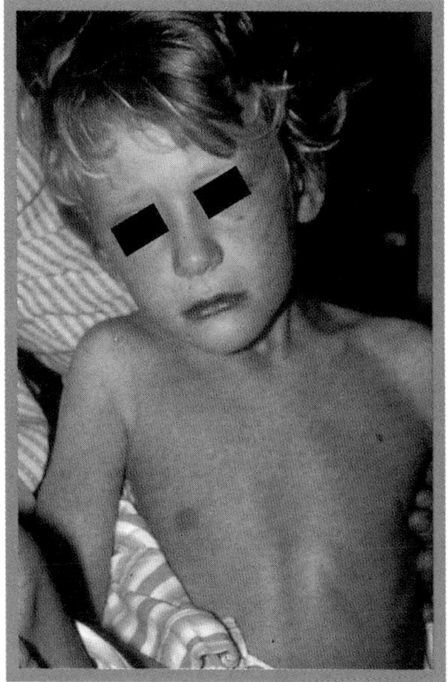

↑ 12.7

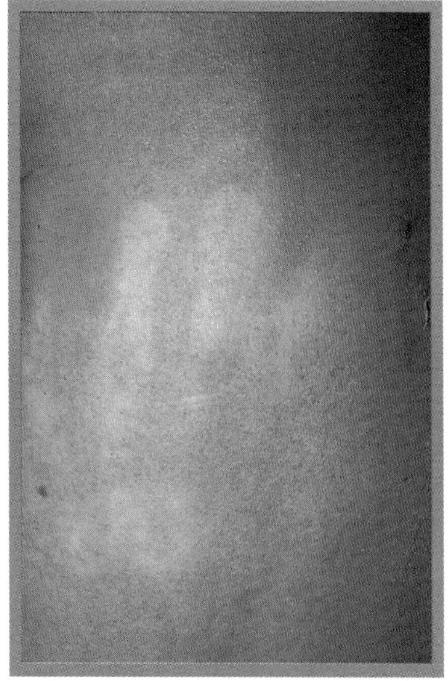

↑ 12.8

Figures 12.9 –12.15 Chickenpox. A range of manifestations and severity of varicella, are shown.

Figures 12.9 –12.10 show a mildly affected child early in the disease process. She looks relatively well, with only a few vesicles present. Note the vesicle on the left lower eyelid and the use of mittens to prevent scratching.

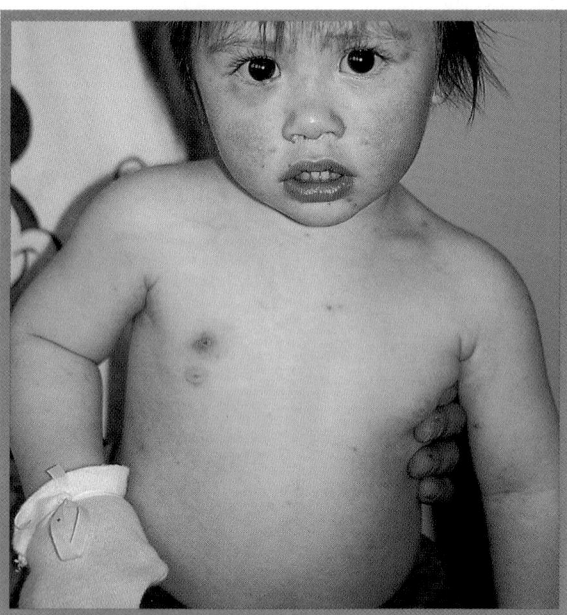

←12.9

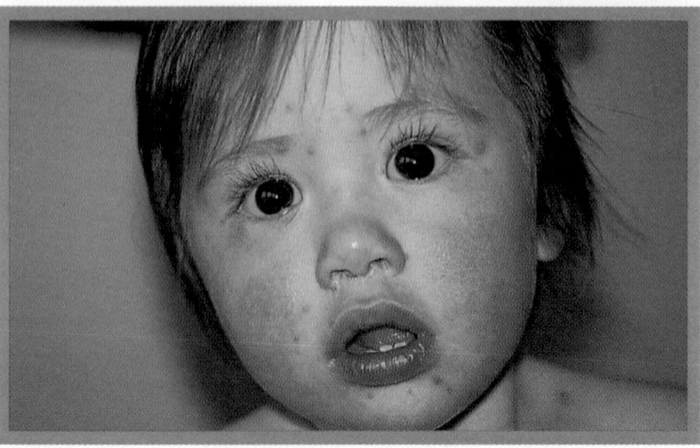

←12.10

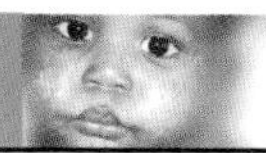

Figures 12.11–12.12 shows a more severely affected child with involvement of the mucosal surfaces. Note the vesicles on the tongue, which interfere with swallowing and feeding. In both this child and that in **Figures 12.9 and 12.10** the vesicles started on the face and scalp, spreading to the trunk, abdomen and limbs.

→12.11

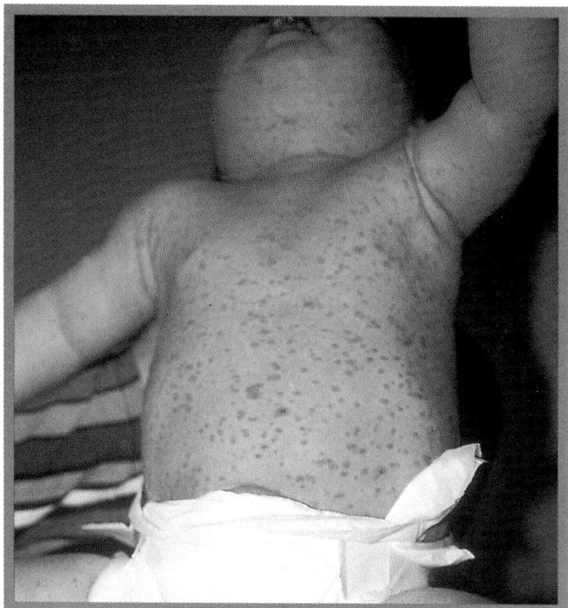

→12.12

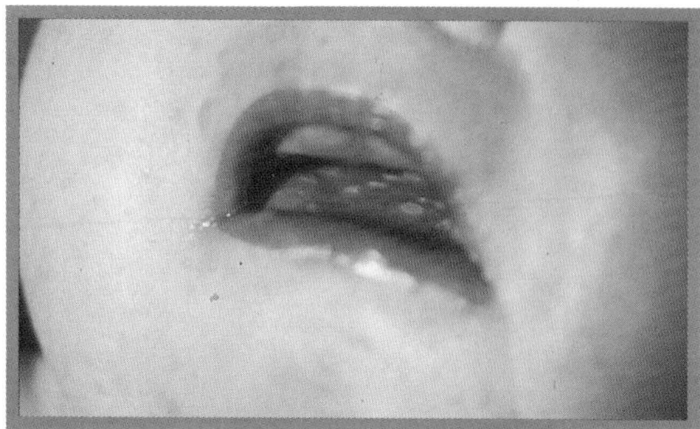

Figures 12.13–12.14 demonstrate some of the complications of chickenpox. Here, secondary infection of the lesions has occurred. The vesicles are erythematous, umbilicated and some hemorrhagic.

Figure 12.15 Purpura fulminans is shown which is a rare complication of chicken pox usually occuring 7–21 days after the onset of the vesicular lesions. The disease is due to widespread venous thrombosis and is associated with acquired protein S deficiency.

Varicella (chickenpox) has an incubation period of 10–20 days. Primary infection results in classic chickenpox, but the virus remains latent in the sensory ganglia. Reactivation, which is commoner in immunocompromised hosts, causes herpes zoster (shingles). Herpes zoster is less infectious than

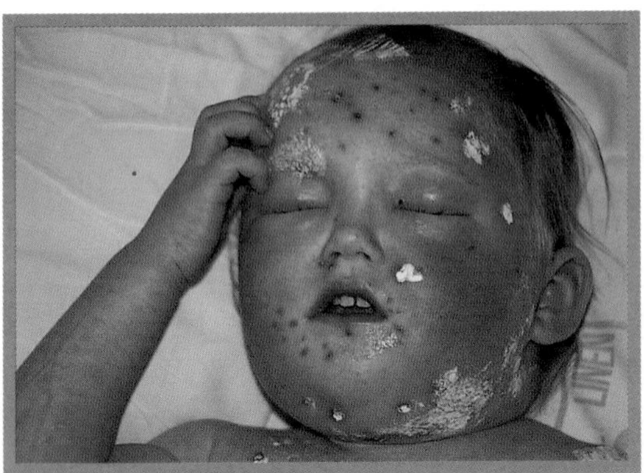

←12.13

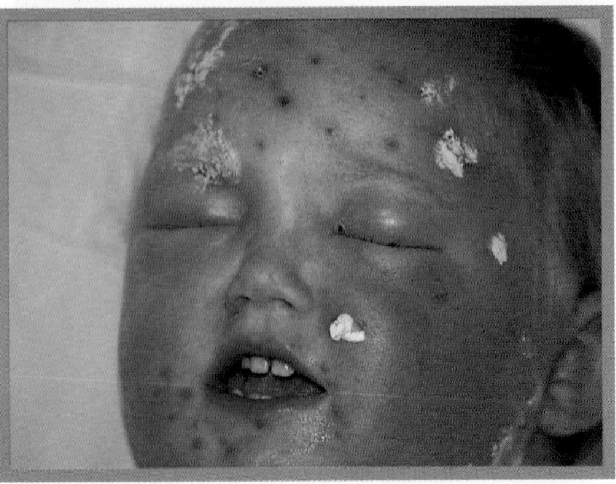

←12.14

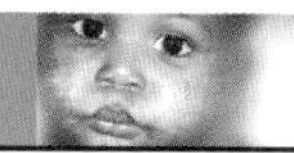

varicella, which is highly contagious. Patients are contagous from 2 days prior to the appearance of the vesicles untill the vesicles are dry.

Complications are:

1. Secondary infection, particularly with *Staphylococcus* and *Streptococcus*.
2. Cerebellar encephalitis.
3. Reye syndrome.
4. Pneumonia.
5. Hemorrhagic lesions that occasionally reflect disseminated intravascular coagulation, but that are more usually due to autoimmune thrombocytopenia.
6. Thrombotic complications, *e.g.* CVA, purpura fulminans
7. Optic neuritis.
8. Transverse myelitis.
9. Orchitis.
10. Arthritis.
11. Disseminated infection in the immunocompromised.

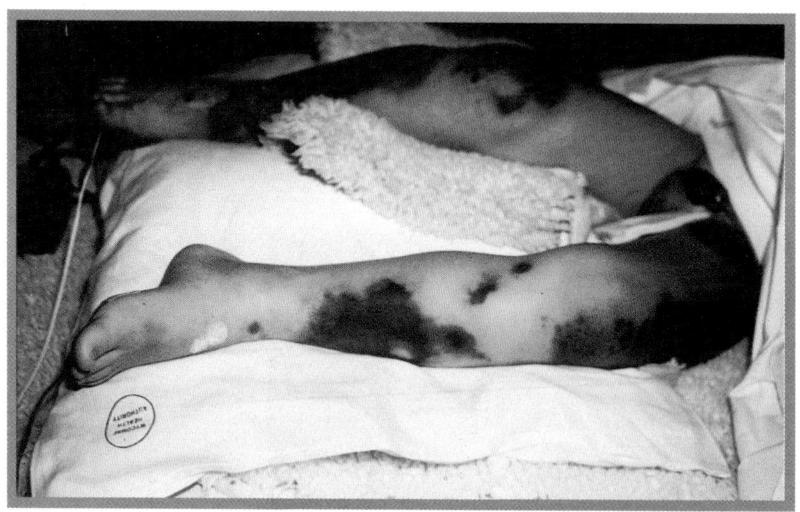

↑ 12.15

Figures 12.16–12.19 Hand, Foot and Mouth Disease. Note the ulcers on the ventral and dorsal aspects of the tongue in **Figures 12.16 and 12.17**. There were also associated ulcers on the oral mucosa. Note the pearly-white vesicles surrounded by red haloes on the soles and palms . There was no associated constitutional upset, but this may occur. This disease is caused by

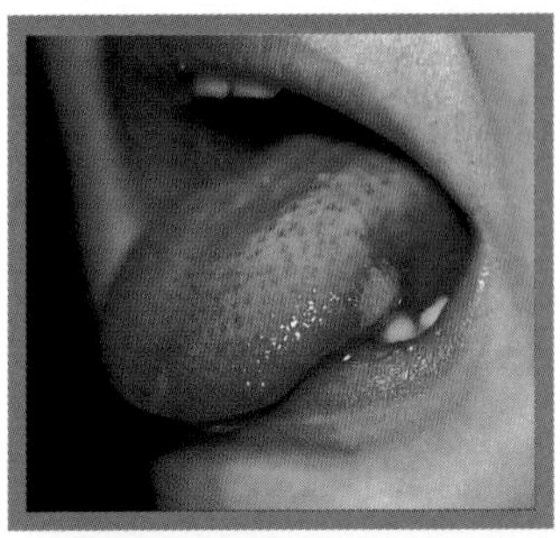

←12.16

→12.17

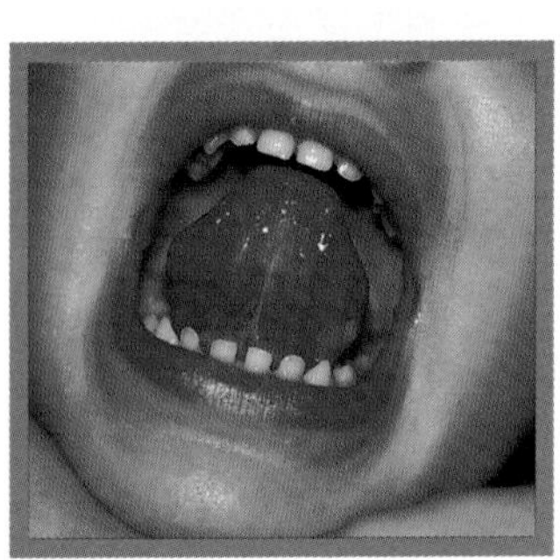

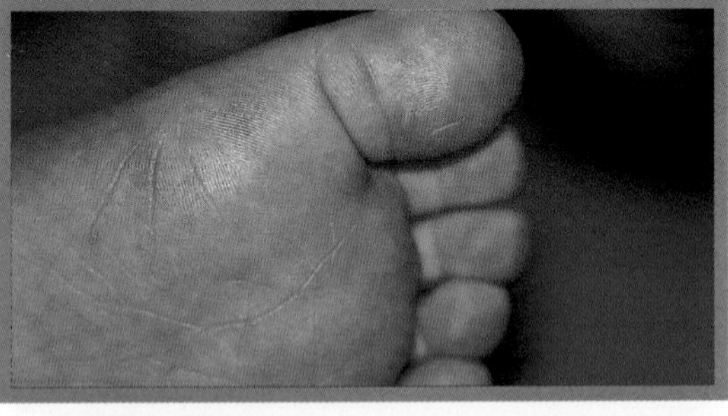

←12.18

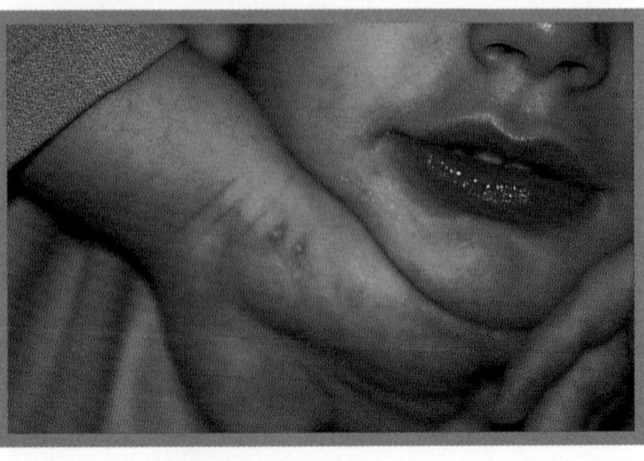

←12.19

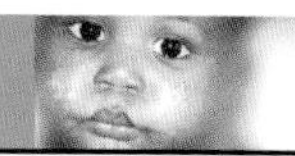

coxsackie viruses A5, A10 and A16. Treatment is symptomatic only, with the use of topical oral anti-inflammatory agents.

Figures 12.20–12.21 Herpes Simplex Virus Type 1 (HSV-1). These figures show infection with herpes simplex. The disease may be particularly severe in the immunocompromised host.

Figures 12.20 and 12.21 demonstrate gingivostomatitis. Note the vesicular lesion and the oral ulceration on the tongue and gingival mucosa, particularly in **Figure 12.21**. The gums are swollen and friable, and bleed easily. In both of these children the condition was accompanied by a high fever and irritability. The condition was treated with analgesia, antipyretics and hydration. Intravenous antiviral therapy is indicated in the immunocompromised child.

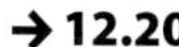

→12.20

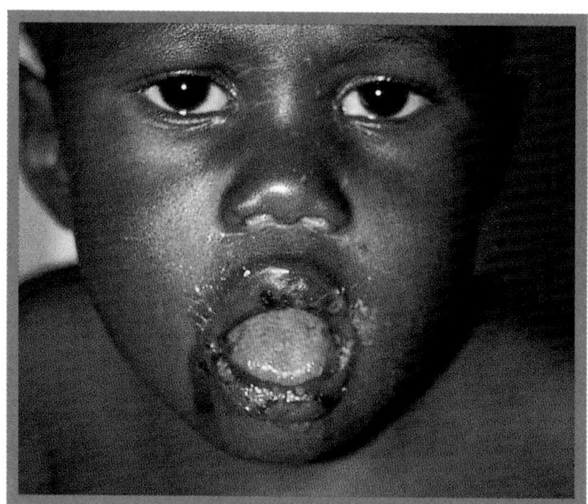

→12.21

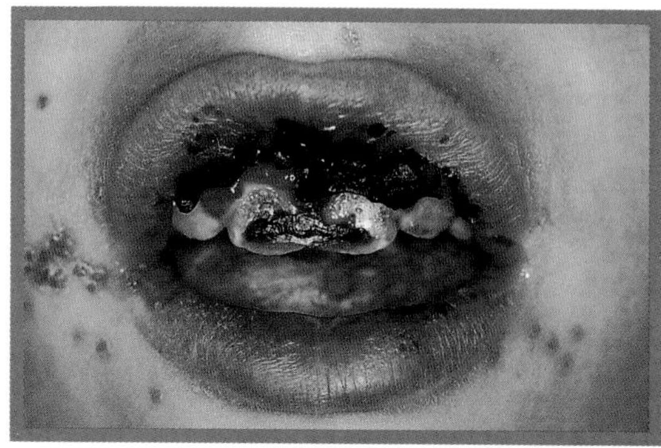

Figures 12.22–12.23 Cutaneous Herpes Simplex Type 2 (HSV-2). The neonate discussed here was infected by the mother. Note the vesicles on the thumb and index finger in **Figure 12.22**.

The skin vesicles can be seen to predominate over a site of trauma where a scalp electrode was sited (**Figure 12.23**).

The disease may disseminate if untreated, particularly if the mother has primary herpes. Intravenous antiviral therapy is indicated and the mother and child should be isolated. Both type 1 and 2 herpes may cause disseminated infection.

Other presentations include:

1. Vulvovaginitis or urethritis.
2. Keratoconjunctivitis, following autoinoculation from the mouth to the eye.
3. Encephalitis, typically involving the frontotemporal region.
4. Eczema herpeticum.

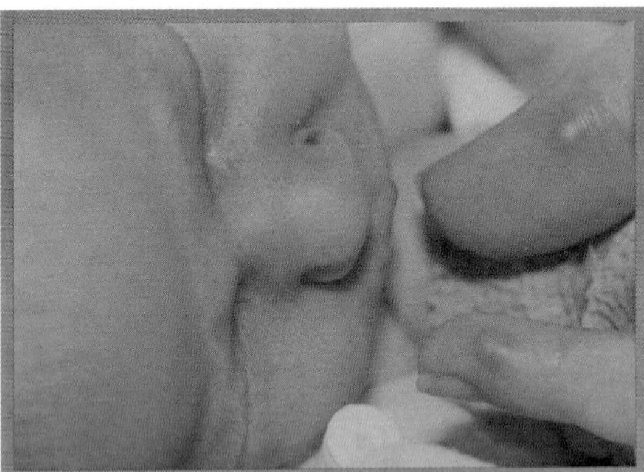

← **12.22**

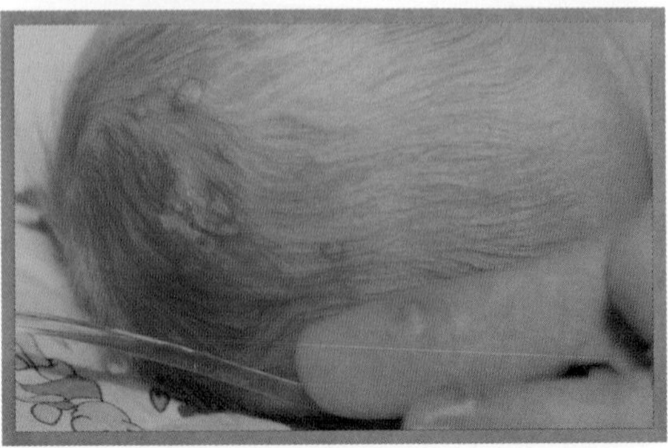

← **12.23**

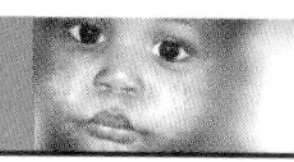

Figure 12.24 Mumps. The child shown here, despite being immunized against mumps, developed a bilateral, tender, parotid swelling associated with fever. Other manifestations of the disease include pancreatitis, orchitis (which occurs in up to one-third of infected post-pubertal males), and meningoencephalitis (which is an important cause of aseptic meningitis).

Complications include sensorineural deafness, myocarditis, transverse myelitis and facial nerve paralysis. The clinical disease is rare in immunized children.

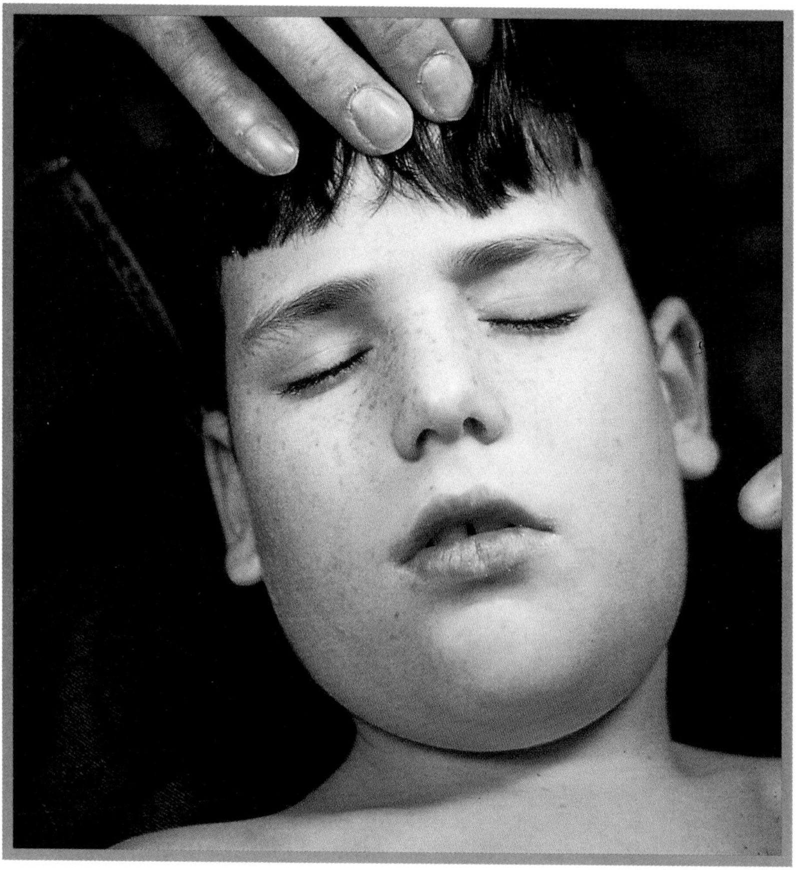

↑ 12.24

Figures 12.25–12.27 Kawasaki Disease. A 4-month-old girl with Kawasaki disease is shown. She presented with a history of high fever of more than 5-days' duration and cervical lymphadenopathy.

Bilateral conjunctival infection and mucous membrane involvement is shown, with dry, cracked, swollen, red lips (**Figure 12.27**). Also shown are edematous, desquamating hands, which developed in the second week of the illness (**Figures 12.25 and 12.26**). She had a polymorphous rash earlier in the disease process.

Investigations showed a neutrophil leukocytosis, thrombocytosis, and a high ESR. Three weeks after the onset of the rash, on echocardiography, the girl was found to have coronary artery involvement, resulting in a myocardial infarction (see Chapter 3, Cardiac Disorders **Figures 3.36 and 3.37**). At diagnosis, the child was treated with high-dose immunoglobulin and aspirin. The aspirin was continued at a high dose until remission of the fever, upon which time the dose was reduced. Histopathological findings are of a vasculitits affecting extraparenchymal muscular arteries.

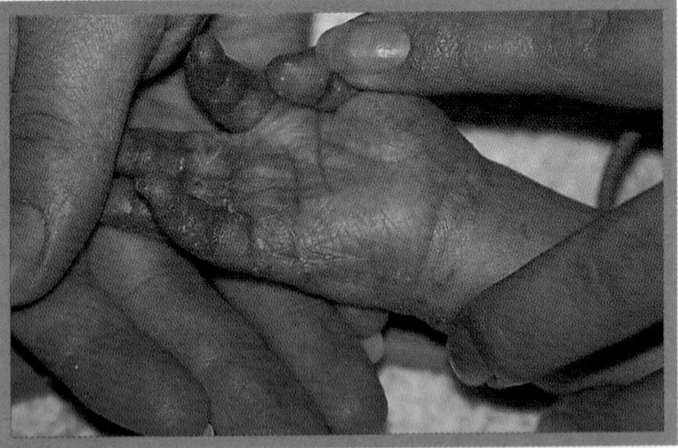

← **12.25**

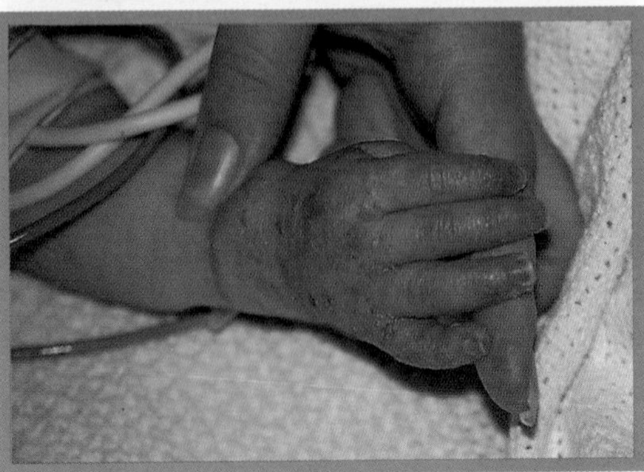

← **12.26**

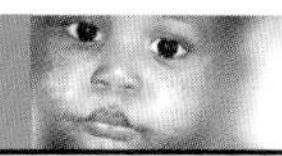

To make the diagnosis, the fever must be present for 5 or more days, and four out of the following five conditions must also be present:

1. Bilateral conjunctival injection.
2. Oral changes: infected pharynx, erythema, fissuring and crusting of the lips, and a 'strawberry tongue'.
3. Lymphadenopathy.
4. A polymorphic nonvesicular rash, primarily on the trunk.
5. Changes in the extremities: edema, erythema and, later, desquamation of the palms and soles.

Other associated complications include arthritis, aseptic meningitis, pericarditis, myocarditis, and hepatitis.

The differential diagnosis includes scarlet fever, erythema multiforme, toxic-shock and toxic-shock-like syndromes, measles, Rocky Mountain spotty fever, and nonspecific viral illnesses.

Although the cause of Kawasaki disease is not known, the epidemiology of the disorder suggests an infective etiology.

Figure 12.28 Desquamation from Viral Illness. The 7-year-old female discussed here has desquamation of the soles of the feet following a viral infection.

→12.27

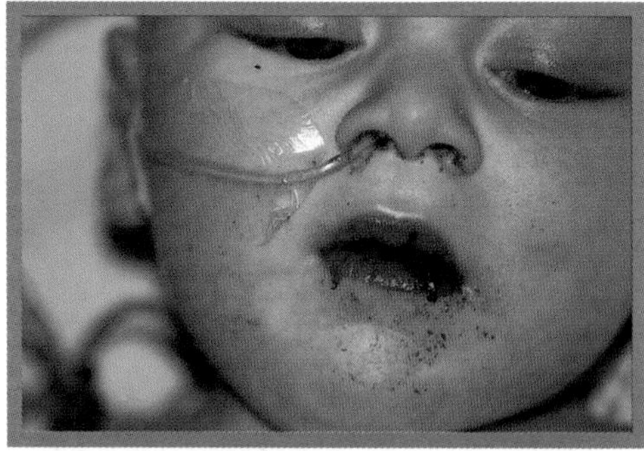

→12.28

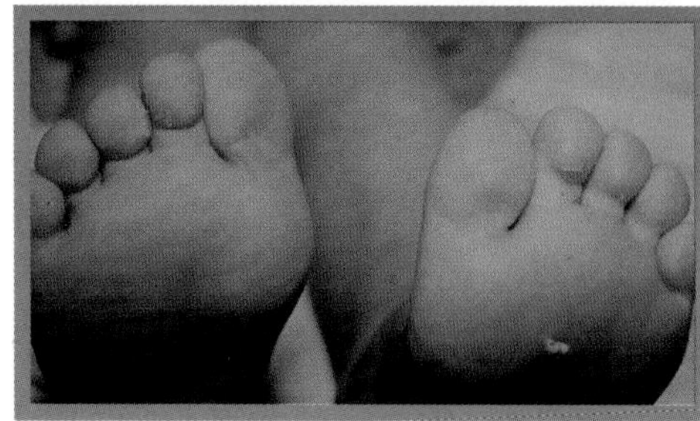

Figures 12.29 and 12.30 Hereditary Angioneurotic Edema. Hereditary angioneurotic edema in a 12-year-old girl following minor injury to the upper right arm, is shown (**Figure 12.29**).

Note the edema of the right arm and hand, which resolved after 2 days following an infusion of fresh frozen plasma.

Investigations confirmed a deficiency of C_1 esterase inhibitor. The disease can also present with painful intestinal edema, and laryngeal edema that may obstruct the airway.

Danazol is an effective prophylactic but is ineffective during an acute attack.

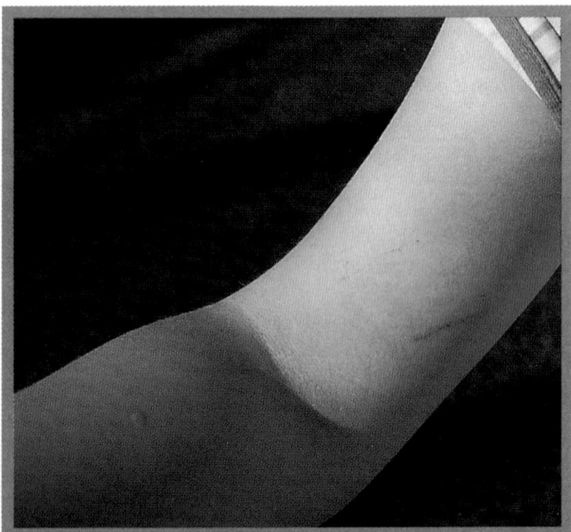

←12.29

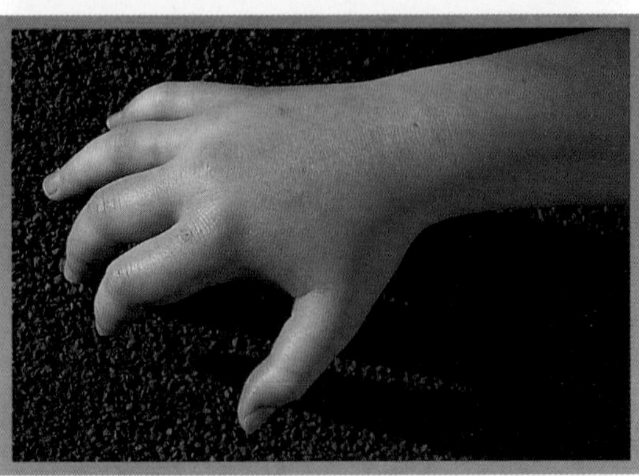

←12.30

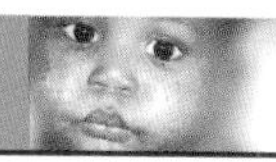

Figures 12.31 and 12.32 Macrophage Dysfunction with Disseminated Mycobacterium. The 9-year-old boy shown here has a macrophage dysfunction – a recently described inherited immunodeficiency caused by gamma interferon receptor deficiency. He has disseminated mycobacterial infection. Cervical lymphadenopathy is shown, as is a marked failure to thrive, and wasting of the limbs, with swelling of the face as a result of superior vena caval obstruction.

Mycobacterial diseases may present with isolated lymphadenopathy or with sinus formation. Treatment of well localized single node disease is by surgical excision. The modern macrolides may be an effective therapy for atypical mycobacterial diseases, that cannot be fully removed surgically.

→12.31

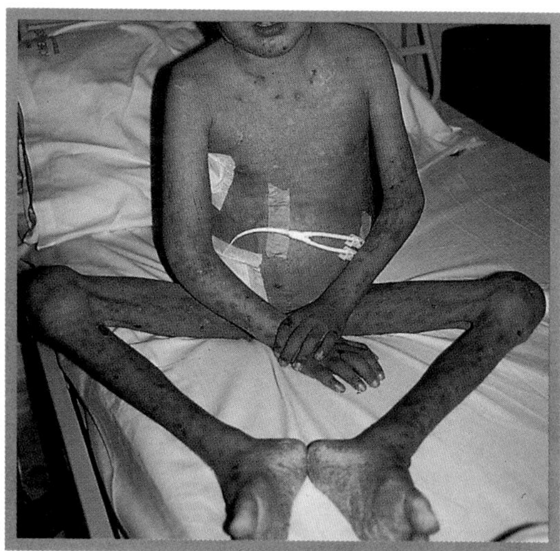

→12.32

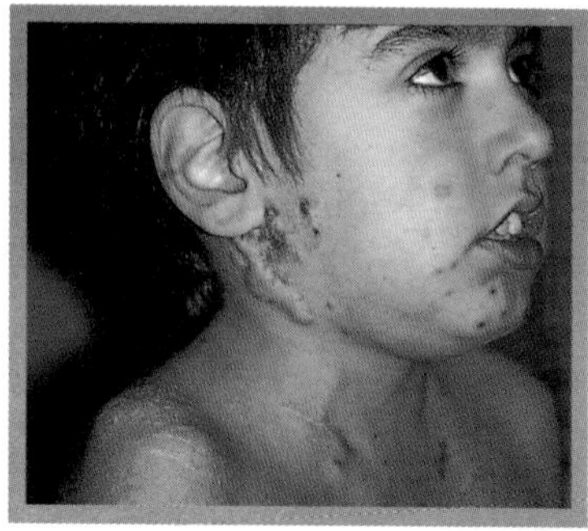

Figures 12.33 and 12.34 Henoch–Schönlein Purpura. Henoch–Schönlein purpura (HSP) is shown in a 4-year-old boy (**Figure 12.33**) and a 3-year-old girl (**Figure 12.34**). Note the petechial lesions on the extensor surfaces of the legs, arms, and face. Note also the girl's orbital hemorrhage with bilateral orbital edema, which is caused by nephrotic syndrome resulting from HSP. Associated symptoms were colicky abdominal pain and polyarthralgia. Both children had had a preceding upper respiratory tract infection.

→12.33

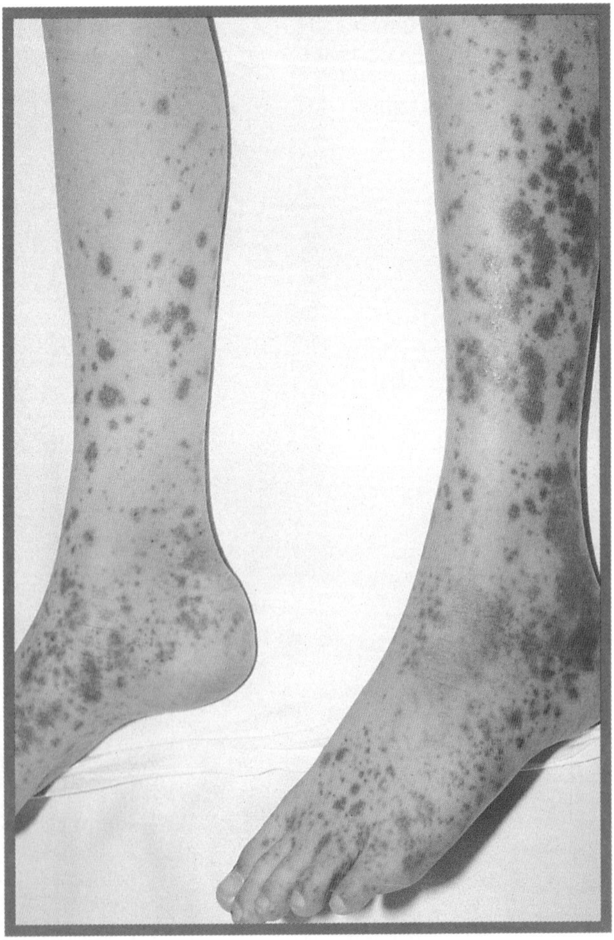

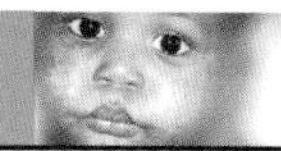

Differential diagnosis includes meningococcal septicemia, idiopathic thrombocytopenia, and non-accidental injury.

Figure 12.35 Insect Sting. A reaction to a bee sting is seen here on the dorsal aspect of the upper arm. Other insects/hymenoptera of medical importance are: wasps, hornets, yellow jackets and some types of ant and scorpion. The ensuing reaction is both immunological and pharmacological, resulting from the release of proteolytic enzymes, peptides and other vasoactive substances.

→ 12.34

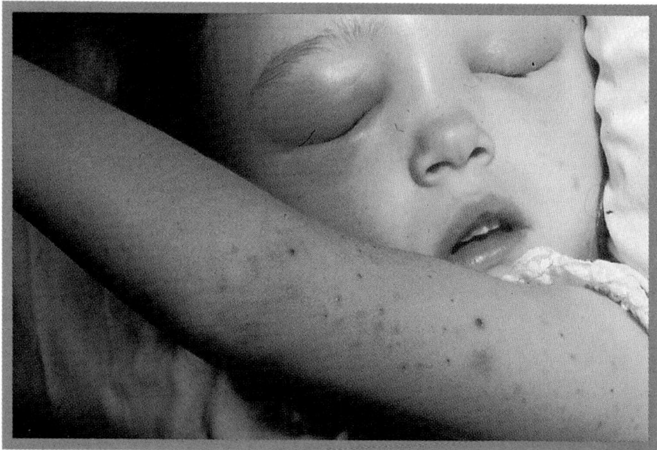

→ 12.35

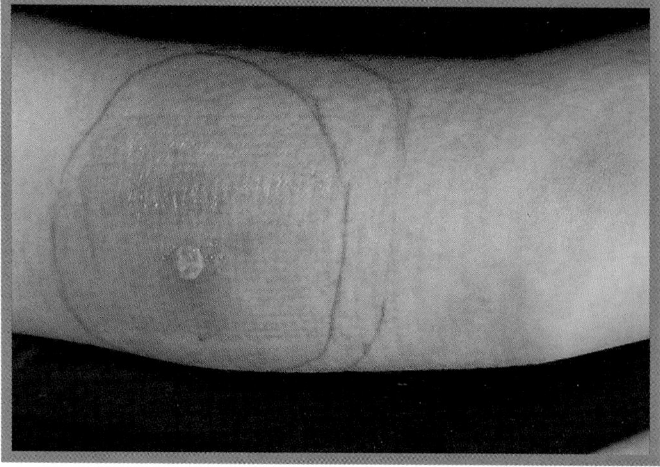

Figures 12.36–12.38 Necrotizing Fasciitis. The 3-week-old female shown here has necrotizing fasciitis of the right mammary area that involves the entire chest wall. She presented with swelling of her right anterior chest wall, and pyrexia, and was systemically unwell.

On examination, the chest wall was found to be red, hot and inflamed. No mass could be identified (**Figure 12.36**). A full blood count showed a neutropenia.

On excision and debridement, liquefied fat, necrotic tissue and pus which later grew *Staphylococcus aureus* was found (**Figure 12.37**).

Necrotizing fasciitis is a rapidly extending erythema of the skin, which is often centrally necrotic. There is systemic upset and a clinically toxic appearance. A high level of suspicion of the disease is required as there may be no specific signs suggesting focal collection of pus. Early surgical exploration is required, and radical surgical excision and debridement with concomitant use of broad spectrum antibiotics is the treatment of choice. *Staphylococcus* and *Streptococcus* are the most commonly isolated organisms.

Figure 12.38 shows another child with the same condition. Note the extent of tissue destruction.

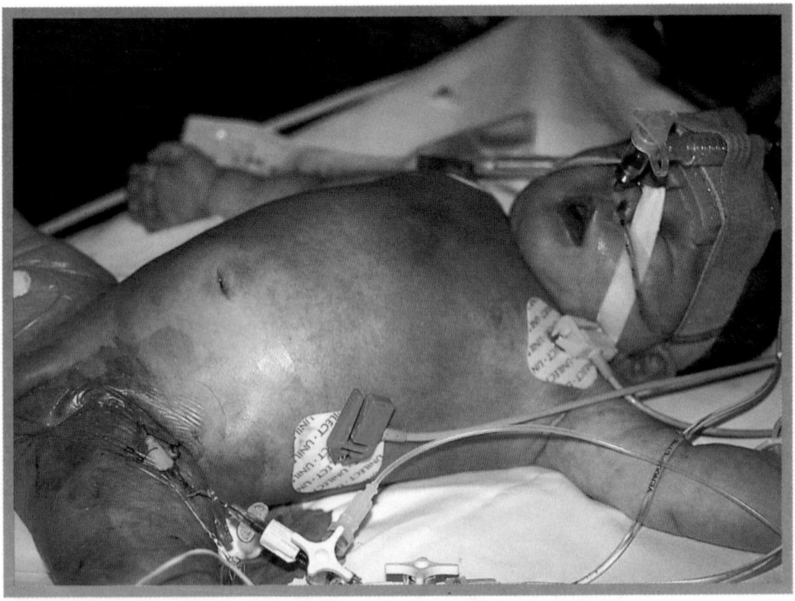

↑ 12.36

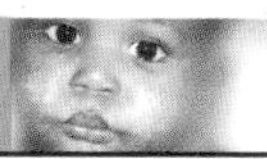

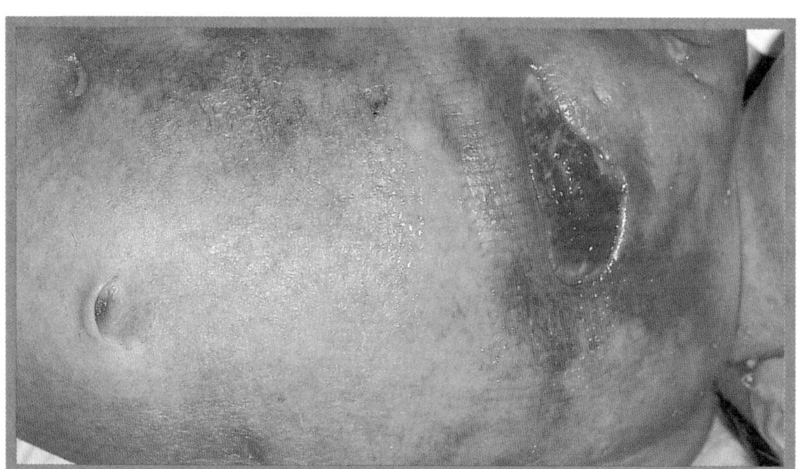

↑ 12.37

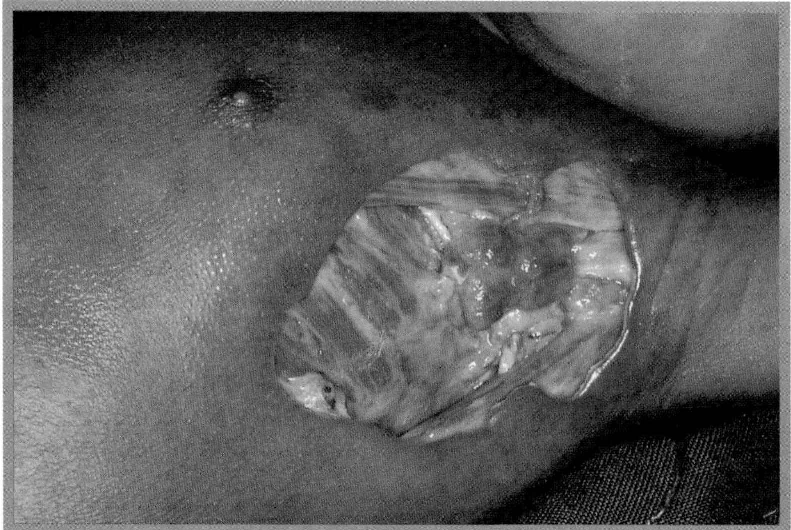

↑ 12.38

Figures 12.39–12.41 Toxic-Shock Syndrome. The 1-year-old child discussed here presented with a high fever, macular rash, confusion, vomiting, right-sided groin lymphadenitis , reduced urine output and shock. On examination she was unable to extend the right leg fully because of the painful lymphadenopathy, and there was poor capillary return with evidence of poor peripheral perfusion.

Note the red, confluent, macular, scarlatiniform rash, particularly over the limbs, the edema of the face and limbs, and the red conjunctivae and lips.

Staphylococcus aureus producing toxic-shock-syndrome toxin 1 was isolated from the infected site.

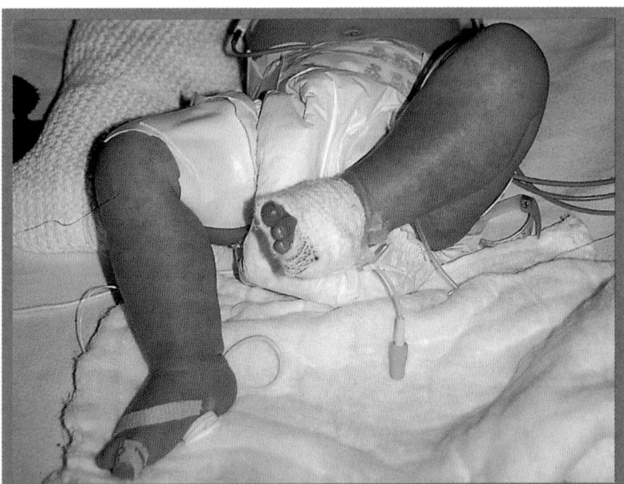

← 12.39

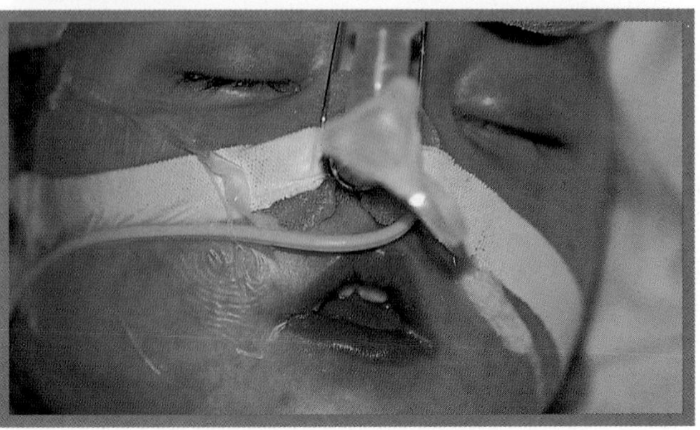

← 12.40

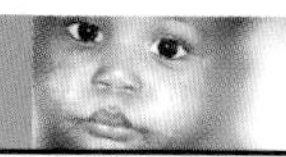

Treatment consisted in aggressive and rapid resuscitation in an intensive care area. It also requires the identification of the site and removal of any focus of infection and administration of antistaphylococcal antibiotics. Intravenous immunoglobulins may also be of benefit.

A similar toxic-shock picture can be produced by toxigenic strains of *Streptococcus.*

Figures 12.42–12.46 Meningococcal Infection. The children discussed here show a range of the manifestations of meningococcal infection. The characteristic non-blanching petechial rash can be seen in either meningitis or septicemia and can range from small petechiae to purpura fulminans.

Figures 12.42 and 12.43 Meningococcal Meningitis. A 4-year-old girl with early features of the disease is shown. This girl presented with the rapid onset symptoms of meningitis: headache, stiff neck, vomiting and a reduced level of consciousness. These were accompanied by a rapidly spreading petechial rash that was non-blanching.

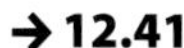

→ 12.41

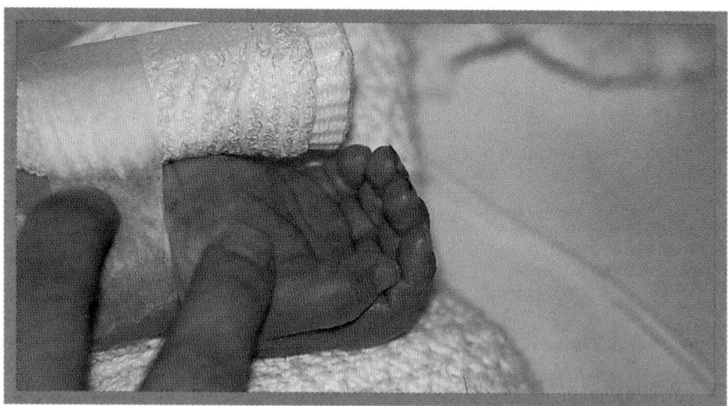

→ 12.42

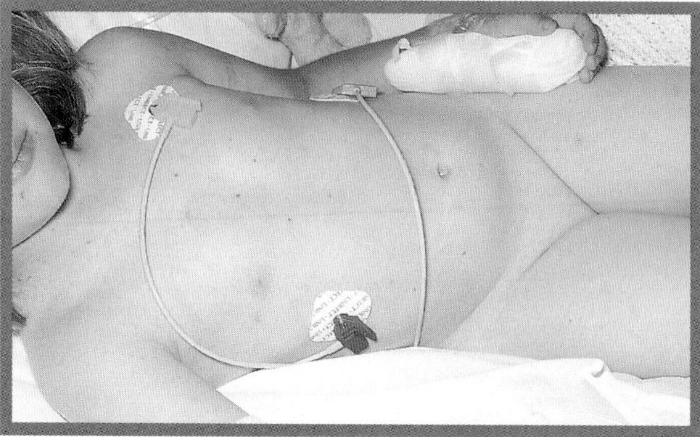

Figures 12.44–12.46 Meningococcal Septicemia. Two children with more severe meningococcal disease are shown here, They had high fever, shock, and hypotension following a prodromal respiratory tract infection. A purpuric, non-blanching skin rash is clearly seen. They subsequently developed a disseminated intravascular coagulopathy, skin and mucous membrane hemorrhages and skin necrosis.

All of the children discussed had positive blood cultures for *Neisseria meningitidis* and were meningococcal-polysaccharide-antigen positive. The majority of the population who carry *Meningococcus* in the nasopharynx are asymptomatic. Fewer than 1% will develop the disease, which presents most

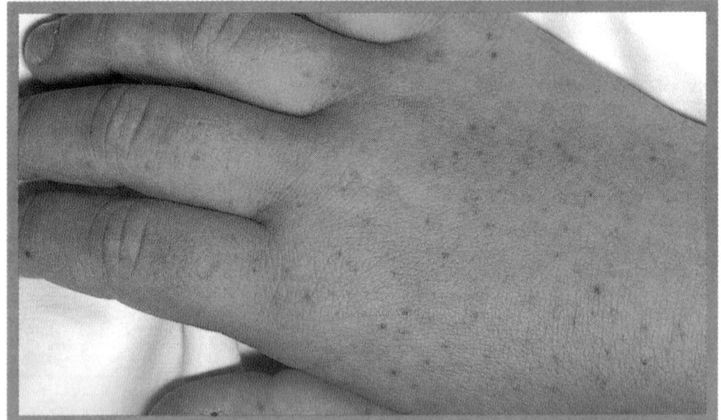

←12.43

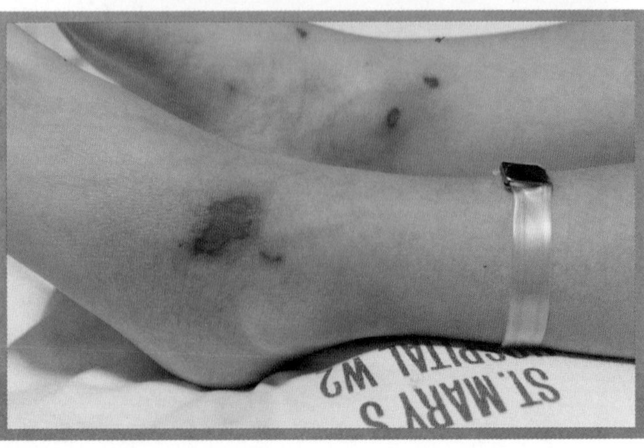

←12.44

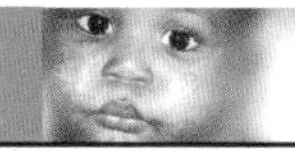

commonly as meningitis and septicemia but also as pericarditis, septic arthritis, pneumonia or otitis media.

Meningococcus can be separated into types A, B and C, Y and W-135. Each strain differs in its virulence and potential for epidemic spread.

Patients deficient in complement C6, 7and 8 and those with reduced splenic function are particularly susceptible. The severity of the disease depends on the amount of an endotoxin present; it causes endothelial damage and disseminated intravascular coagulation.

Treatment involves antibiotics, resuscitation and intensive care unit cardiopulmonary and hematological support. Rifampicin prophylaxis should be given to household members and kissing contacts.

→ 12.45

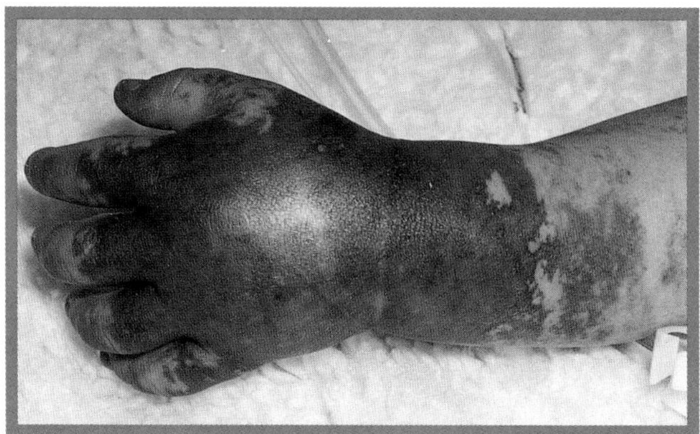

→ 12.46

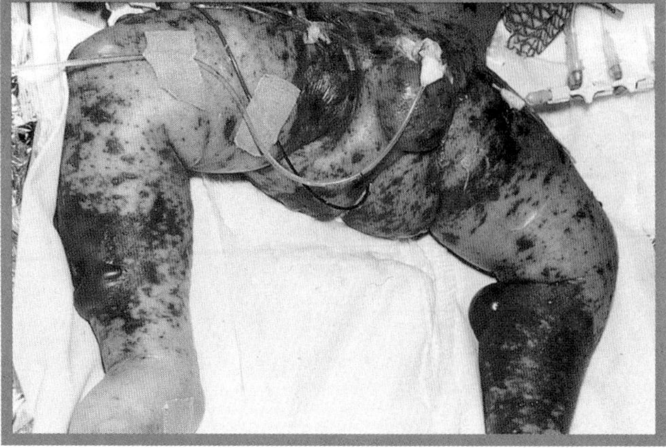

Figures 12.47 and 12.48 Impetigo. Impetigo is shown on the face and chest of a 3-year-old girl (top), and bullous impetigo is shown over the right elbow at the site of an eczematous patch of skin on a 5-year-old boy (bottom). Note the annular

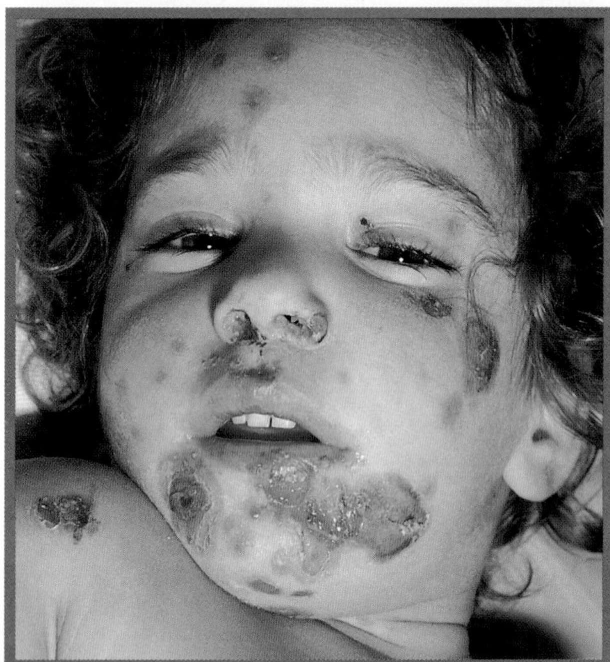

← **12.47**

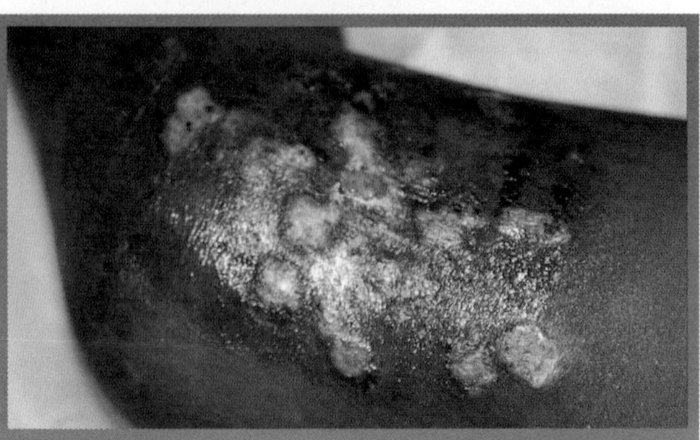

← **12.48**

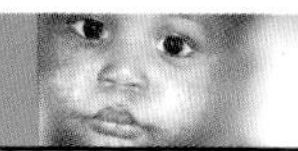

erosions with honey-colored crusts and hyperkeratosis of the flexural surfaces. The cases were treated using anti-staphylococcal antibiotics and isolation.

Impetigo can also result from group A *Streptococcus,* when it is possible to get nephritogenic strains resulting in glomerulonephritis in endemic areas.

Impetigo is an intraepidermal lesion that does not leave scarring.

Figure 12.49 Submandibular Abscess. The 4-week-old boy had a 5-day history of swelling over the left submandibular area. The swelling was 2 cm × 2 cm in area. The lesion was tender, fluctuant, hot and inflamed. Ultrasound showed the prescence of a fluid-filled mass. Aspirated pus grew *Staphylococcus* and the lesion was incised and drained. Antibiotic treatment was initiated.

Figure 12.50 Whitlow. Whitlow of bacterial origin is shown on the right thumb in a 1-month-old infant. It was treated with antibiotics. Whitlow can often be chronic and are then usually caused by fungi, *e.g., Candida.* Whitlow may also be viral, *e.g.,* herpetic.

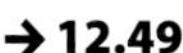

→ 12.49

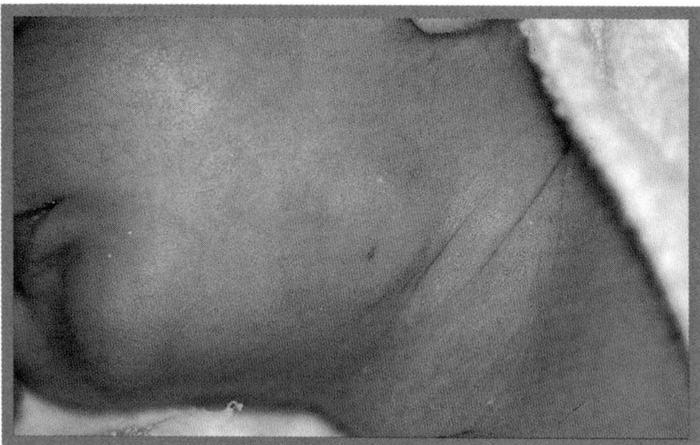

→ 12.50

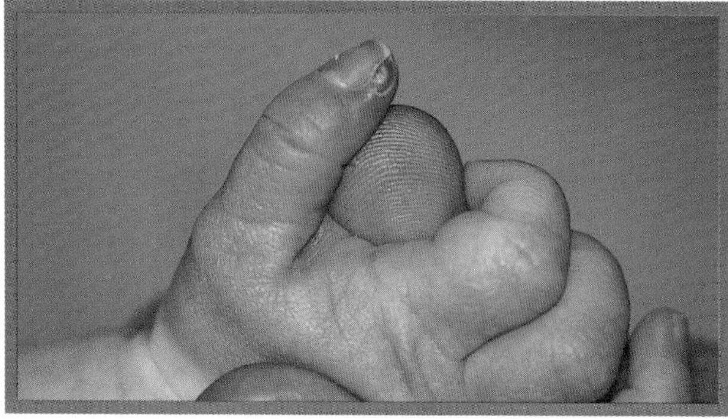

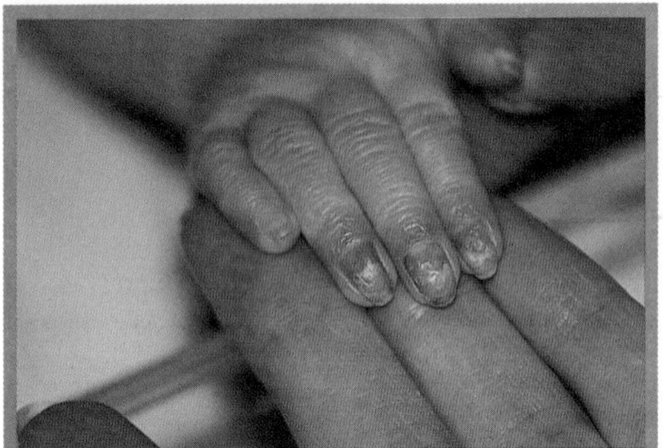

← 12.51

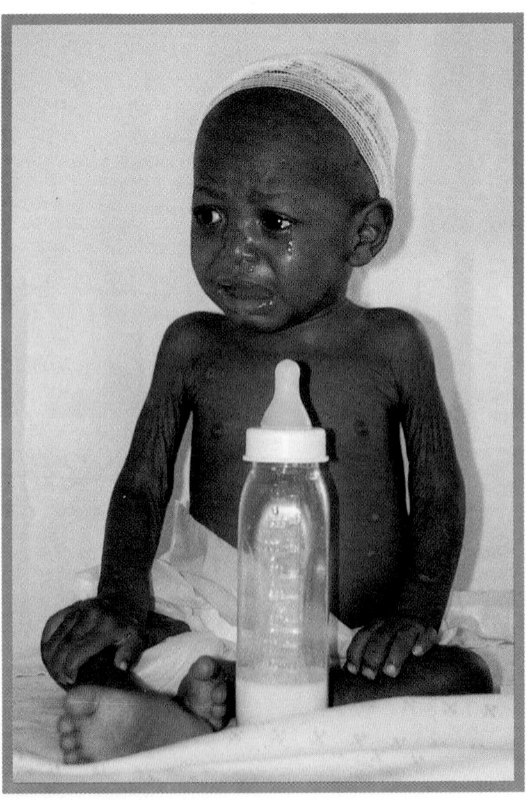

← 12.52

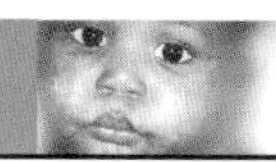

Figure 12.51 Cutaneous Candidiasis. The clinical features of cutaneous candidiasis can be seen, particularly at the terminal ends of the finger nails. The differential diagnosis is Beau lines resulting from arrested nail growth during acute illness.

Candidiasis occurs classically in the skin, mouth and groin. Extensive involvement of the nail bed as shown here may be associated with T- cell abnormalities. Treatment is application of topical and sytemic antifungal agents.

Figures 12.52–12.58 Human Immunodeficiency Virus (HIV) Infection. HIV is a major problem worldwide. It may present with failure to thrive or as any of a wide range of opportunistic infections, *e.g., Pneumocystis* carinii, cutaneous candidiasis, focal infections, and other viral infections.

Figure 12.52 Failure to Thrive. The 2-year-old girl shown here had marked failure to thrive. There is extreme muscle wasting and the child has a miserable affect. She had chronic diarrhea and gross motor, speech and language delay.

Figures 12.53–12.54 HIV and Chickenpox. Figure 12.53 shows chickenpox with secondary infection due to invasive fungi.

Figures 12.54 Non-healing Ulcers following Chickenpox. Varicella may be life threatening in the immunosuppressed patient, often progressing to pneumonia, encephalitis and hepatitis requiring parenteral antiviral treatment as well as antibiotic treatment of secondary infections.

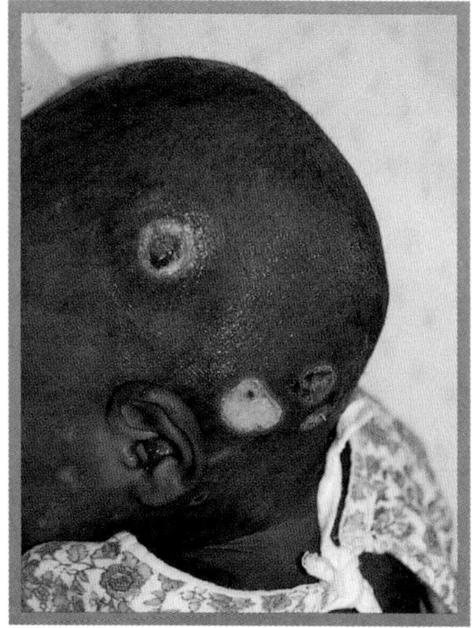

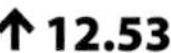 **12.53**

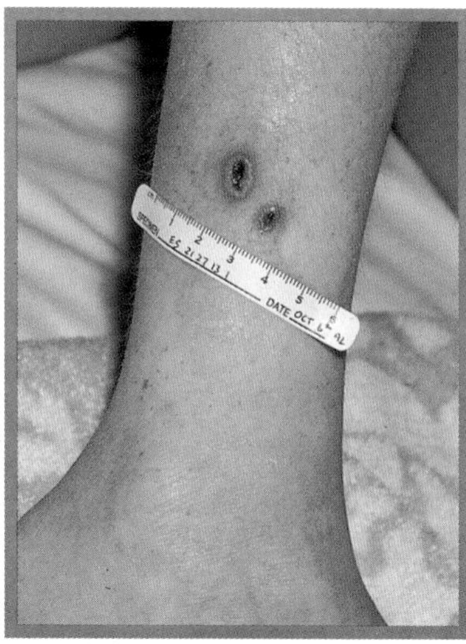

↑ 12.54

Figure 12.55 Herpes Zoster in an HIV-Infected Child. Reactivation along the C3 dermatome of latent varicella in a child with HIV is shown. The left shoulder is affected. The child initially suffered from pain over this area followed a few days later by clusters of papules over the area of pain, some of which have crusted over. There is associated regional lymphadenopathy.

Treatment consists of admininstration of intravenous antiviral drugs.

In the HIV-positive patient there is additional risk of dissemination, secondary infection, herpes encephalitis, or peripheral neuropathy .

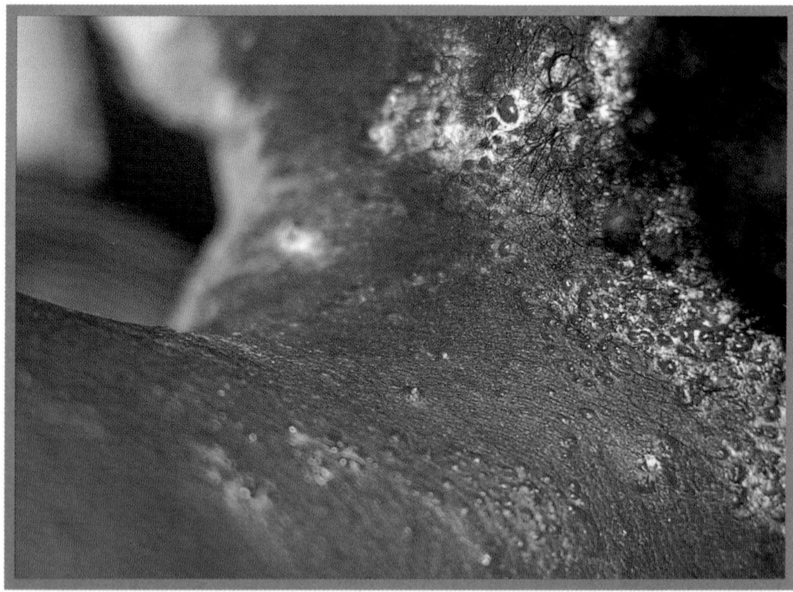

↑ 12.55

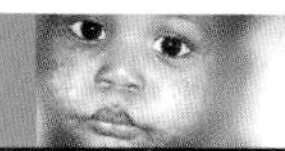

Figure 12.56 Fluorescent Antibody Staining of Varicella Used to aid diagnosis.

Figure 12.57 Kaposi Sarcoma. Kaposi sarcoma is uncommon in childhood and rarely manifests as a cutaneous lesion. A skin lesion in an adolescent is shown. The lesion presents as a red, raised nodule.

Kaposi sarcoma is a vascular multifocal malignant tumor. Although rare, Kaposi sarcoma in childhood is aggressive and fulminant and is found in the liver, lymph nodes, lungs and intestine.

Treatment consists of radiotherapy or chemotherapy.

→12.56

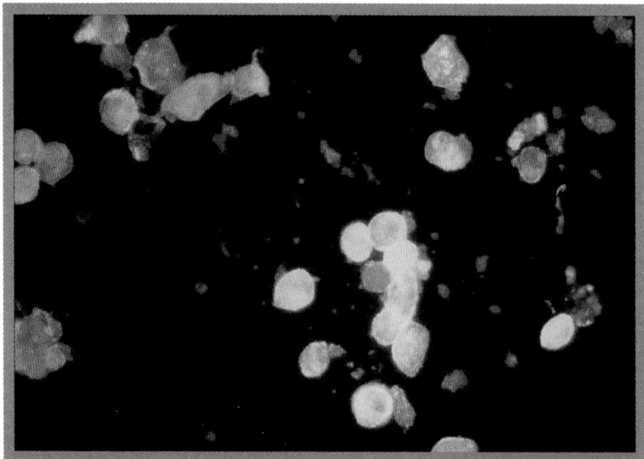

→12.57

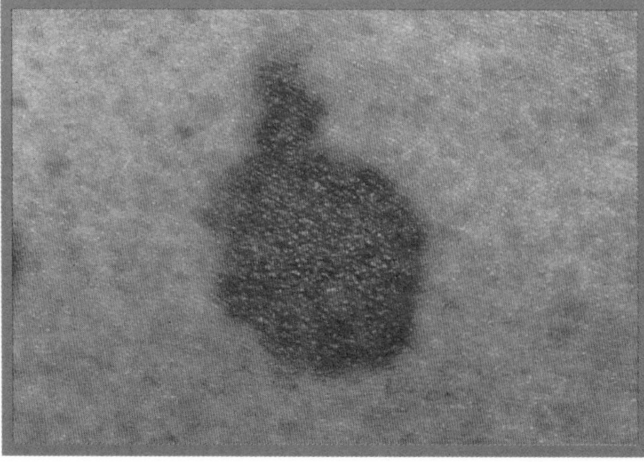

Figure 12.58 Folliculitis. Acneiform eruption is shown in a patient with AIDS. Treatment involves the use of disinfectant cleansing solutions with prolonged courses of low-dose antibiotics.

Pulmonary and ophthalmological manifestations of HIV infection are illustrated in chapters 4 and 15.

Figure 12.59 Congenital Syphilis. Syphilis is shown in a newborn female. A number of features of infection by spirochetes of the fetal skeleton are shown. There is a diffuse diaphysitis present with a hyperplastic cortex. Additionally, metaphysitis can be seen as transverse bands sandwiching areas of diminished density at the ends of the shafts of the long bones. Lateral metaphyseal defects are seen bilaterally at the proximal and medial ends of the tibia (Wimberger sign).

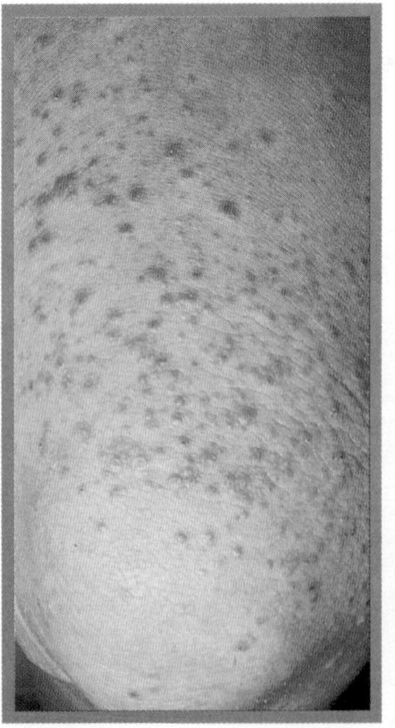

↑ **12.58**

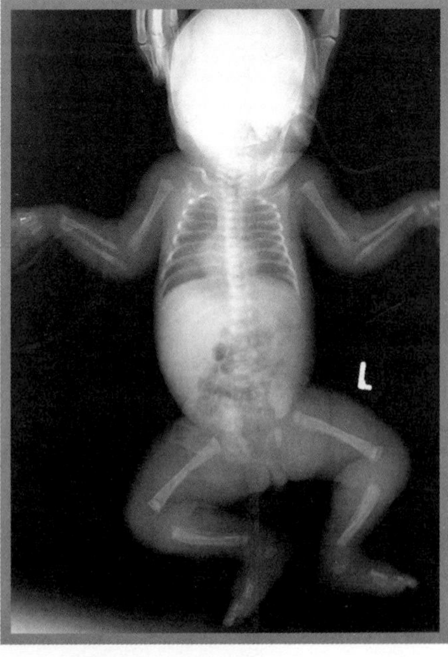

↑ **12.59**

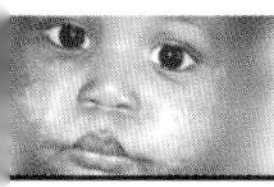

13 Non-accidental injury and neglect

This chapter is included to emphasize the importance of the clinical features of non-accidental injury to the general practitioner and expert alike. The pictures demonstrate how important it is to examine all parts of the child routinely. The format is designed to give an overview of the nature of the clinical features that are more frequently found.

The reader is advised that this is one of the most contentious areas of pediatrics in terms of the interpretation of clinical signs. The radiological features are also subject to interpretation, and this section of the book must not be considered an expert guide to the radiological findings of non-accidental injury.

Figure 13.1 Facial appearance. 'Frozen awareness' associated with profound and prolonged deprivation.

Figure 13.2 Same child as in **Figure 13.1** shown 1 year after reception into foster care. Ultimately the child was returned to his own family after agreement with the social services.

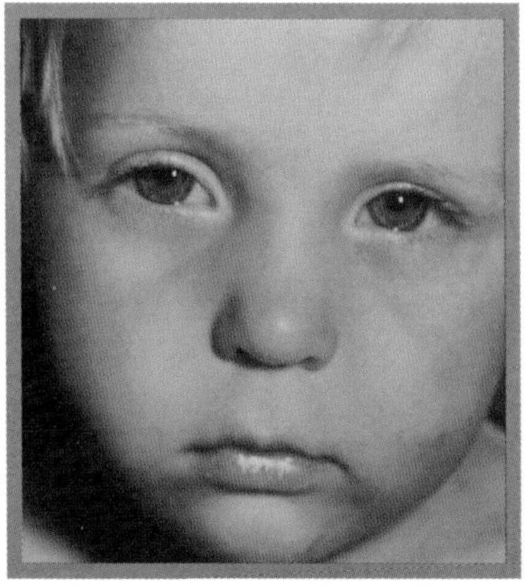

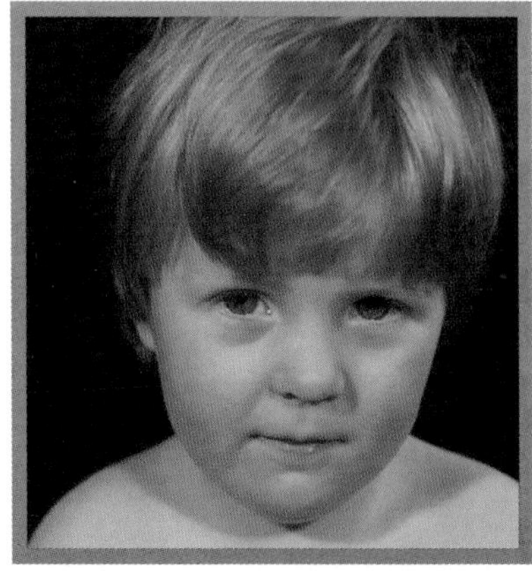

↑ 13.1

↑ 13.2

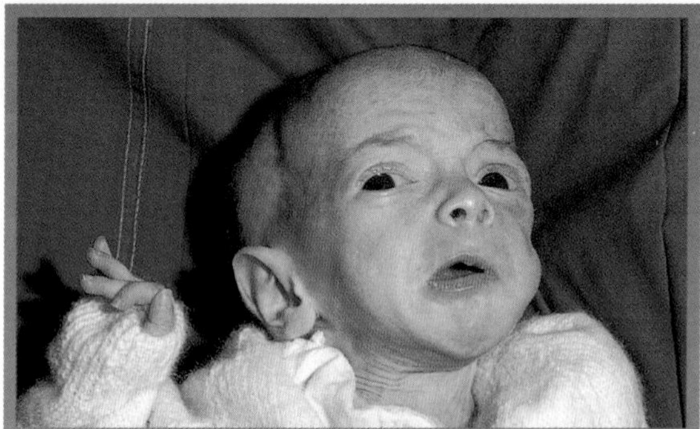

←13.3

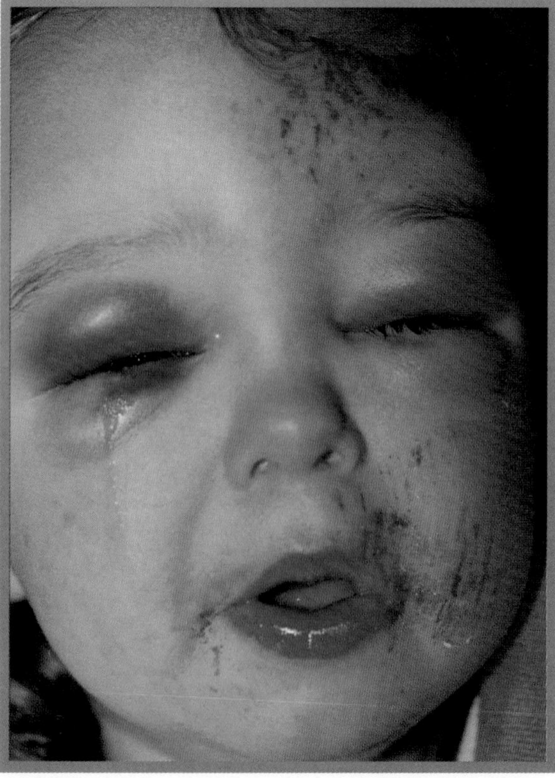

←13.4

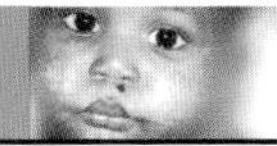

Figure 13.3 Gross Failure to Thrive. This child had been left in the care of a sibling. Access by health visitors had been denied and the police were required to forcibly enter the house to gain access to the infant.
Figure 13.4 Bilateral Periorbital Hematoma. Black eyes* and facial abrasions are shown in this 2-year-old. At presentation there was an alleged history of 'falling out of the cot'. Note the linear scratches on the face . On later enquiry it emerged that the child had been dropped from a first floor window.

There was bilateral orbital bruising suggestive of an anterior fossa skull fracture. This was confirmed on X-ray. A full skeletal survey showed no other fractures.
Figure 13.5 Facial Bruising. The 8-month-old child shown here has facial bruising due to a slap. Note the multiple purpuric elements to the bruise, as opposed to the confluent redness of slapped-cheek disease.
Figure 13.6 Facial Bruising (in a Slightly Older Child). The bruising is more confluent in this child and has a bluish tinge. The handprint can just be identified.

→13.5

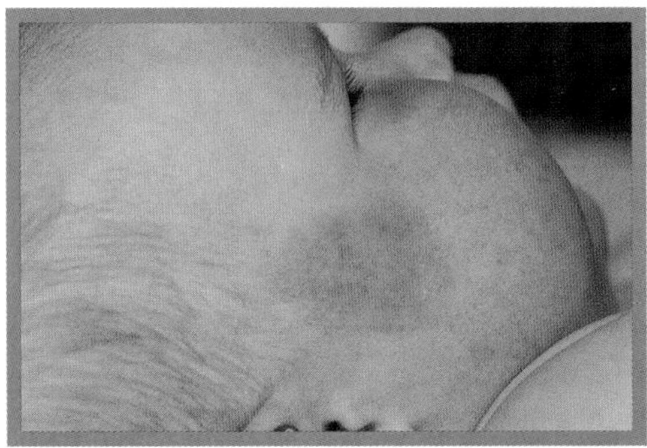

→13.6

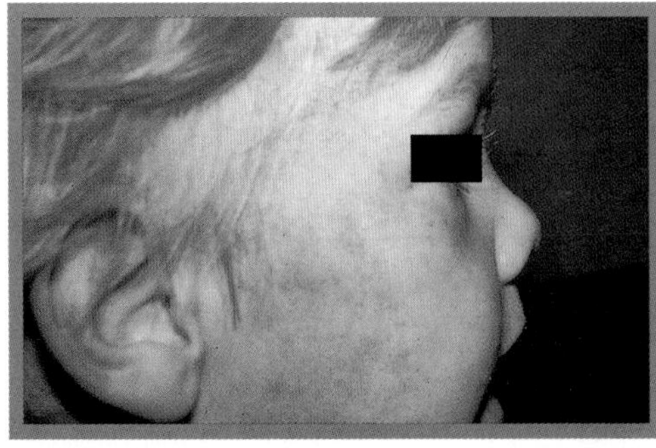

*One must be careful when using the term 'black eye'. 'Bruise around the eye' which is often used to replace it, may be a more sensitive term, but does not raise sufficient anxiety.

Figure 13.7 Linear Facial Bruises. The bruise seen here was caused by a slap. The linear bruises on the cheek correspond to the fingers.
Figure 13.8 Finger Tip Bruising. The 1-year-old shown here sustained finger tip bruising of the chest resulting from being grabbed forcefully. This bruising is commonly associated with a shaking injury and underlying rib fractures caused by the forceful compression.

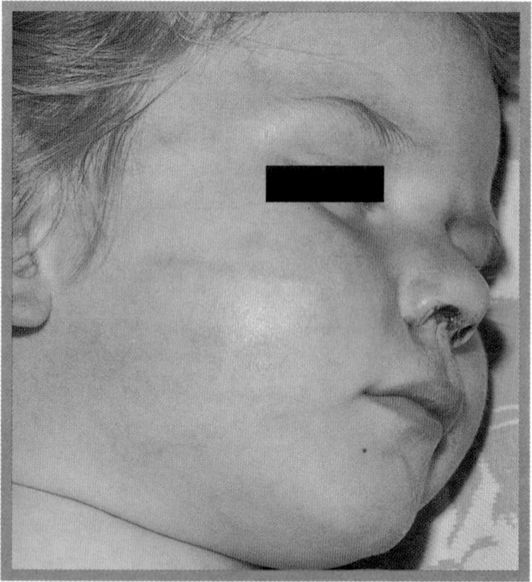

←13.7

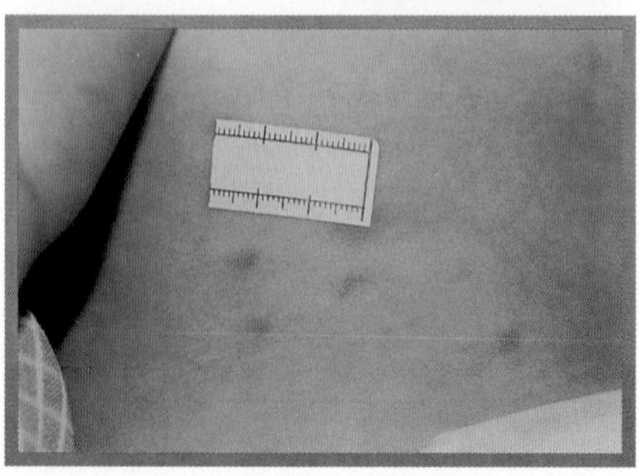

←13.8

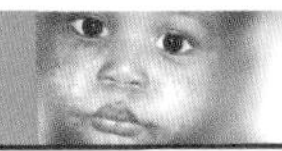

Figure 13.9 Unilateral Periorbital Hematoma (Black Eye). In this case the injury was caused by a punch. Unilateral black eyes should always raise the suspicion of a non-accidental injury, especially in the absence of any other damage to the scalp or forehead. The orbit is a relatively well protected site and is rarely accidentally injured in the young child. Note that blood extravasation does not always occur straight away.

Figure 13.10 Thigh Bruising (Ultraviolet Photograph). This 12-year-old girl had been the victim of a sexual assault. Bruising of the right inner thigh resulted from a human bite.

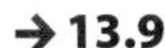

→ 13.9

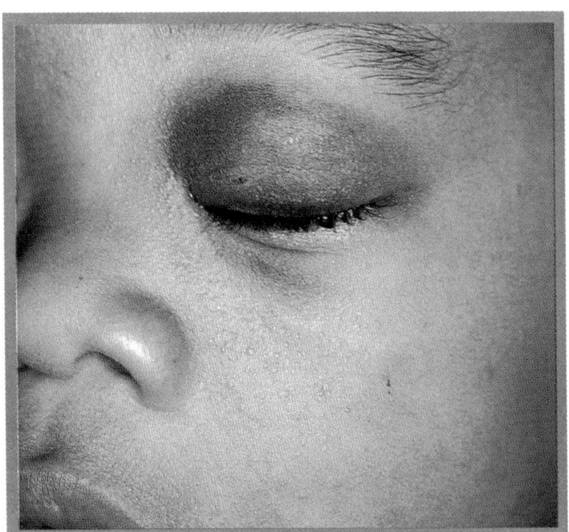

→ 13.10

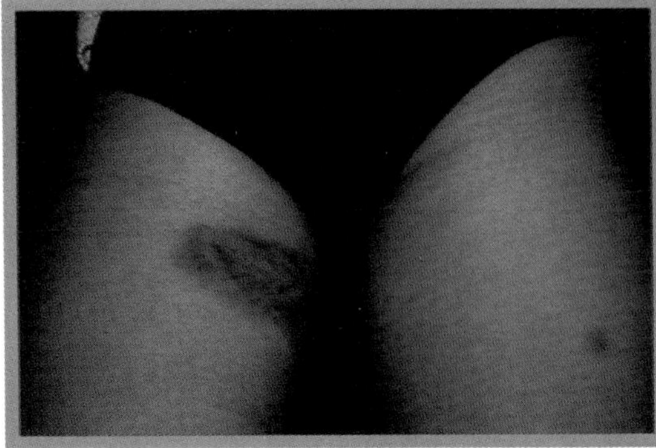

Figures 13.11 and 13.12 Bruising on the Forearm. No explanation was found for this bruising initially. On closer examination, all the bruises were found to be of the same age and corresponded to the grip of an adult hand (**Figure 13.12).**

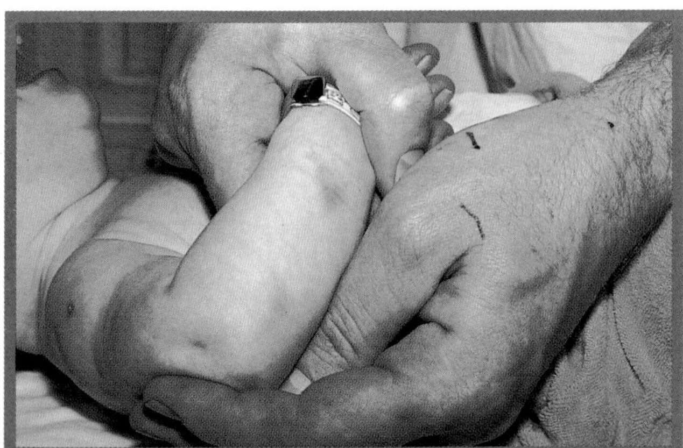

←13.11

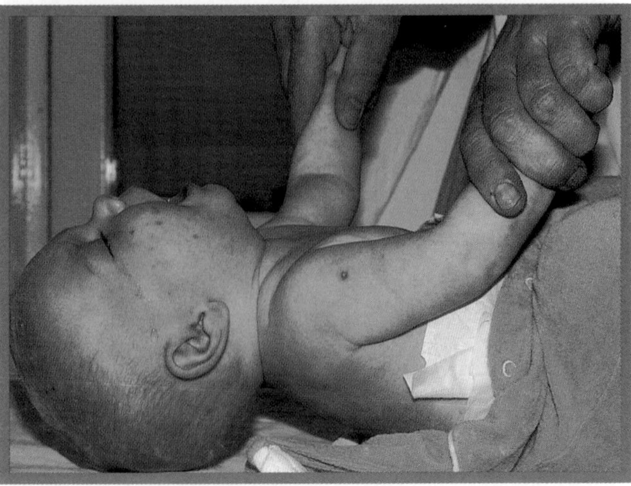

←13.12

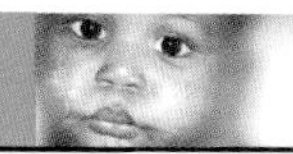

Figure 13.13 Apparent Bruising on the Trunk and Buttocks. The apparent bruising shown here was on the trunk and buttocks of a newborn Asian baby. The bruises seen are extensive **Mongolian blue spots,** which are quite normal, but easily confused with bruising.

Figure 13.14 Finger Tip Burns. The child discussed here had had her hand forcibly pressed against a hot electric cooking ring. The burns are confined to the finger tips as she had tried to prevent her hand being flattened against the ring.

→13.13

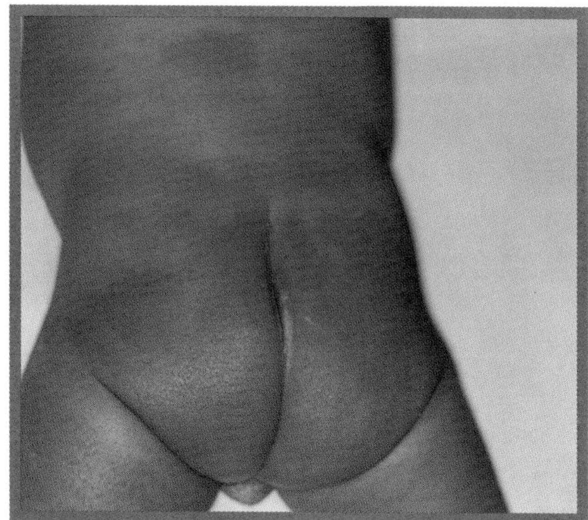

→13.14

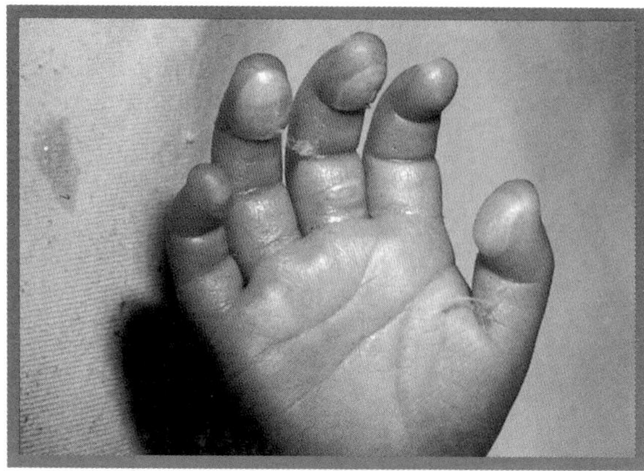

Figure 13.15 Burns. Superficial and full-thickness burns are seen here on the thigh of a child who had burning rags thrown at her. The lesions are discrete but there are no satellite lesions due to splashes that would be expected with a scald from hot liquid.

Figure 13.16 Superficial Blisters. The superficial blisters seen here are from a scald with hot liquid — a 9-month-old spilt a cup of hot tea onto her hands. This was an accidental injury.

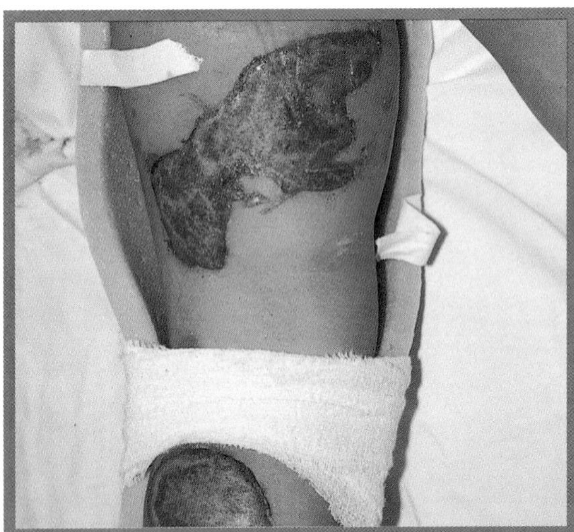

←13.15

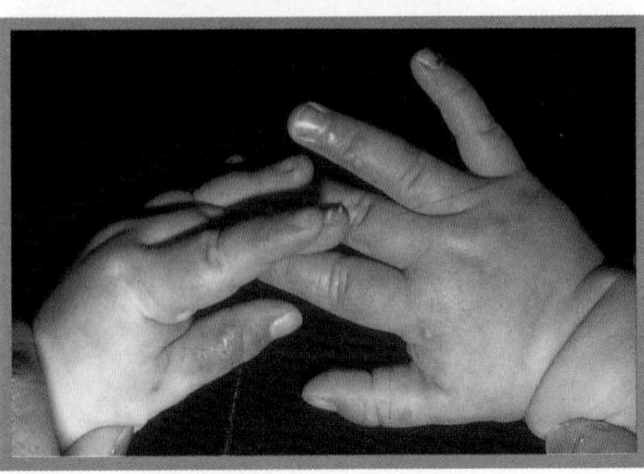

←13.16

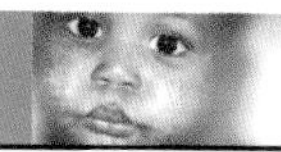

Figures 13.17 and 13.18 Cigarette Burns. The well-circumscribed lesions with blistering seen here are the result of a cigarette burn.
Figure 13.18 shows the same child as in **Figure 13.17**. The well-circumscribed lesions seen here were initially thought to be due to impetigo. The child herself gave a history of being deliberately burnt by a carer while her mother was away.

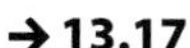

→ 13.17

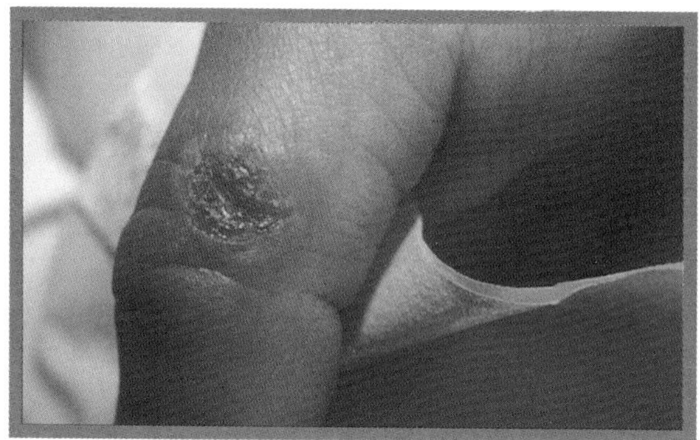

→ 13.18

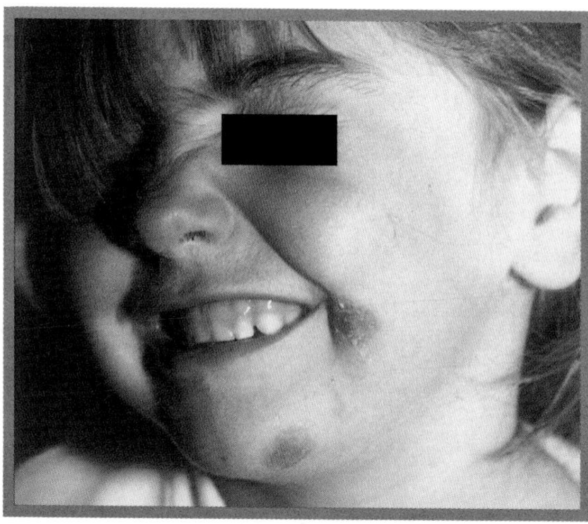

Figure 13.19 Abrasion Caused by a Ligature. Ligature marks are very variable and depend on the tightness of the ligature and the effects of abrasion as the child struggles. In this case, the elder sibling had tied the child to the cot with a tie from the cot bumper.
Figure 13.20 Carpet Burns. Carpet marks are seen here on the forehead of a 9-year-old who had been forcibly pushed on to a carpeted floor. She attended school with these marks, which were unexplained at the time.

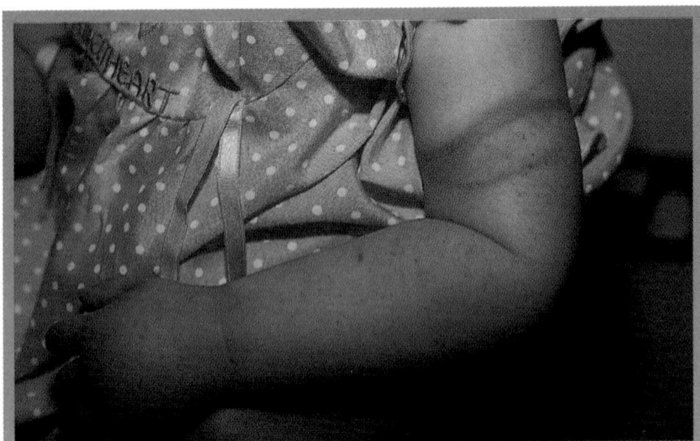

←13.19

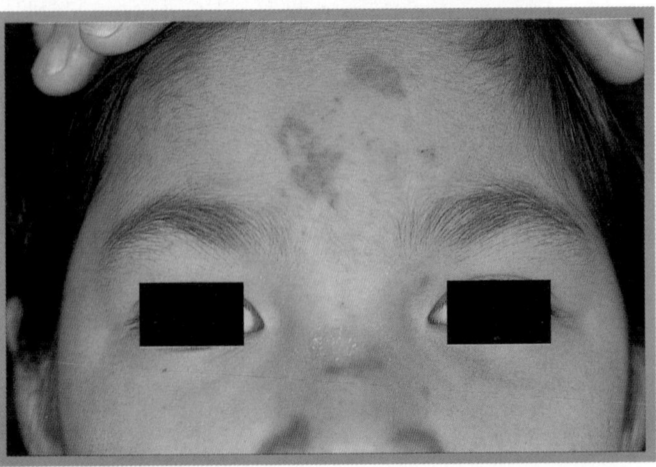

←13.20

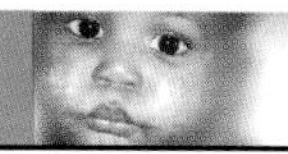

Figure 13.21 Depressed Left Parietal Fracture (Skull X-ray).
Figure 13.22 Tibia and Fibula in a 4-week-old Infant (X-ray). The X-ray shows a very marked subperiosteal reaction and epiphyseal fractures. Other fractures appeared over a period of time with no adequate explanation. The optimal time for observing changes on X-ray is between 10 and 14 days after being injured. Nevertheless, X-rays must be taken on the day of presentation in case there is a fracture that is in need of urgent treatment. A second X-ray should be taken between days 10 and 14.

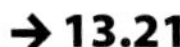

→ 13.21

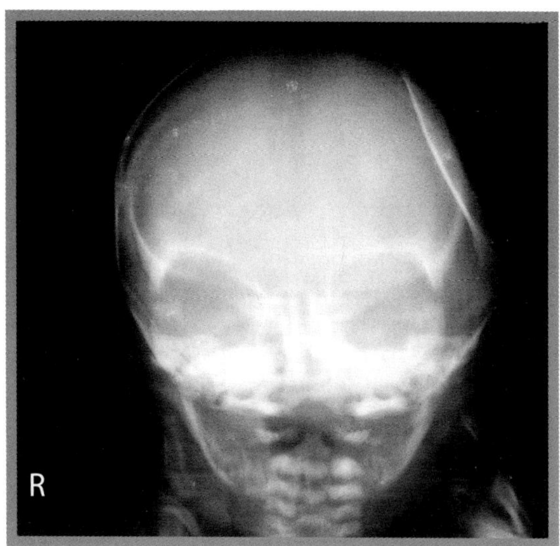

→ 13.22

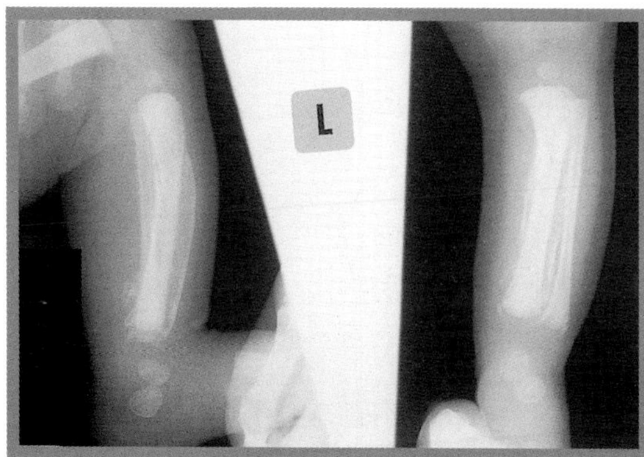

Figure 13.23 Gonococcal Conjunctivitis. Gonococcal conjunctivitis is shown in a boy who had been sexually abused.

Figure 13.24 Vulval Warts. The 2-year-old girl discussed here had no relevant history. Her distressed mother presented to her GP with the finding shown below. The mother was noted to have warts on the hands but there were no genital warts in either parent. The girl's warts were ultimately presumed to have occurred by digital spread. Treatment consisted in ablation under general anesthetic.

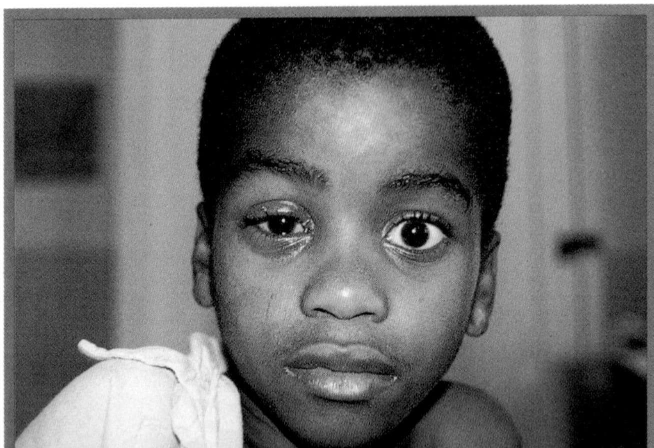

← 13.23

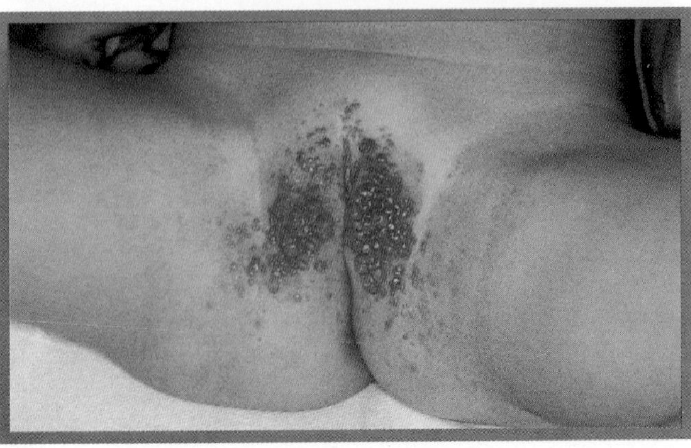

← 13.24

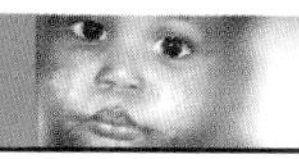

Figure 13.25 Torn Frenulum. The 8-month-old shown here presented with bleeding from the mouth. The frenulum was found to be the source of the bleeding, and was torn. On enquiry, a history was found of being hit by a young babysitter. Torn frenulums heal very quickly. They should always be looked for at presentation or one risks missing this important sign.
Figure 13.26 Superficial Scalds to Buttocks. The baby discussed here had been sat in a bath of hot water. Note the circumferential nature of the scald. In this case, the scald was very superficial and healed well.

→ **13.25**

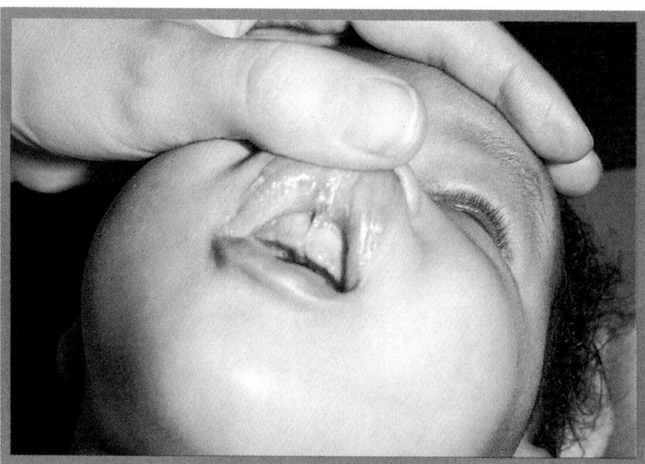

→ **13.26**

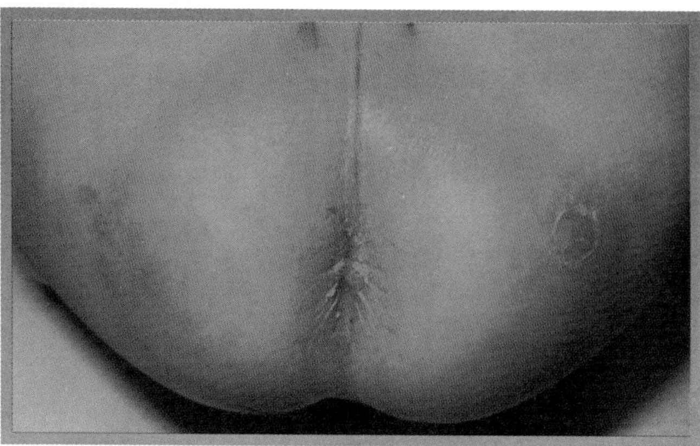

Figure 13.27 Pinch Marks on the Ear. Careful examination is the key to successful collection of medical evidence . The bruises seen here could easily have been missed if the hair covering the ears had not been drawn back.

Figure 13.28 Spiral Fracture of Shaft of Femur (X-ray). The isolated spiral fracture shown was secondary to an external rotatory force. A spiral fracture in a non-ambulant child raises high suspicion of non-accidental injury. However, in ambulant toddlers, such a fracture may occur if the foot becomes trapped.

Suspicious X-ray signs are:

1. Multiple epiphyseal fractures (this finding is pathognomonic of abuse).
2. Multiple asymmetric fractures in various stages of repair.
3. A bucket-handle fracture.
4. Corner fractures secondary to a sudden twisting motion of an extremity.
5. Extensive periosteal reaction from subperiosteal hemorrhage.
6. An avulsion fracture of ligamentous insertion.
7. Skull fracture (particularly of a linear nature).
8. Posterior rib fractures.
9. Irregularities in the outline of a healing periosteum (this may indicate that the child had sustained further trauma).

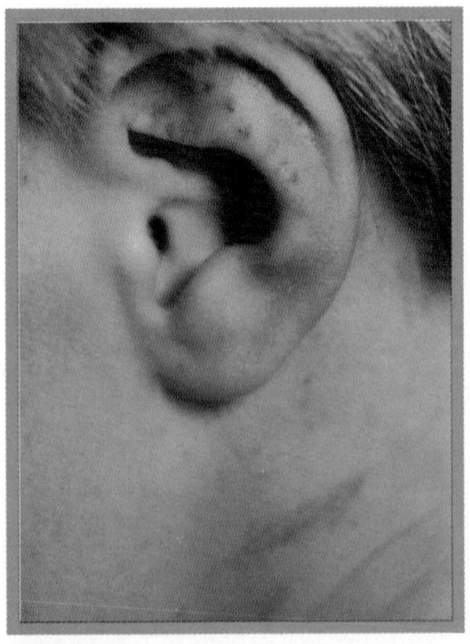

↑ 13.27

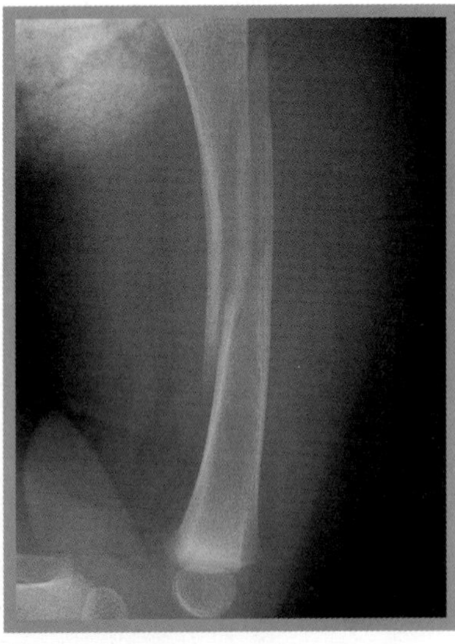

↑ 13.28

14 Pediatric surgery and ENT

In this chapter some of the more important and common general surgical, urological, plastic, orthopedic, ENT and trauma disorders are illustrated. Some are presented elsewhere if relevant.

Figure 14.1 Postaxial polydactyly of the fingers in a newborn child. There is an extra digit on the ulnar side of the hand. It arises postaxially, is poorly formed, and is of type B. If the extra digit is on the radial or thumb side, *i.e.*, preaxial, it will have arisen earlier in embryogenesis and is therefore more likely to have other associated abnormalities.

Postaxial polydactyly is associated with:

1. Ellis-van Creveld syndrome.
2. Laurence–Moon–Biedl syndrome.
3. Infantile thoracic dystrophy.
4. Hydrocephalus and polycystic kidneys.

Preaxial polydactyly is associated with:

1. Carpenter syndrome.
2. Orofacial digital syndrome type II.
3. Polydactyly with peculiar skull shape.

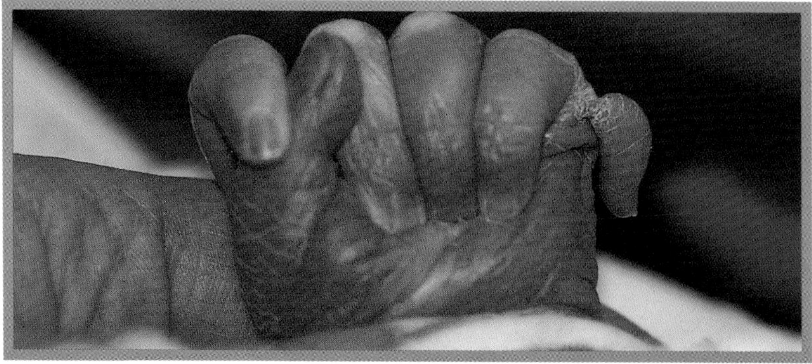

↑ 14.1

Figure 14.2 Postaxial polydactyly of the feet. Here, the extra digit is more normally fixed and contains bone. X-ray investigation should be used to indentify bony structures.

Figure 14.3 Syndactyly of the Fingers. Syndactyly is complex fusion of the digits, *i.e.*, involving the fusion of bone and soft tissue. This is the most common of the digital abnormalities and in its simplest form involves only soft-tissues fusion.

Syndactyly has a number of associations:

1. Absent pectoralis major muscle (Poland's anomaly).
2. Acrocephalosyndactyly type 1 (Apert's syndrome), type II (seen in Vogt syndrome), type III, type IV (seen in Waardenburg syndrome), and type V (seen in Pfeiffer syndrome).
3. Oculodactylodigital dysplasia.

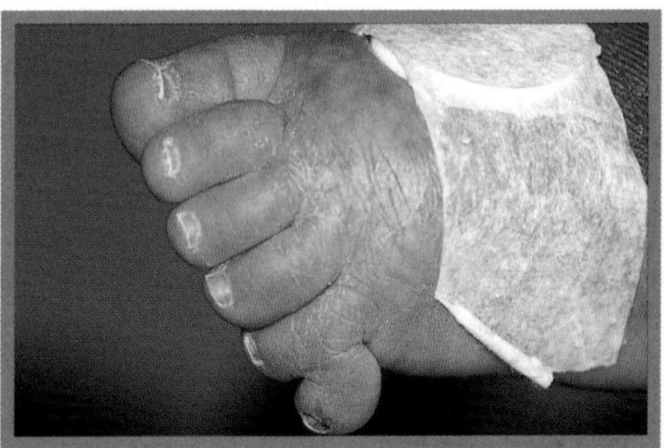

←14.2

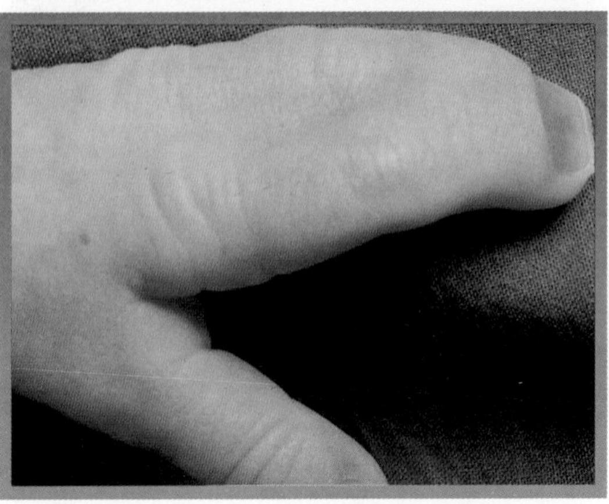

←14.3

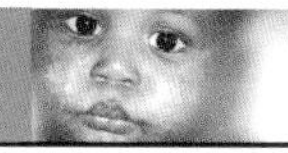

Figures 14.4 and 14.5 Fixed Contractures. Figure 14.4 shows fixed contractures of the digits in a newborn infant. The condition may be isolated, or may occur as a feature of a syndrome, *e.g.*, trisomies 17 and 18, of a congenital muscular dystrophy or of arthrogryposis.

Figure 14.5 Talipes Equinovarus (Club Foot). Club foot is shown in a newborn boy. Both feet were affected. There is fixed plantar flexion (equinus) with inversion of the heel and hindfoot, and forefoot varus and adduction.

The incidence is 1 per 1000 live births, and the condition occurs more commonly in boys. It is bilateral in 50% of cases. There is a familial tendency, with a 5% chance of recurrence in a sibling. It may occur in association with or secondary to neuromuscular disorders such as spina bifida, cerebral palsy and poliomyelitis. Treatment should be commenced soon after birth, using physiotherapy, stretching and splinting before starting operative orthopedic management.

→14.4

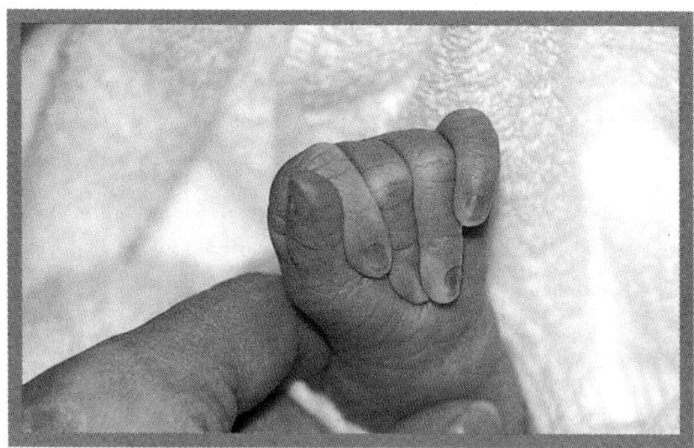

→14.5

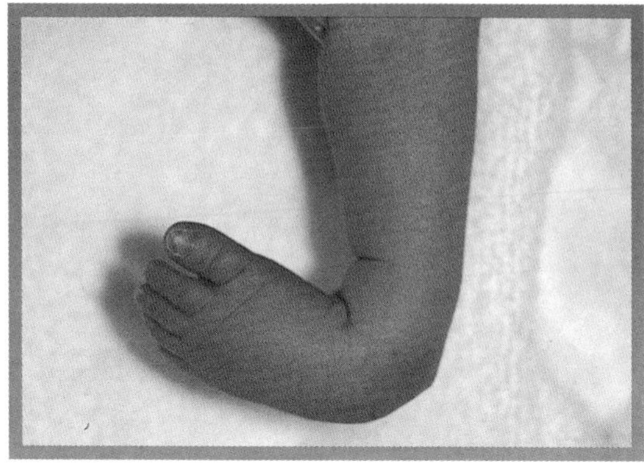

Figures 14.6 and 14.7 Examination of the Hip Joint. Barlow modification of Ortolani test is shown.

All hips should be carefully examined in the neonate for the presence of dislocation. Even in the best hands, however, this test will fail to detect up to 50% of cases, and ultrasound examination may be a better way to screen for this important condition.

The classic method is shown. The baby is placed on a firm surface on its back. The hips and knees are flexed, placing the examiner's index and middle fingers over the greater trochanter and the thumbs across the knees on the inner side of the thighs as shown. Only one hip at a time is examined. First (see **Figure 14.6**) the femoral head is pushed downwards and if the hip is dislocatable the femoral head will be posteriorly displaced out of the acetabulum. Then with the hip abducted, upward pressure is applied (see **Figure 14.7**). A dislocated hip will return with a 'clunk' into the acetabulum. Limited abduction of an affected hip suggests that the hip is anteriorly dislocated and will not relocate. Variable degrees of dysplasia account for many cases of so-called missed dislocation.

There is an incidence of hip dislocation in 1–2 per 1000 live births.

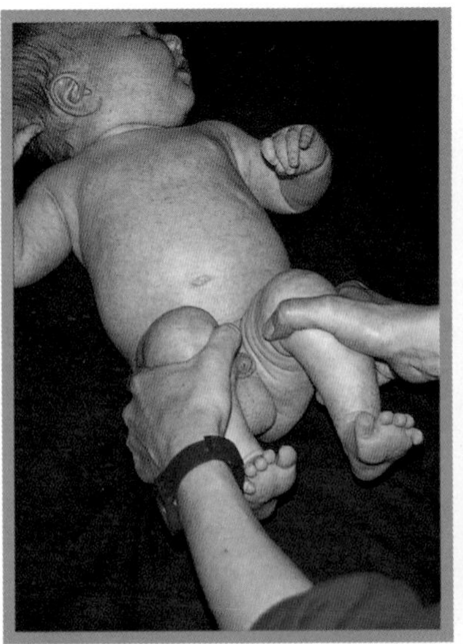

↑ 14.6

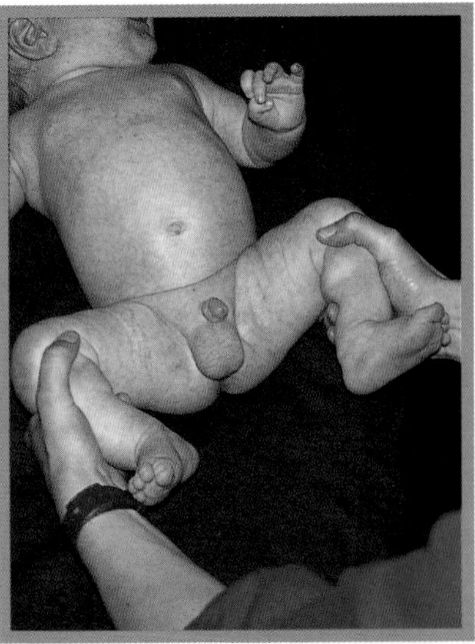

↑ 14.7

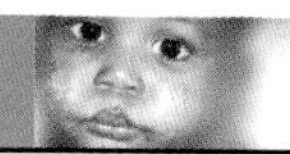

The following are indications for screening:

1. Indicative family history.
2. Breech presentation.
3. Mediterranean origin.
4. Females.
5. First born.
6. Oligohydramnios.
7. Other congenital abnormality.

Figures 14.8 and 14.9 Dislocation of the Knees in a Newborn. The figures show anterior dislocation of the right knee (**Figure 14.8**), and anterior subluxation of the left knee (**Figure 14.9**). There was no other associated abnormality such as hip dislocation, spina bifida, talipes or arthrogryposis. Treatment is usually conservative, and should be started in the first week of life. Physiotherapy with splinting or immobilization by traction or plaster is usually successful and operative correction is rarely required.

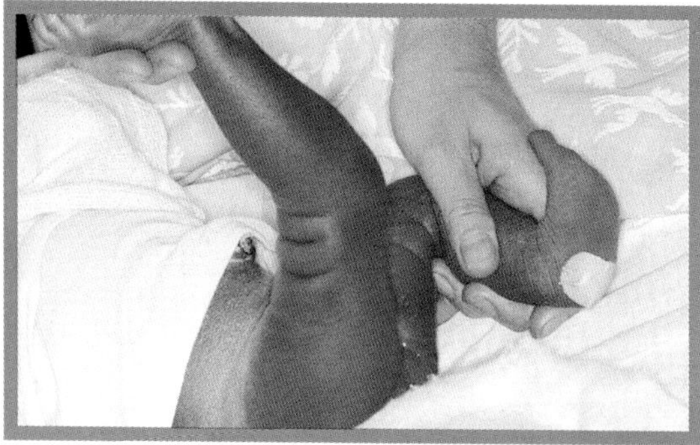

← **14.8**

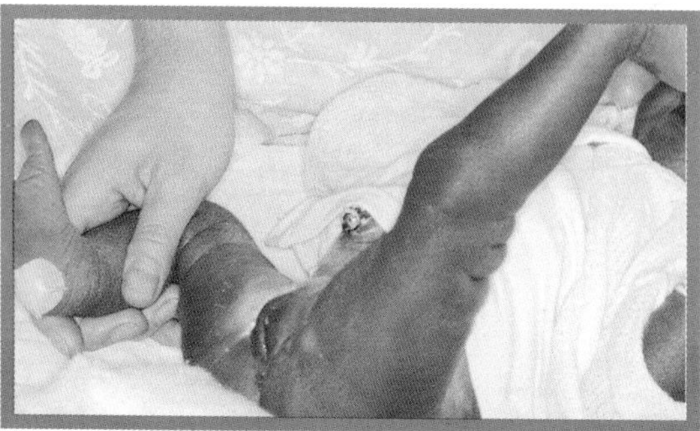

← **14.9**

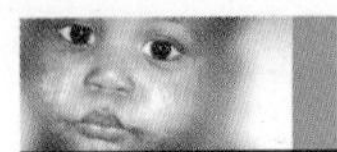

Figure 14.10 Compound Fracture of Tibia. A wound is shown in communication with a fracture of the tibia. All compound fractures carry a risk of infection and external hemorrhage.

The risk of infection here is further increased as the causal force has broken the skin. The risks are greater in this type of compound fracture because:

1. Dirt may be driven into the wound.
2. The skin is frequently damaged, with skin loss leading to skin closure difficulties.
3. Muscle damage may exacerbate the problem.
4. Hemorrhage and shock may be quite significant.

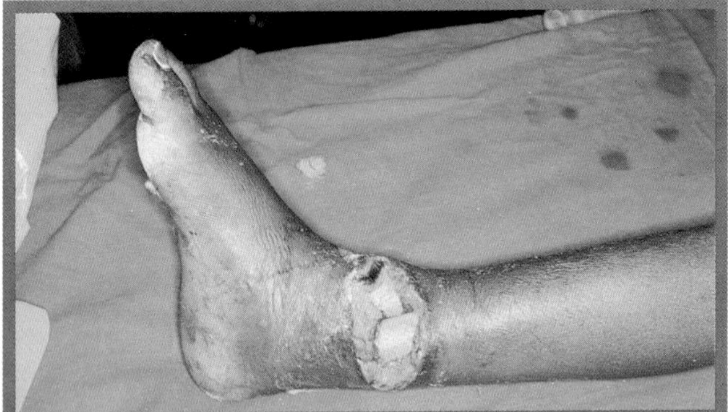

←14.10

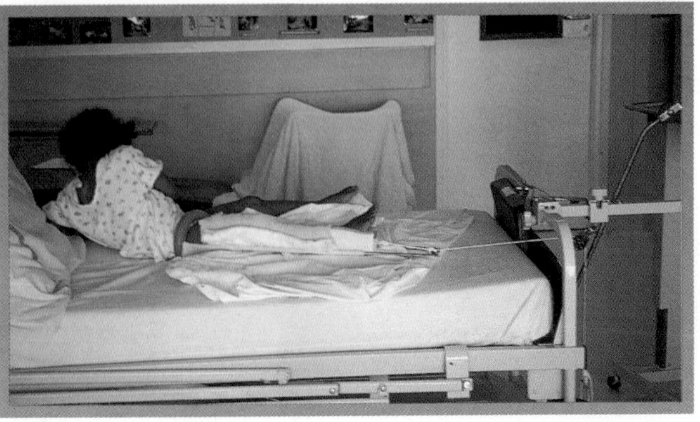

←14.11

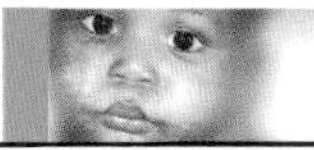

Figures 14.11 and 14.12 Treatment for Femoral Shaft Fracture. Skin traction (St Thomas splint) is shown. The aim is to achieve and maintain alignment of the fractured ends of the femur, and to achieve some correction of the shortening. Approximately 1–1.5 cm of overlap of the fracture is allowed in young children, in anticipation of the stimulation of growth by the fracture.

The splinting can be continued at home in suitable cases, and is usually applied for 4–6 weeks. On removal, gentle mobilization with physiotherapy is required for restoration of confidence (see **Figure 14.12**).

→ 14.12

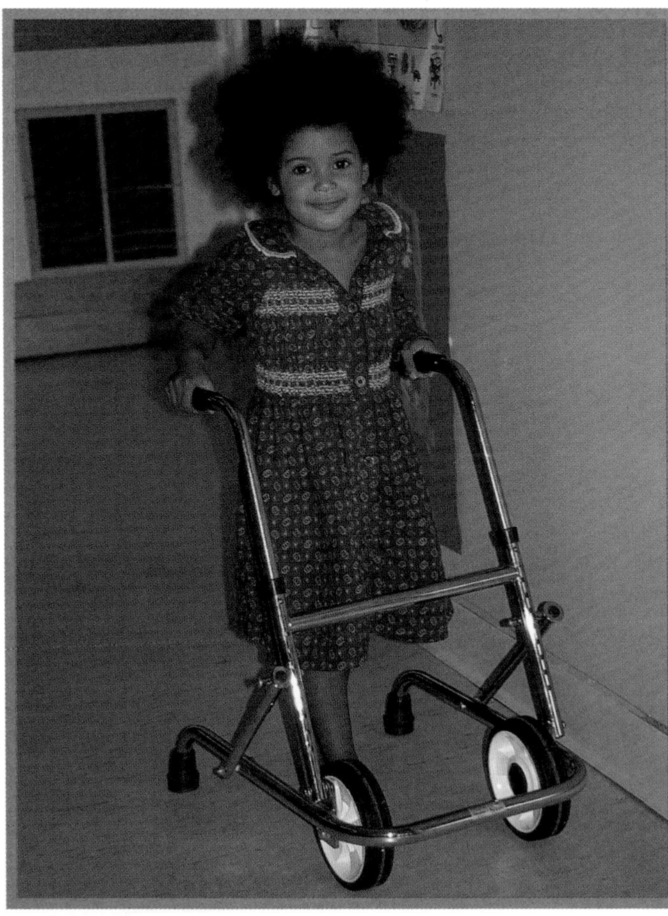

Figure 14.13 Osteogenic Sarcoma. This is a rare tumor, but is the most common primary malignant tumor in bone. It occurs primarily in the long bones of the lower limbs, with 75% occurring age 10–25 years.

The tumor tends to occur in the metaphysis of the long bone, mainly in the lower end of the femur or the upper end of the tibia.

In this case, the child presented with knee pain and a hard, warm, tender mass was found. The X- ray shows an infiltrative, poorly demarcated tumor located predominantly in the tibial metaphyseal region. There is angulation due to pathological fracture.

Figure 14.14 Ewing Sarcoma of Left Femur. The child shown here presented with bone pain and swelling of the femur. A mass could be felt on examination. The X-ray shows an expansile region of the mid-diaphyseal region of the left femur. There is a periosteal reaction and new bone formation is prominent, predominantly in a lamellar configuration.

Ewing Sarcoma is a malignant neoplasm arising in the medullary tissue in the diaphysis of a long or flat bone, *e.g.*, the ilium. It presents in late childhood,

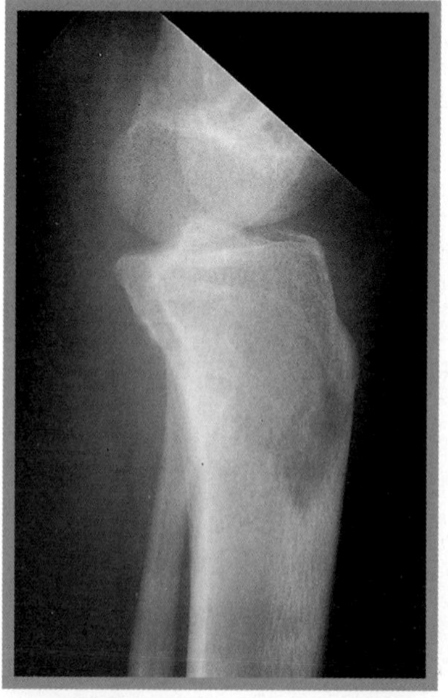

↑ 14.13

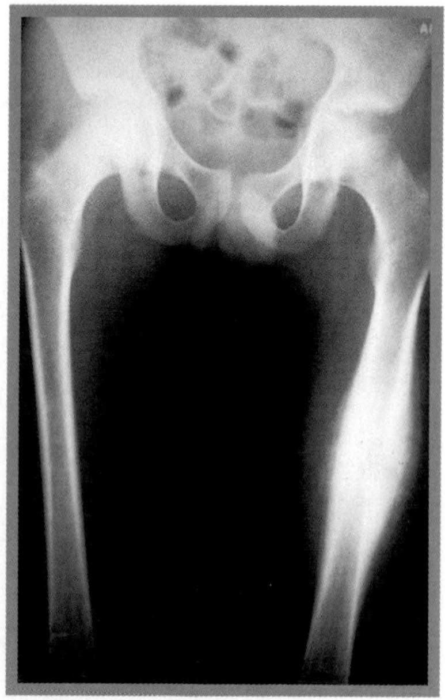

↑ 14.14

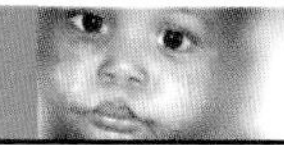

typically between the ages of 10 and 20 years, with fever, pain, swelling and tenderness.

Metastasis to other bones and lungs is the presenting feature in up to a third of cases. Treatment includes a combination of chemotherapy and radiation. Surgical resection may be considered if this would not result in loss of function.

Figure 14.15 Histiocytosis of Shaft of Right Femur (Class I). The 6-year-old girl shown here presented with pain and a limp in the right leg despite having no history of trauma. On examination, the right midfemoral region was found to be tender and a mass could be felt. The chest X-ray and bone scan were normal, Mantoux was negative, and biopsy showed eosinophilic granuloma. Class I histiocytoses are proliferations, not malignancies, and are probably secondary to defects of immunoregulation. Minimal intervention is needed for non-progressing, single lytic bone lesions like this one. The condition resolved spontaneously 18 months later. The differential diagnosis includes Ewing sarcoma and chronic infection, *e.g.*, tuberculosis.

→ 14.15

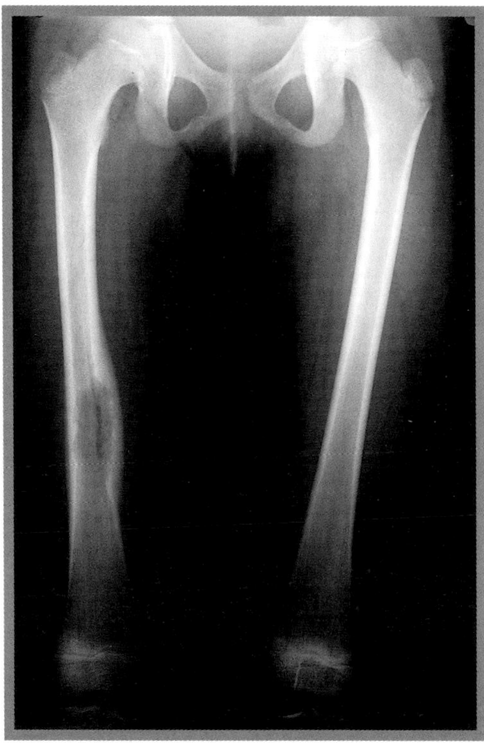

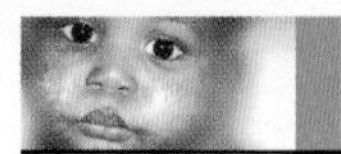

Figure 14.16 Cystic Hygroma. Cystic hygroma is shown arising from the left side of the neck in an infant. It was noted on an antenatal scan at 21 weeks' gestation. There is a large, transilluminating, skin-covered mass arising from the posterior triangle of the neck.

A cystic hygroma is a lymphatic malformation of anomalous channels and cysts. The abnormality is frequently present at birth, with 90% having presented by the second year of life, mainly in the neck, but also in the axilla, groin and retroperitoneum.

Complications include:

1. Obstructed labor or delivery.
2. Upper airway obstruction.
3. Infection.
4. Hemorrhage into the cyst.
5. Esophageal obstruction.

Treatment consists of surgical excision.

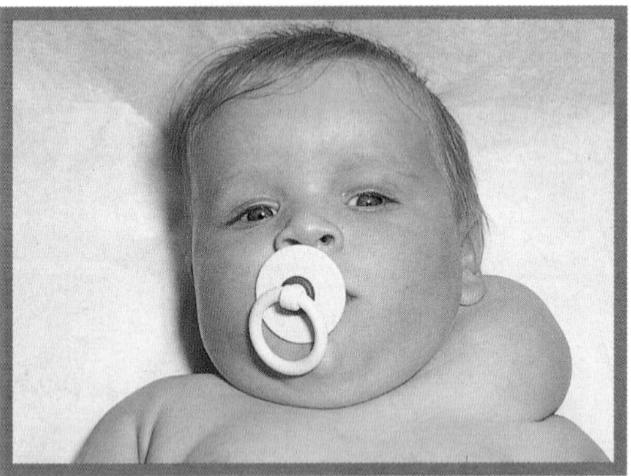

← **14.16**

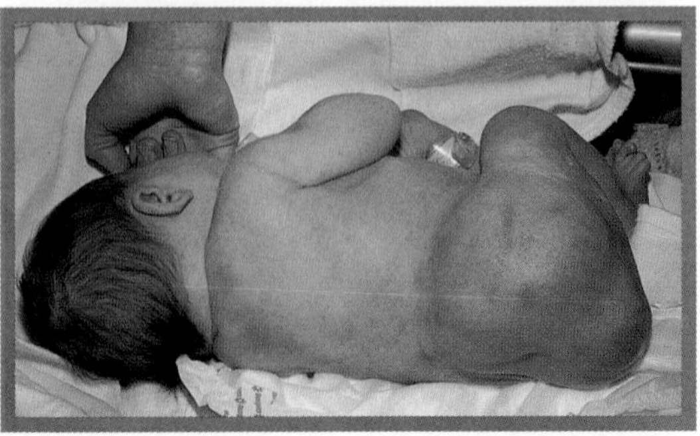

← **14.17**

Figures 14.17–14.19 Sacral Mass (Lipoma). A mass arising asymmetrically from the sacrum is shown. It was not diagnosed antenatally, and there was no obstruction of labor. Despite a full range of movement there was evidence of postural abnormalities as a result of intrauterine movement being reduced by the mass.

Postnatal ultrasound scanning showed a homogeneous mass arising to one side of the midline. X-ray revealed no evidence of calcification, but it did show vertebral, sacral and rib abnormalities. The differential diagnosis is sacral teratoma.

In view of the skeletal abnormalities the mass is more likely to be a lipoma. This was confirmed on surgical excision.

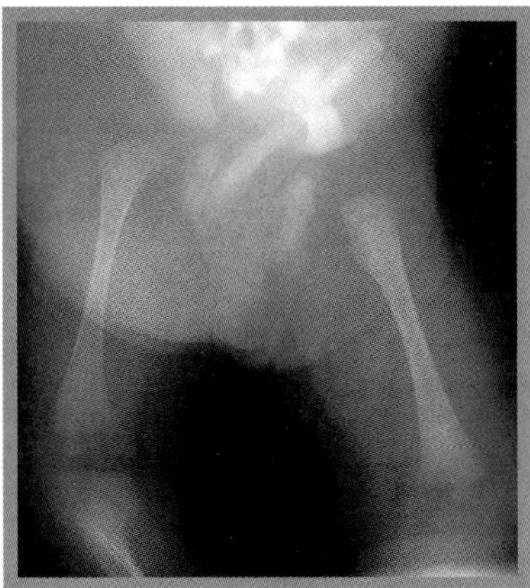

↑ 14.18

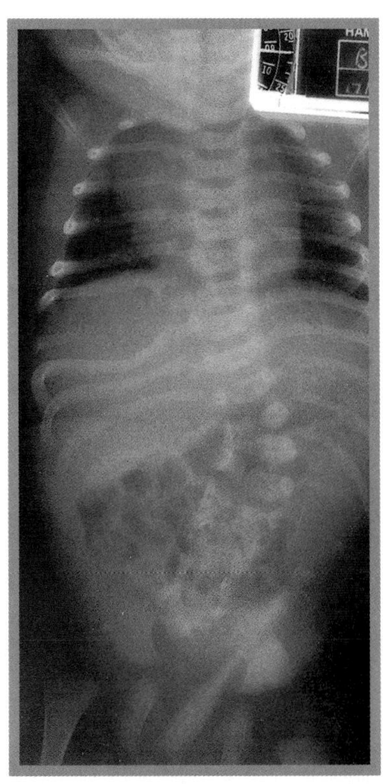

↑ 14.19

Figure 14.20 Exomphalos. Herniation of intra-abdominal contents through the umbilical ring into the umbilical cord is shown. The exomphalos is covered by a sac made up of fused layers of the amniotic sac and peritoneum.

Exomphalos can be classed as major and minor. Exomphalos minor tends to be less than 5 cm in diameter and there are rarely any associated abnormalities. In the major forms, the defect is greater than 5 cm and in addition to herniated intestine the sac may contain liver, spleen, stomach and bladder. The defect lies in the upper abdomen, with the umbilical cord being attached to the apex. Malrotation of the small bowel is frequently associated, as are cardiac defects, anencephaly and Beckwith–Wiedemann syndrome (exomphalos, macroglossia and giantism).

Treatment consists of surgery. Small defects can be closed by direct primary closure, but larger defects may require a staged closure using a dacron-reinforced silastic patch as a temporary covering. The patch is reduced in size over time and closure of the abdominal wall is then performed. Post-operative ventilation may be required after primary repair.

Figure 14.21 Gastroschisis. A neonate with gastroschisis is shown. The condition was diagnosed on antenatal ultrasound scanning. In this case it is associated with atresia of the bowel. The figure shows a temporary enterostomy following resection of the atretic loop. Closure was accomplished at a later date. Gastroschisis is a complete defect running through all layers of the anterior

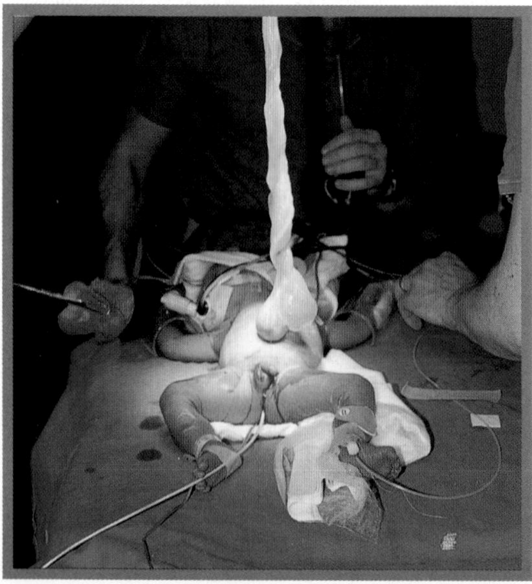

← 14.20

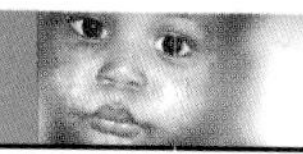

abdominal wall, usually lying to the right of the umbilical cord. Ten to fifteen percent of cases are complicated by intestinal atresia due to volvulus or interruption of the blood supply to segments of exposed intestine.
Following delivery, an affected child requires intravenous fluids and decompression of the obstructed bowel with a large-bore nasogastric tube. The exposed bowel is covered in a waterproof dressing to minimize desiccation of the exposed tissues. Fluid management and control of infection are essential if the infant is to survive. Postoperative maintenance of nutrition is essential, sometimes requiring total parenteral nutrition (TPN) because of associated bowel problems including motility disorders.
Figure 14.22 TPN Associated Hepatitis. This infant aged 4 months developed jaundice following prolonged TPN for postgastroschisis-repair-associated ileus.The hepatitis results from both biliary cholestasis and from a direct hepatocellular effect of the TPN on the liver. Treatment consists of the introduction of oral feeds.

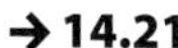

→ 14.21

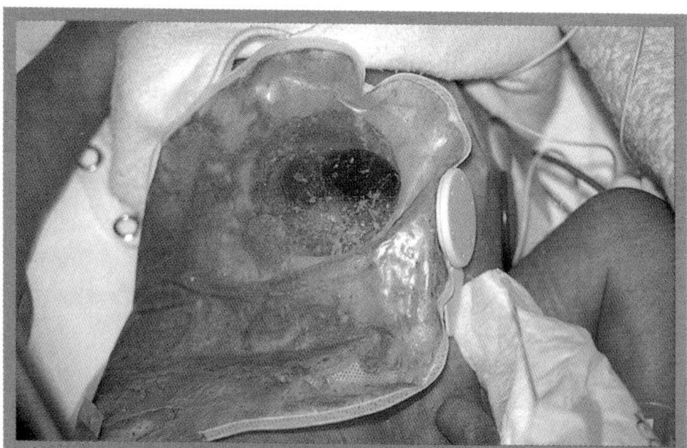

→ 14.22

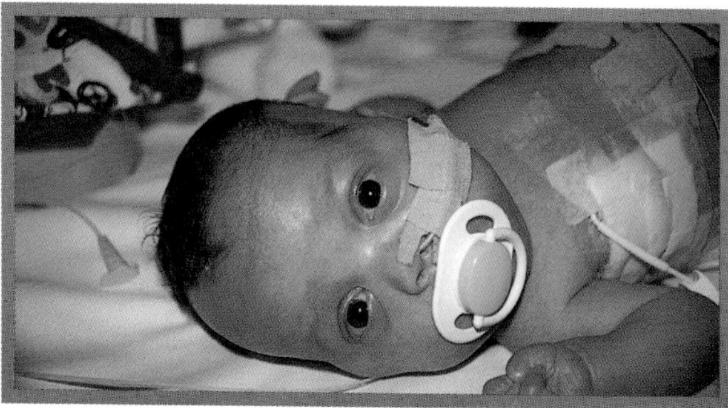

Figures 14.23 and Figure 14.24 Imperforate Anus. The child shown here was noted at birth to have a dimple but no anal orifice. There was no vomiting. Structural malformations of the urinary tract are frequently associated with this anomaly. The baby also had a cystic kidney and a hydroureter.
Figure 14.24 shows a lateral shoot-through with an anal marker at the anal dimple (image on left). Gas rises to the apex of the blind bowel but does not reach the anus.

The anomaly is refered to as a low defect imperforate anus when an orifice is seen at the perineum (cutaneous perineal fistula). When there is no obvious fistula at perineal level a high defect is suspected, in which there is often a fistula with the bladder or uretha in males, and vagina in females.

The term 'low vaginal fistula' should not be considered indicative of a low type of defect. It simply means that the fistula opens into the lower part of the vagina but this defect is still considered as a high defect.

Low anomalies are usually repaired using the perineal approach in the newborn. High anomalies are treated by preliminary sigmoid colostomy; at a later date one of many reconstructive procedures is carried out and the colostomy is closed. There may be associated abnormalities of the sacrum with neuromuscular and genitourinary anomalies. The urinary tract should be investigated with ultrasound very early to ensure that any hydronephrosis is detected and treated.

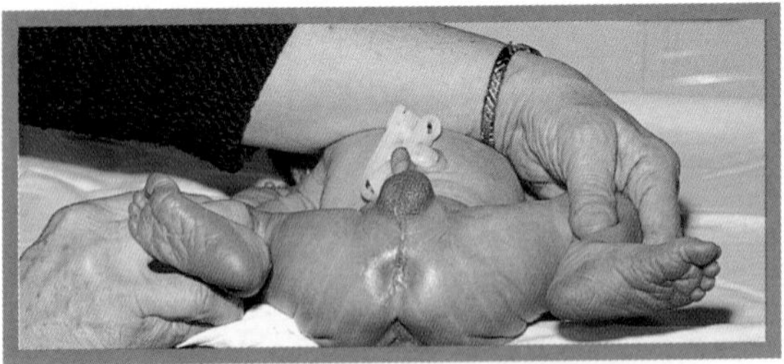

← 14.23

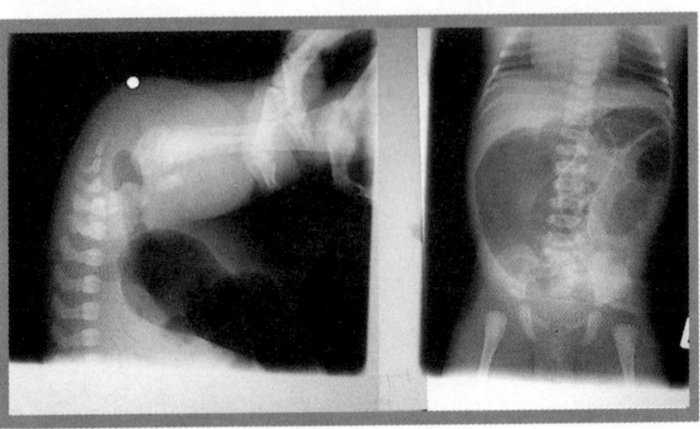

← 14.24

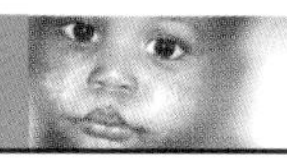

Figure 14.25 Supraumbilical Hernia and Umbilical Hernia. A supraumbilical hernia is present superiorly, and an umbilical hernia is present inferiorly. There is a higher incidence of umbilical hernia in Afro-Caribbeans than in Caucasians; it occurs in Beckwith-Wiedermann syndrome, Hurler syndrome and trisomies 13 and 18. The vast majority of such hernias resolve spontaneously within the first 4 years of occurrence and do not need intervention. A supraumbilical hernia requires surgical repair as it will not close spontaneously.

Figure 14.26 Ectopia Vesicae. Failure of the anterior abdominal wall to fuse below the umbilicus results in the bladder opening onto the anterior abdominal wall. A male infant is shown here with complete bladder extrophy, epispadias, bifid scrotum and undescended testes. This is a major malformation that is more common in males.

Urgent referral to a pediatric urological surgeon is indicated as the renal tract is at risk of damage from sepsis. Decisions concerning reconstruction depend upon a team approach. Late complications are urinary incontinence, infertility and impotence.

→ 14.25

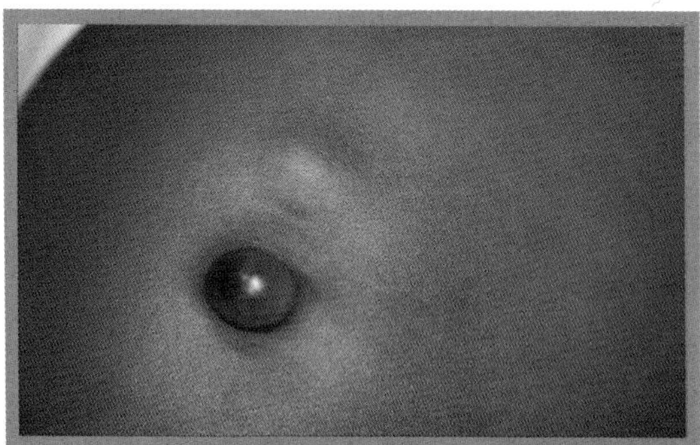

→ 14.26

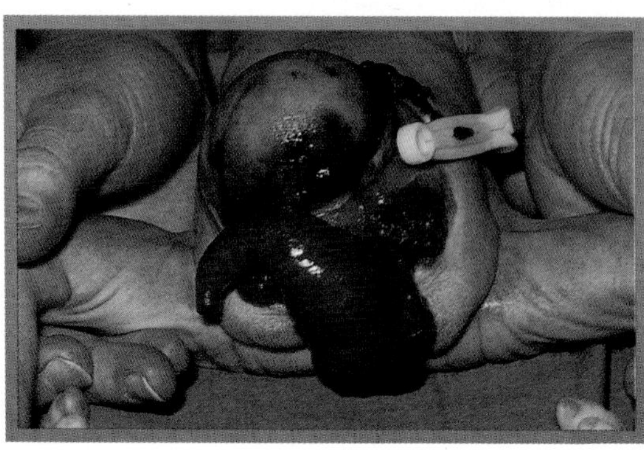

Figure 14.27 Undescended Testes. Cryptorchidism is shown here in a 5-year-old boy. Undescended testes is a common condition in boys. Three percent of term and 30% of preterm infants have undescended testes at birth. In over half these cases the testes will descend by 2 months of age, and in 80%, by 1 year.

Considerable debate exists over whether there is an increased risk of malignancy if the testes remain intra-abdominal into puberty. Nonetheless, relatively early referral (before 1 year of age) to a pediatric surgeon is advisable. In bilateral undescended testes a trial of HCG may bring about descent. Intra-abdominal testes are located by laparoscopy. Failure of spermatogenesis is more common in these patients, even when early orchidopexy is undertaken.

Undescended testes should be differentiated from retractile testes.

Figure 14.28 Hypospadias. Hypospadias is shown in a newborn boy. Note the urethral meatus, which is displaced ventrally onto the coronal aspect of the penis. The urinary stream is displaced downward.

Hypospadias occurs in 1 in 300 males. The urethral meatus may be located anywhere from the glans to the perineum. The more proximal the hypospadias, the more likelihood there is chordee (longitudinal curvature) of the penile shaft. The prepuce is frequently hooded or bifid in its ventral aspect and circumcision should not be undertaken before expert pediatric surgical advice has been obtained.

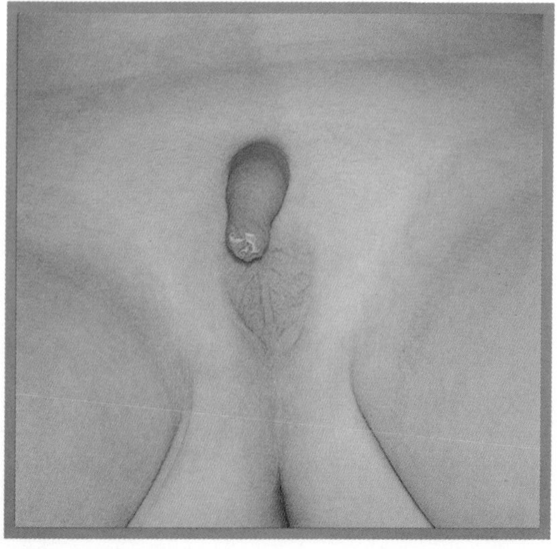

← 14.27

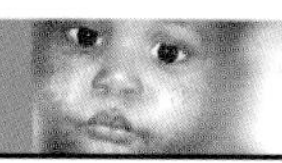

Surgical repair is performed as a single stage or multi-stage procedure and aims to provide a functional urethra with a meatus at the tip of the penis, and to release any associated chordee. This is best undertaken by an expert pediatric urological surgeon.

Figure 14.29 Torsion of Testes. Neonatal torsion, which presumably occurred antenatally, is shown. At operation, the testicle was nonviable and required excision. Fixation of the opposite testicle is indicated.

Note the spread of edema across the scrotum, anterior abdominal wall and inner thigh. This may occur in the absence of torsion and is called idiopathic scrotal edema.

Torsion of the testicle occurs during two periods: neonatal and pubertal. In the neonate, the torsion occurs outside the tunica vaginalis (extravaginal torsion) and is due to faulty scrotal fixation. This results in an infarcted testicle. Some studies suggest that early removal of the infarcted testicle may prevent functional damage to the opposite testicle. The contralateral testicle must be fixed, to avoid torsion and infarction at a later date. At puberty, intravaginal torsion occurs and presents as a painful, hard, swollen erythematous testicle. This is a surgical emergency and exploration, untwisting and fixation is required. Young boys may present with vomiting and few localizing signs.

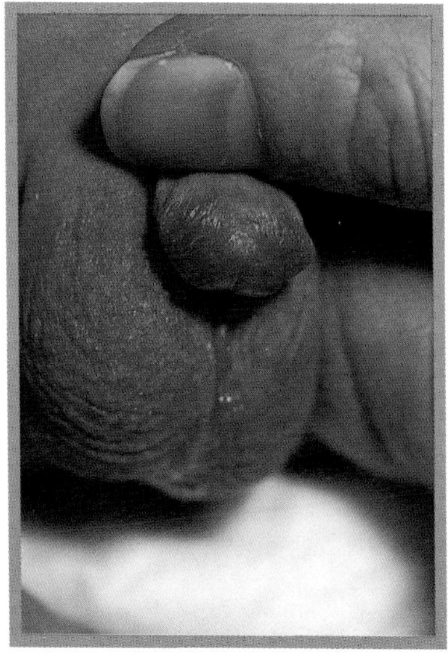

↑ **14.28**

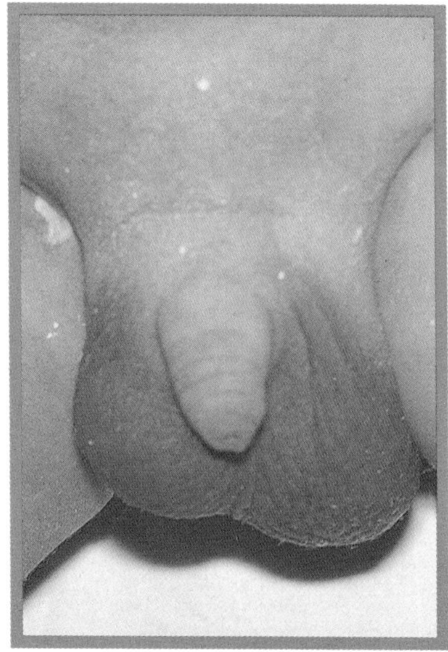

↑ **14.29**

Figure 14.30 Barium Enema of Ileocolic Intussusception. The 1-year-old shown here presented with paroxysmal screaming attacks, vomiting and drawing up of the knees. A sausage-shaped mass could be felt in the right hypochondrium. A barium enema view is shown here. There is a filling defect of the advancing intussusception that is displacing and obstructing the passage of barium at the hepatic flexure. A hydrostatic reduction (air or barium can be used) was carried out following resuscitation of the child.

Intussusception is the invagination of one part of the bowel into the lumen of an adjoining part, and occurs most commonly at the ileocecal valve as in this case. Seventy percent of cases occur before the age of 1 year. In older children, an abnormality may be the leading point of the intussusception, *e.g.*, Meckel diverticulum.

Indications for operative reduction are:

1. Shock or collapse.
2. Peritonitis.
3. Barium reduction failure.
4. The child is outside the typical age group, *i.e.*, less than 2 months or more than 2 years of age.

Figure 14.31 Barium Enema Demonstrating Hirschsprung Disease. A narrowing of the rectum and sigmoid colon can be seen. This aganglionic segment fails to dilate and transmit peristalsis, resulting in proximal bowel dilatation

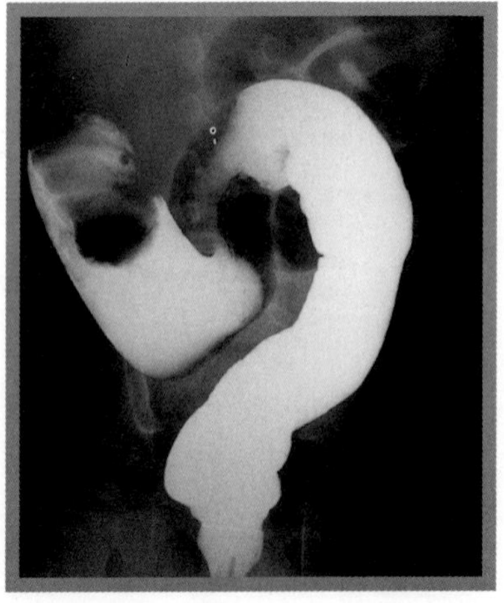

↑ **14.30**

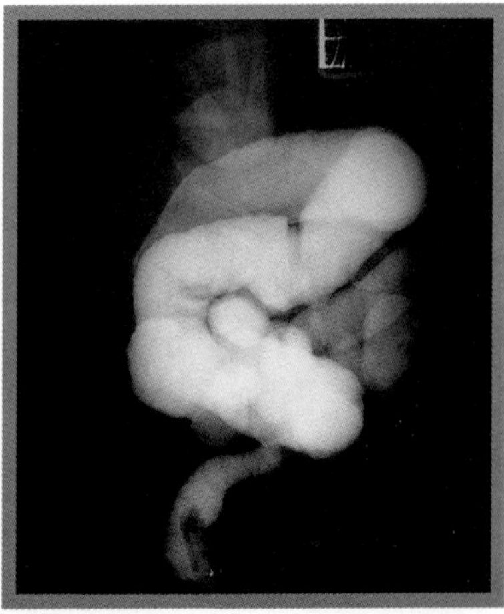

↑ **14.31**

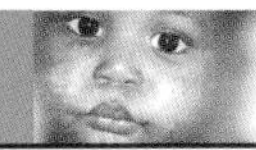

and distal contracted colon. This baby presented in the first few weeks of life with intestinal obstruction. The gold-standard test is rectal biopsy showing aganglionosis (absence of ganglion cells).

Figure 14.32 Dental Abscess. The 5-year-old girl shown here presented with a dental abscess. Findings included a diffuse, fluctuant, erythematous, painful swelling on the left mandible. An incision was made and the pus was drained off. The pus grew a mixed culture of anaerobic and aerobic organisms. The underlying cause was a decayed tooth, which was removed.

Figure 14.33 Peritonsillar Abscess (Quinsy). This child presented with a right-sided cervical swelling. Fever, pain, trismus and drooling were noted. In view of the inability to examine the upper airway and tonsils, an ENT opinion was sought. At examination under anesthesia a large peritonsillar abscess was noted. The tonsils and associated structures were displaced medially and were edematous. At incision, more than 60 ml of green pus was drained off. Treatment consisted of antibiotics, given intravenously for 48 hours and then orally.

Complications of quinsy include lateral pharyngeal abscess, which may cause airway obstruction or erode into the carotid artery.

→14.32

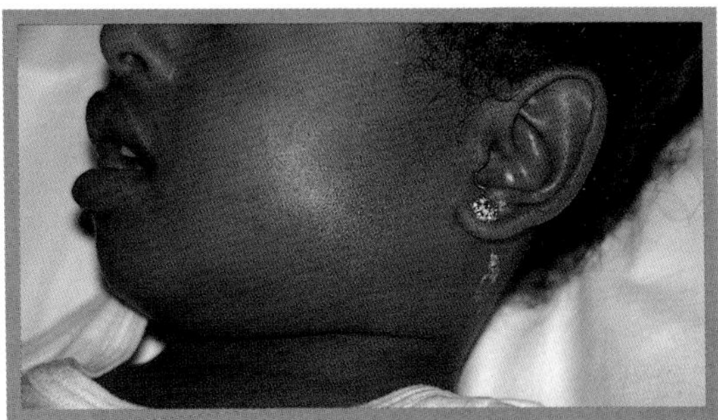

→14.33

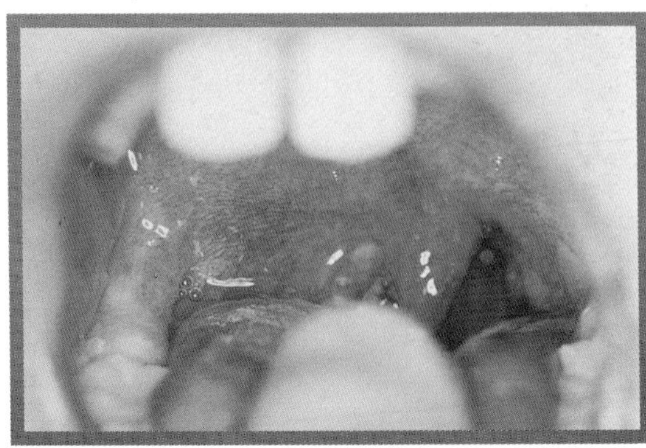

Figure 14.34 Tracheostomy. A tracheostomy in a 1-year-old is shown. In this case, the child presented at 4 months of age with severe croup. The child was intubated and ventilated for 72 hours, but extubation was not possible due to obstruction of the airway. Laryngoscopy revealed a vascular hemangioma and a tracheostomy was performed. This child subsequently had significant morbidity from recurrent infection and mucus-plug obstruction.

Indications for tracheostomy due to upper airway obstruction are:

1. Congenital: tracheal stenosis, laryngeal web, hemangioma of the larynx, tracheo-esophageal anomalies, and bilateral cord palsy.
2. Infectious/inflammatory: epiglottitis, laryngotracheobronchitis, bacterial tracheitis, and diphtheria.
3. Trauma: prolonged intubation, inhalational injuries, radiation injury, and foreign bodies.
4. Neoplastic: benign and malignant laryngeal tumors.

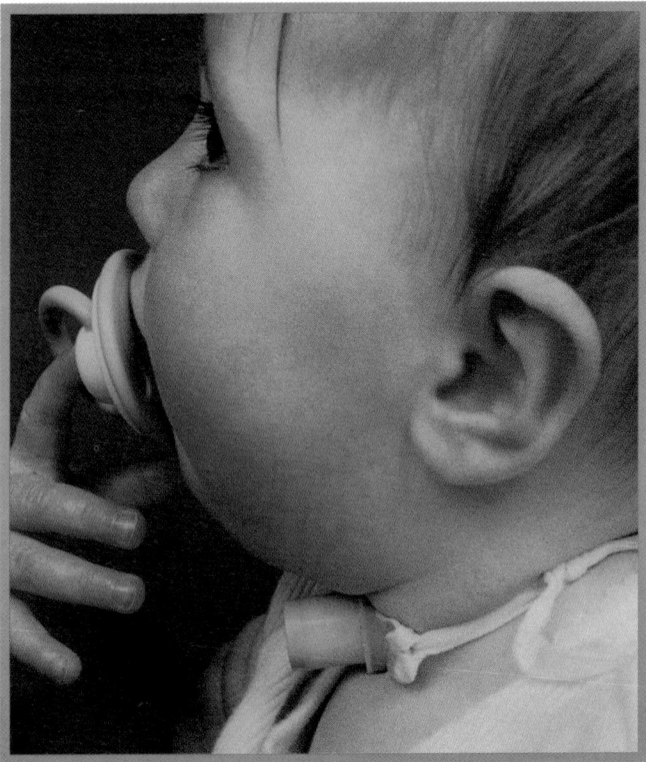

← **14.34**

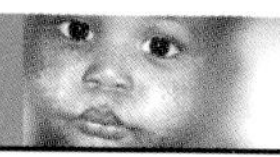

Indications for tracheostomy for protecting of the airway are neurological conditions predisposing to recurrent aspiration, *e.g.*, severe cerebral palsy, Guillain–Barré syndrome, poliomyelitis, and tetanus.

Indications for tracheostomy for prolonged ventilation are spinal cord lesions and neuromuscular diseases.

Complications of tracheostomy include:

1. Obstruction.
2. Displacement.
3. Infection.
4. Tracheal stenosis.
5. Speech delay.

Figure 14.35 Sinusitis. A unilateral right-sided maxillary sinusitis is shown. The child discussed here presented with an upper respiratory tract infection, with pain over the maxillary antrum. The pain was throbbing in nature and was exacerbated by bending over and coughing. There were findings of a unilateral nasal obstruction and a persistent cough.

On examinatiion, she was found to be pyrexial, with tenderness over the maxillary antrum, and there was a mucopurulent nasal discharge. The X-ray shows complete opacity of the right maxillary antrum.

Most cases of sinusitis are secondary to one of the following:

1. Infection, viral or bacterial.
2. Dental infection.
3. Barotrauma.
4. Skull fracture.

Treatment consists of administration of analgesics, decongestants and antibiotics. Sinusitis is generally bilateral.

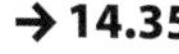

→14.35

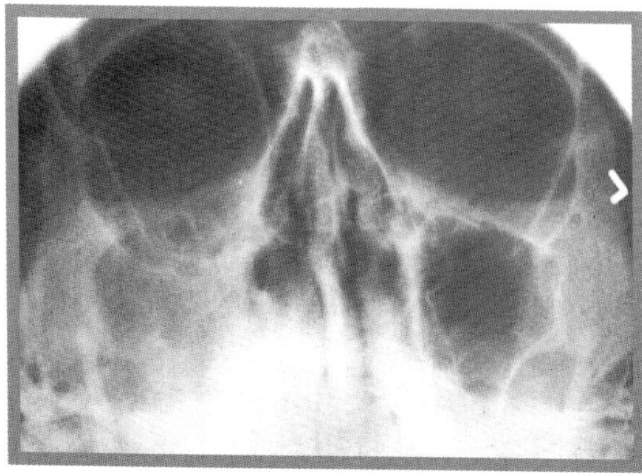

Figures 14.36 and 14.37 Burns. This girl aged 2 years has burns to both legs following an accidental scald injury from hot water. The thickness of the burn determines its management. Full-thickness burns, *i.e.*, those leaving no viable dermis, require grafting. Partial-thickness burns, *i.e.*, those leaving a residual dermis, are usually healed by the regeneration of healthy skin across denuded areas.

The severity of burns is determined by:

1. The degree of damage, *i.e.*, partial- or full-thickness.
2. The area damaged as a percentage of the total body area.
3. The site of the burns, *i.e.*, involvement of the face and hands.
4. Associated injuries, *e.g.*, inhalation.

Fluid loss from burned areas can be enormous, as can heat loss through bare tissues. Infection, especially staphylococcal sepsis and toxic shock can rapidly complicate management.

Figure 14.37 shows an autograft of split skin used to cover a burn.

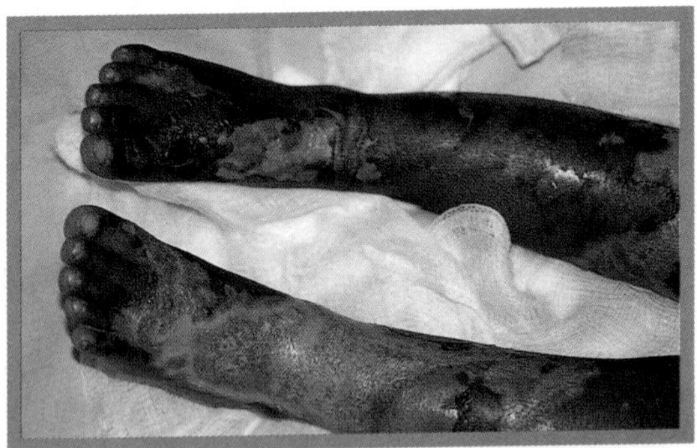

← 14.36

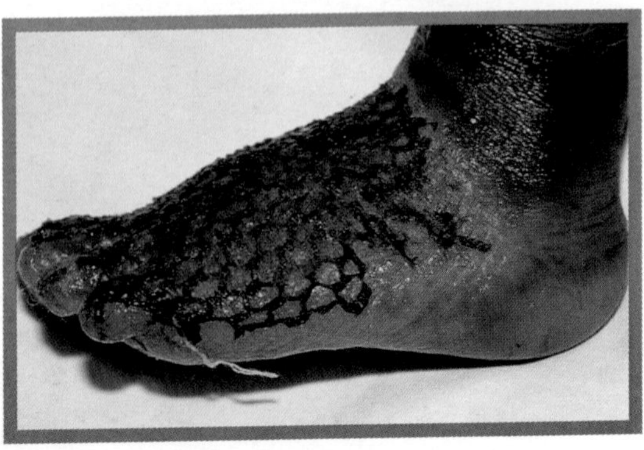

← 14.37

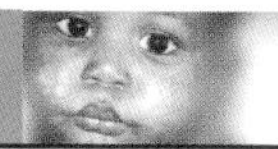

Figures 14.38 and 14.39 Siamese Twins. One-year-old Siamese twins are shown. These twins are joined at the abdomen, pubic areas and upper thigh, having one urethra, one anus, two umbilical cords and two vaginas. CT scans of the chest, abdomen and pelvis showed them to have separate livers, kidneys, bladders and small bowel, with a shared large bowel.

The X-ray in **Figure 14.39** shows them to be fused at the pelvis.

→ 14.38

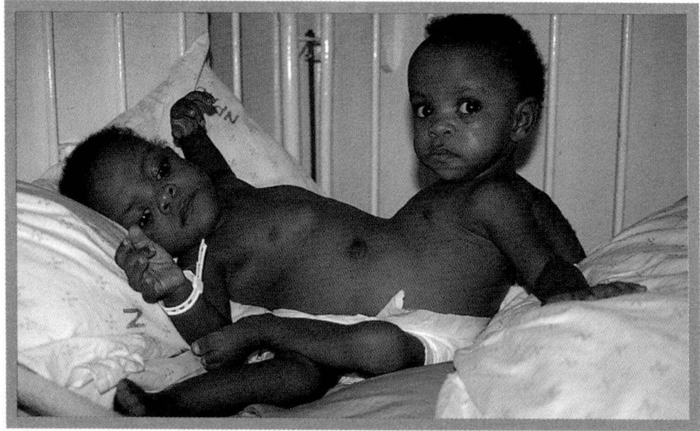

→ 14.39

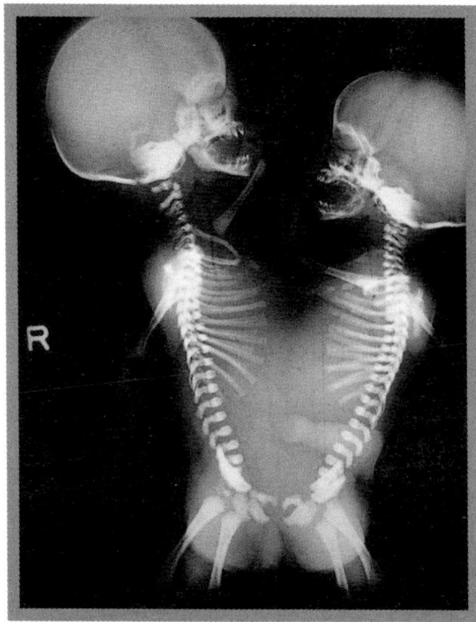

Figure 14.40 Cecal Volvulus. A bowel obstruction caused by *Ascaris lumbricoides* is shown. There is a dilated, gas-filled bowel loop that is orientated away from the right iliac fossa. The outlines of large, round worms of *Ascaris lumbricoides* are seen within the loop. The child was resuscitated, and this was followed by operative repair.

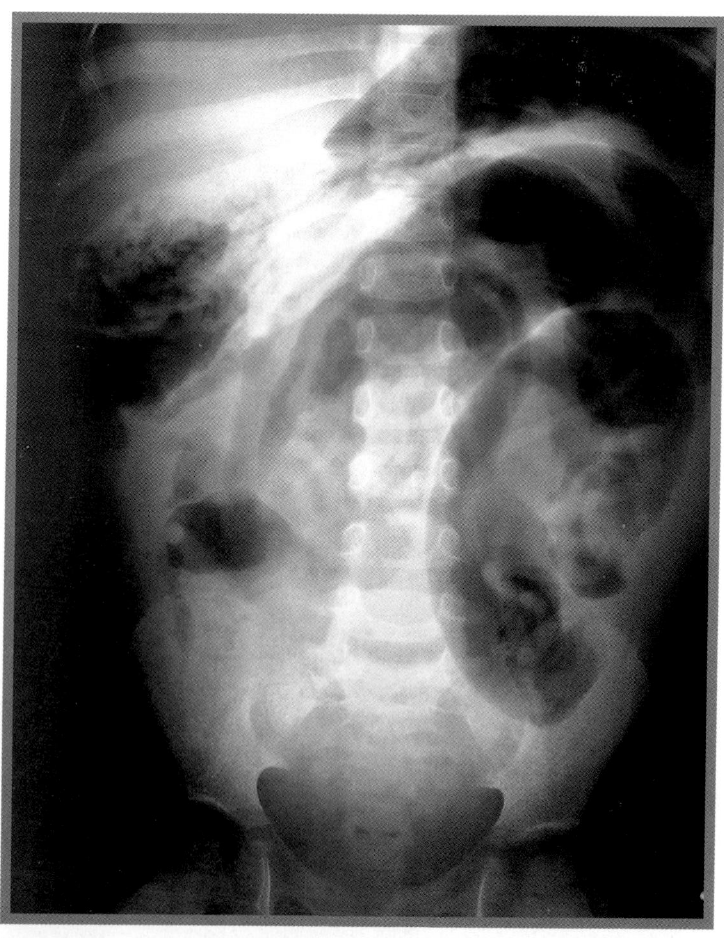

↑ **14.40**

15 Ophthalmology

Strabismus

Strabismus, or squint, is present when the fovea of each eye is not simultaneously fixating the object of regard. There are two important types:

1. Nonparalytic strabismus: this occurs when the angle of the squint remains constant in all directions of gaze.
2. Paralytic strabismus: this occurs when the angle of squint varies, being maximum when looking in the direction of action of the paralyzed muscle.

The principal causes of concomitant squints are impairment of the sensory afferent visual pathways, due to cataract, retinal disease, myopia and other refractory errors, and impairment of the motor efferent pathways .

Figure 15.1 Divergent Squint. A divergent (exotropic) nonparalytic squint is shown in a 12-year-old boy. The right eye is turned outwards. The squint was treated surgically.

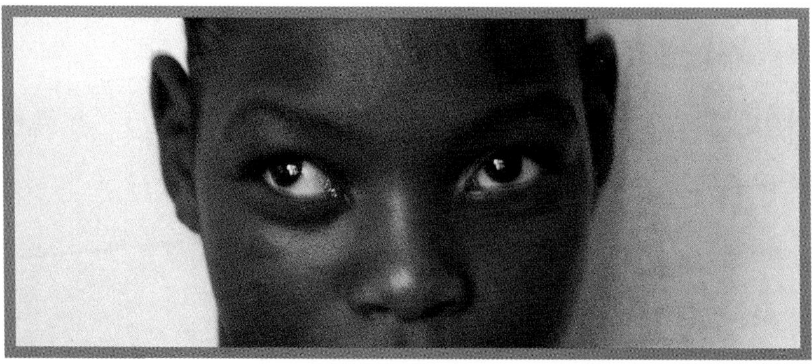

↑ 15.1

Figure 15.2 Right Convergent Squint. The convergent squint (esotropia) shown here in a 2-year-old boy was first noticed when he was looking at a detailed object nearby. The right eye is turned inward. Note the epicanthic fold, which may lead to an incorrect diagnosis of a squint. In this case the asymmetric position of the corneal light reflexes confirmed the presence of an esotropia. Convergent squints are four times more common than the divergent variety.

It is important to diagnose squints early so that:

1. An abnormality of the squinting eye is diagnosed early, *e.g.*, cataract or retinoblastoma.
2. Amblyopia (central suppression of vision) of the squinting eye is prevented/treated.
3. Glasses can be prescribed to correct refractive errors (hypermetropia is common in children with esotropia).
4. Appropriate surgery may be carried out to straighten the eyes and improve the cosmetic appearance.

Treatment involves achieving the best possible vision by reversing suppression and amblyopia where possible, and attempting to improve

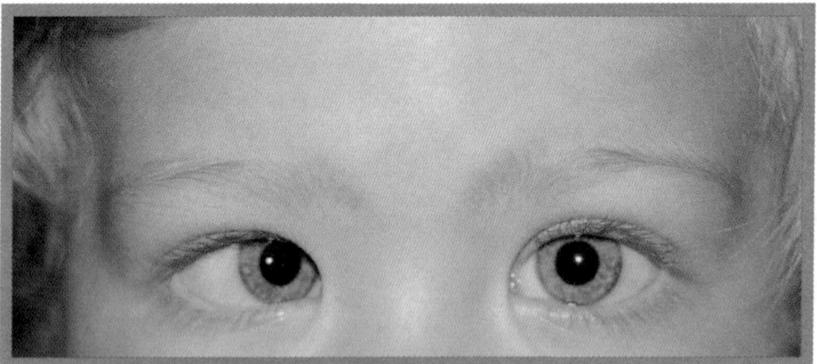

←15.2

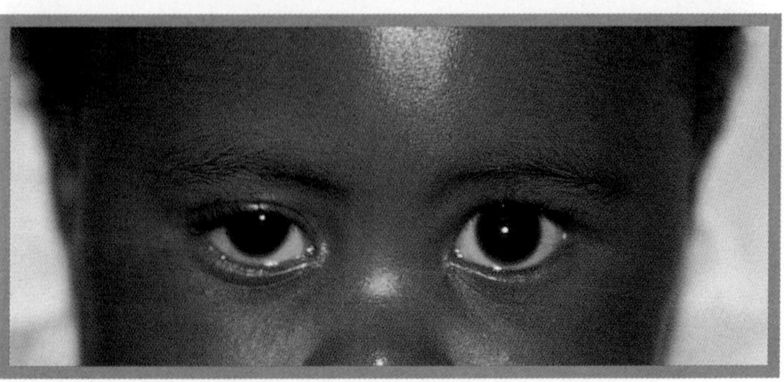

←15.3

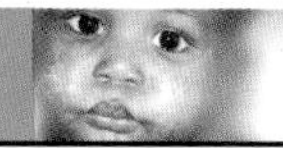

stereoscopic vision by straightening the eyes. This is done by correcting refractive errors, occlusion of the non-squinting eye, orthoptic exercises where appropriate, and finally, surgical correction. Surgery is frequently performed for cosmetic reasons only.

Figure 15.3 Unilateral Pseudoptosis. A 9-month-old girl with amaurosis (blindness) in the right eye. The apparent ptosis is due to micropthalmia of right globe an association of congenital blindness. She was observed to have nystagmus and to rub and poke her eyes frequently (oculodigital phenomenon).

Figure 15.4 Bilateral Congenital Ptosis. Bilateral congenital ptosis in a 10-year-old boy is shown. There is drooping of both upper eyelids and absent elevation of both eyes. This common congenital defect is due to incomplete development of the levator palpebrae superioris muscle. This defect is commonly associated with a reduced action of the superior rectus muscle which prevents elevation of the eye. It can be seen that the patient has attempted to overcome the ptosis by contracting the frontalis muscle causing the forehead to wrinkle. Tilting the head back is another commonly observed strategy. Surgical procedures to elevate the eyelids are usually successful.

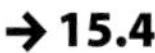
→15.4

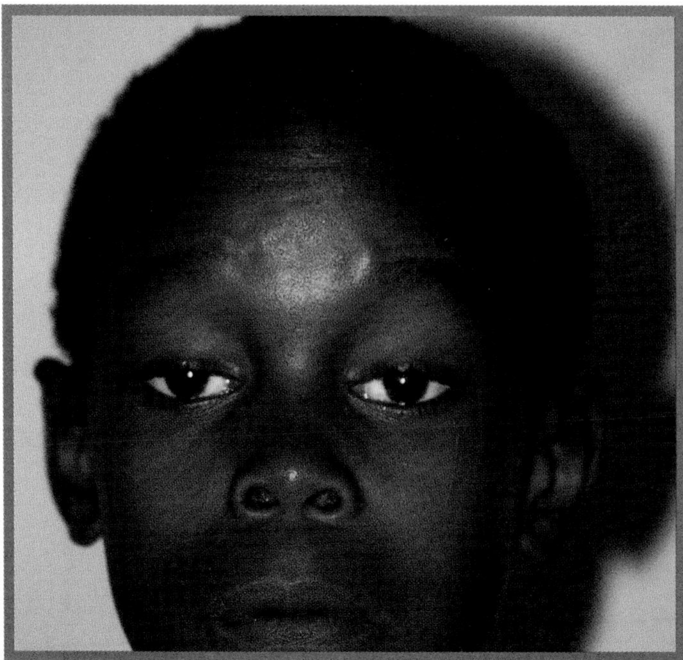

Figures 15.5–15.7 Developmental Ocular Motility Defect (Duane Retraction Syndrome). Type I, left Duane retraction syndrome is shown. The syndrome is characterized by limitation of abduction with normal adduction.
Figure 15.5 shows the eyes looking straight ahead.
Figure 15.6 shows the defective abduction of the patient's left eye and widening of the patient's left palpebral fissure.

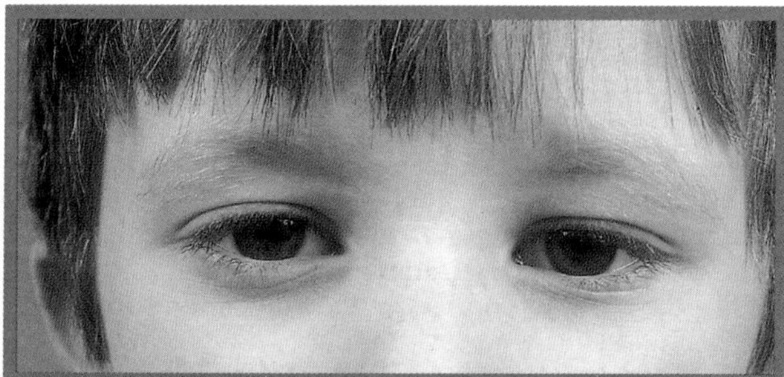

←15.5

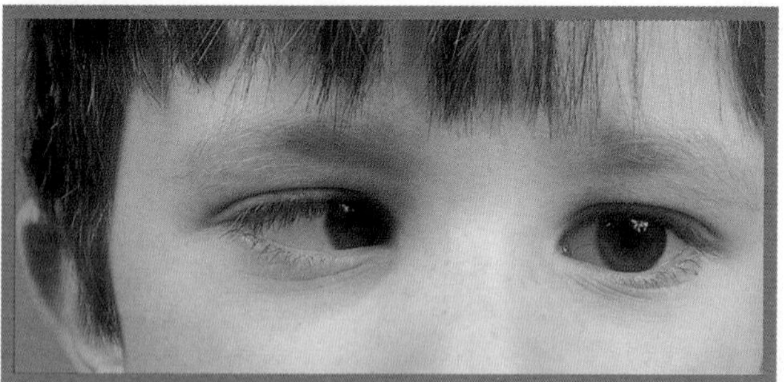

←15.6

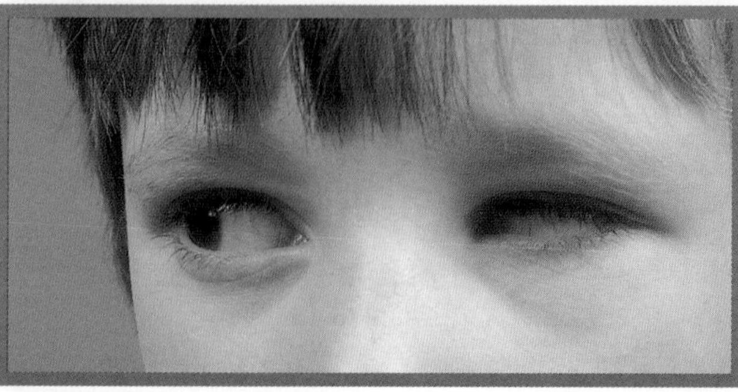

←15.7

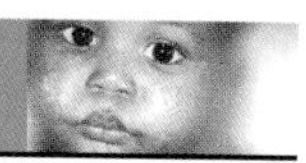

Figure 15.7 shows retraction of the patient's left eye into the orbit on adduction. This is effected by co-contraction of the medial and lateral recti muscles, and results in narrowing of the palpebral fissure. Surgery is indicated only if the eyes are not straight in the primary position or the child has to adopt an abnormal head posture to maintain binocular vision.

Figure 15.8 Cataracts. Congenital cataracts in a neonate are shown. The true incidence of cataract is not known and there are multiple causes. Inherited forms are usually autosomal dominant and some are associated with genetically or chromosomally determined conditions. On examination they are easily seen as opacities against the red reflex. It is important to look for signs of visual impairment, nystagmus, squint, failure of fixation and to examine the fundi. Tests of visual function that are used are the acuity card test, preferential looking, the Catford drum and visually evoked responses.

The differential diagnosis of the etiology of congenital cataracts is:

1. Metabolic, *e.g.*, galactosemia (central 'oil droplet' cataract), galactokinase deficiency, Löwe (oculo-cerebro-renal) syndrome and hypercalcemia syndromes.
2. Associated with dermatoses, *e.g.*, ectodermal dysplasias, ichthyosis and incontinentia pigmenti.
3. Intrauterine infections, *e.g.*, rubella, toxoplasmosis and cytomegalovirus infection.
4. As part of a recognized syndrome: *e.g.*, Down syndrome and other trisomies.
5. Embryopathy associated with maternal drug ingestion, *e.g.*, thalidomide and steroids.
6. Secondary to other abnormalities of the eye, *e.g.*, retinopathy of prematurity.

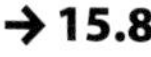
→15.8

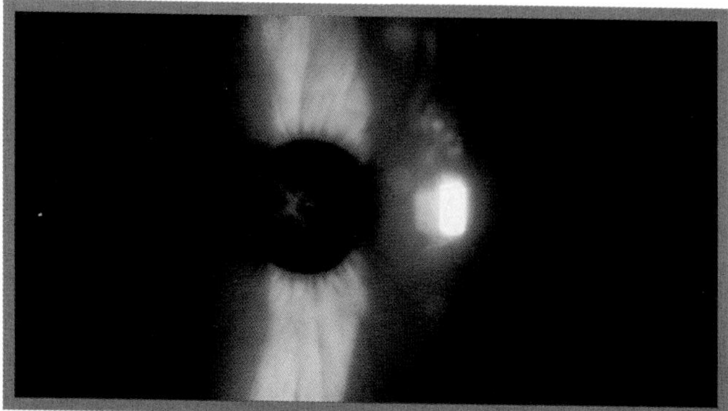

Figure 15.9 Rubella Cataract. Bilateral cataract is shown in a child with positive serology who had had viral isolation of rubella. Infection occurred at 12 weeks gestation. There is associated microphthalmos of the right eye.

Other features associated with congenital rubella are:

1. Growth retardation.
2. Cardiac abnormalities.
3. Other ocular abnormalities.
4. Deafness.
5. Hematological features, *e.g.*, thrombocytopenia.
6. Hepatitis.
7. Neurological abnormalities, *e.g.*, encephalitis.

Figure 15.10 Coloboma of Upper Eyelid. Eyelid coloboma is due to failure of normal eyelid development. Colobomas affecting the globe are caused by failure of fusion of the optic cup, and may occur anywhere from the optic nerve

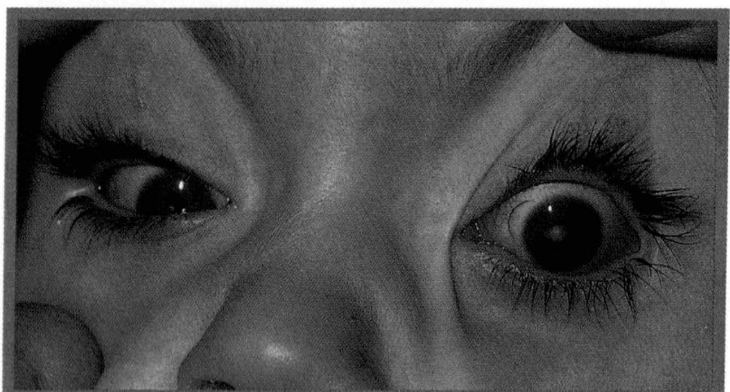

←15.9

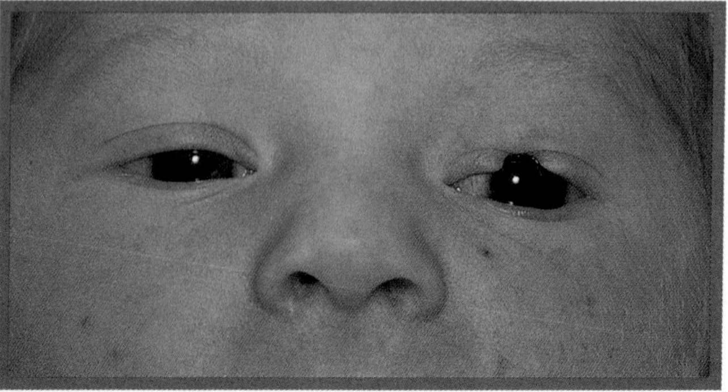

←15.10

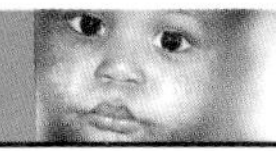

to the iris. There is often associated microphthalmos. Colobomas may occur as part of several syndromes, *e.g.*, CHARGE, Treacher–Collins, and Goldenhaar syndrome.

Figures 15.11 and 15.12 Conjunctivitis. Acute conjuctivitis is shown in a 1-month-old baby and a 15-year-old boy. Note the increased lacrimation, injected and edematous conjunctiva (chemosis), swelling of the eyelids and copious purulent discharge.

The culture grew *Staphylococcus* and the condition responded well to topical antibiotics.

The differential diagnosis is viral or chlamydial infection, which is associated with a persistent cough and marked lid edema. In infants, conjunctivitis is less frequently due to allergens or chemical irritants. In ophthalmia neonatorium it is vital to exclude transvaginally acquired infection by *Neisseria gonorrheae* as a cause, as it is one of the few organisms capable of penetrating the cornea and causing blindness.

→15.11

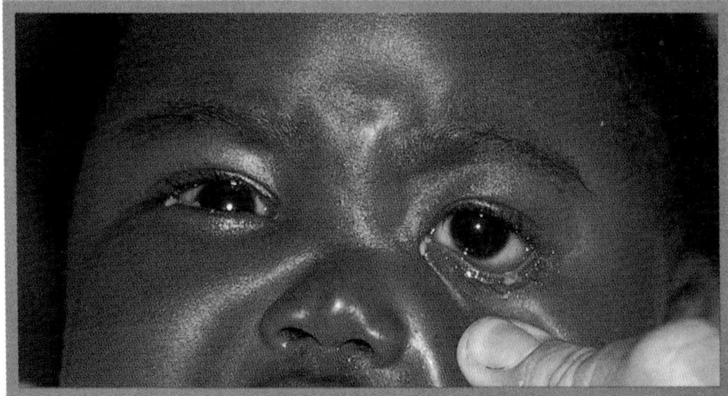

→15.12

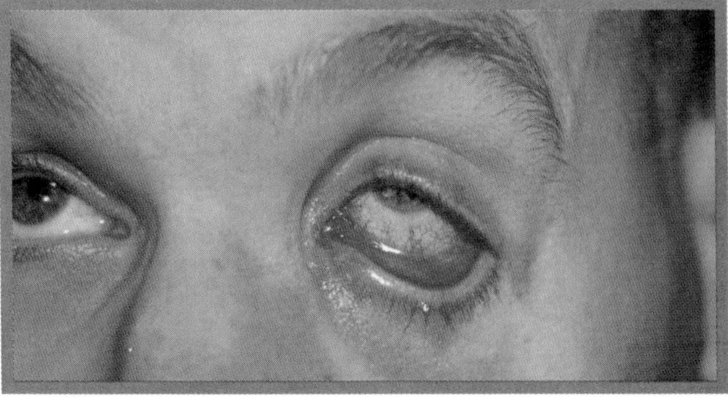

Figure 15.13 Acute Gonococcal Conjunctivitis. Acute purulent conjunctivitis is shown in a 7-year-old boy. This child presented with a 2-day history of a painful, profusely dicharging, red right eye. Severe conjunctival injection and chemosis can be seen with lid edema and tenderness. In addition there was blepharospasm and pre-auricular lymphadenopathy. Cultures grew *Neisseria gonorrheae* that was sensitive to penicillin given orally. In view of his age this child was investigated for possible sexual abuse.

Figure 15.14 Anterior Uveitis. The child shown here presented with pain, photophobia, redness, reduced vision and lacrimation in both eyes. Examination revealed ciliary vessel hyperaemia, reduced visual acuity and swelling of the eyelids. Uveitis is associated with juvenile chronic arthritis (the pauciarticular form), sarcoidosis and, less frequently, with tuberculosis. Other infections that may produce uveitis include syphilis, toxoplasmosis and viral infections. Uveitis also occurs in Reiter and Behçet disease.

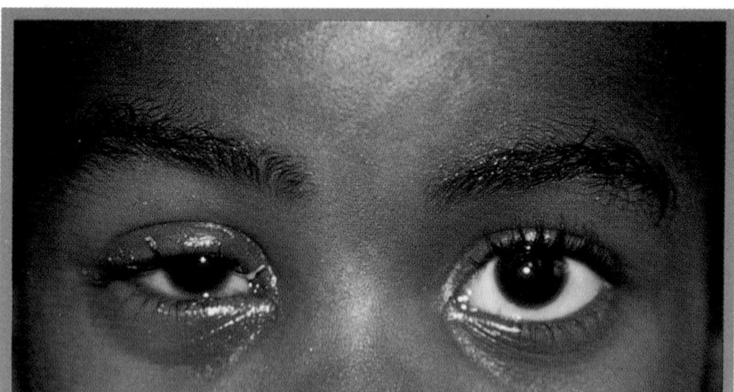

←15.13

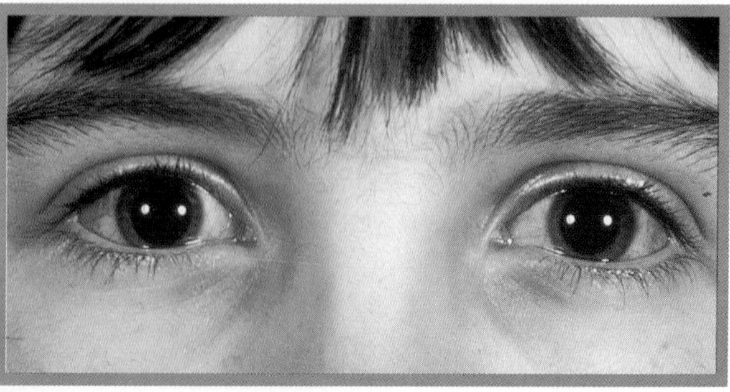

←15.14

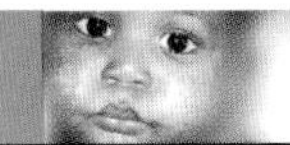

Figure 15.15 Stye (Hordeolum). A stye is shown on the lower left eyelid. The eyelid had been painful and swollen for 2 days. On inspection, a swelling was seen around the lash follicle. A stye is an acute staphylococcal infection of an eyelash follicle. Local heat may allow the stye to point and drain. In children with recurrent styes, a history of chronic nose picking and eye rubbing is common. Less common is the finding of diabetes or immune deficiency as a cause.

Figures 15.16–15.17 Cellulitis. Figure 15.16 shows preseptal cellulitis involving the eyelids of the left eye of a 3-year-old boy. Note the absence of proptosis, and the white bulbar conjunctiva. There is no history of pain on eye movement or diplopia. On examination, the pupillary reflexes were normal, as was the visual acuity. Cellulitis is usually due to spread of infection from skin lesions or from the ethmoid sinuses. The fibrous orbital septum dividing the anterior eyelid structures from the orbital contents is not well developed in children. Intravenous antibiotics for 24 hours is recommended followed by oral treatment.

→15.15

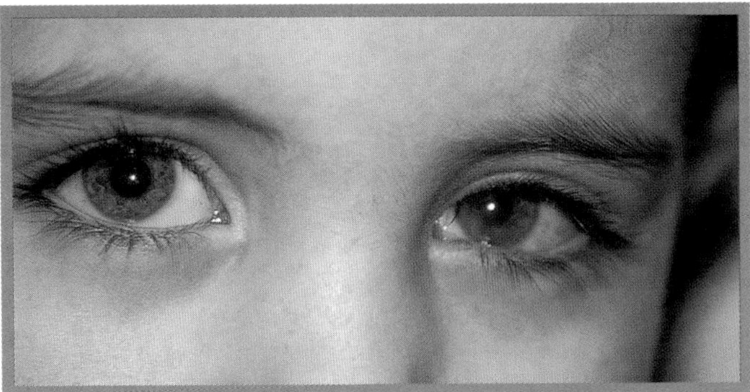

→15.16

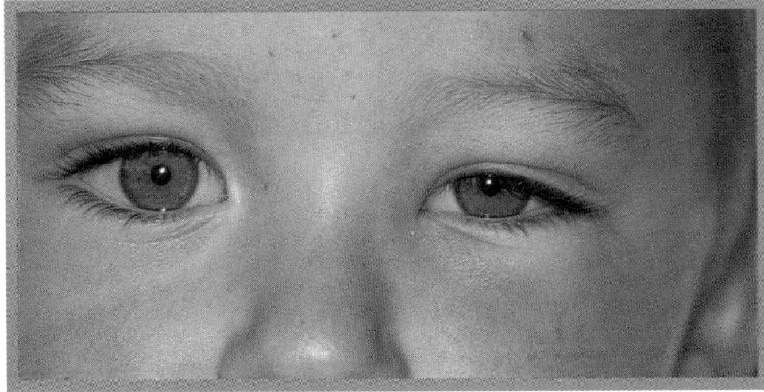

Figure 15.17 Right-sided orbital cellulitis in a 4-year-old boy. The cellulitis was of rapid onset. The conjuctiva is injected, there is chemosis, and the eye is proptosed laterally and downwards. The eyelids are swollen, and were tender on palpation. Ocular movements were restricted and there was systemic upset.

The above is usually due to the spread of infection from the ethmoid sinuses; it is a life- (and sight-) threatening condition and requires immediate treatment because of the risk of intracerebral spread and cavernous venous sinus thrombosis. The focus of infection can be identified by CT. Loss of vision is usually due to pressure on the optic nerve. Treatment consists in administration of intravenous antibiotics, including agents against anaerobic bacteria, and surgical drainage where necessary.

Possible causes are:

1. Sinus infection: the most common cause.
2. Spread from adjacent structures, *e.g.*, dental, or dacryocystitis.
3. Hematogenous spread.
4. Post-traumatic, *e.g.*, a penetrating orbital injury.
5. Post-squint surgery.

Potential complications are:

1. Intracranial: this occurs in approximately 4% of cases and includes meningitis, subdural/cerebral abscess, and cavernous sinus thrombosis.
2. Orbital abscess.
3. Ocular complications, *e.g.*, raised intraocular pressure, occlusion of the central retinal vessels, and pressure effects on the optic nerve.

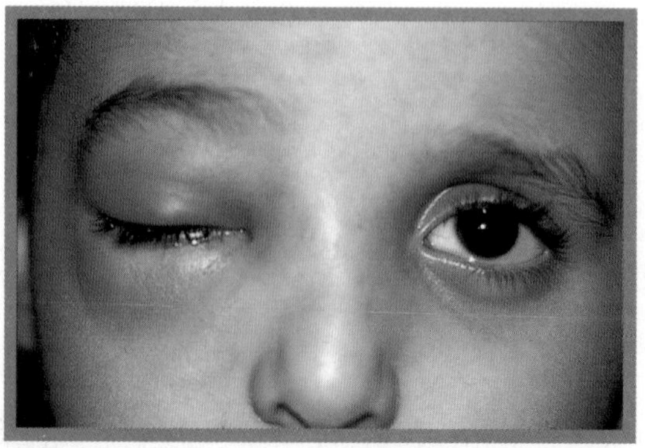

← 15.17

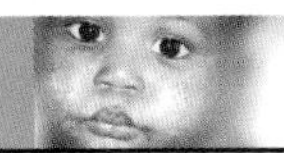

Figure 15.18 Herpes Simplex Blepharoconjunctivitis. The 5-year-old boy shown here presented with herpes simplex blepharoconjunctivitis that had become secondarily infected with *Staphylococcus,* resulting in orbital cellulitis.

The herpes vesicles can be seen well on the medial aspect of the lower lid and periorbital areas, and have formed crusts. This condition should be treated with antiviral drugs as well as antibiotics.

Figure 15.19 Herpes Zoster Ophthalmicus. The 6-year-old boy shown here has a history of chickenpox. He presented with a prodrome of fever, malaise, headache and facial pain, and then developed cutaneous vesicles. The rash is distributed over all three divisions of the ophthalmic branch of the trigeminal nerve, *i.e.,* the frontal, lacrimal and nasociliary divisions. Treatment consists in administration of topical and systemic antiviral agents. Post-herpetic neuralgia is rare in children. Ocular involvement should be suspected in those with involvement of the nasociliary division that supplies the side of the nose (Hutchinson sign).

→15.18

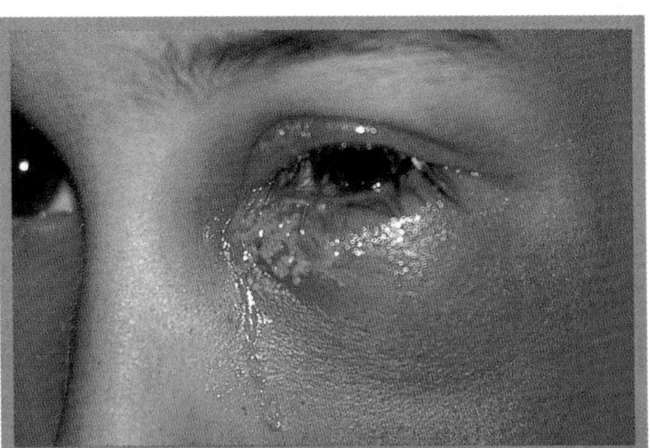

→15.19

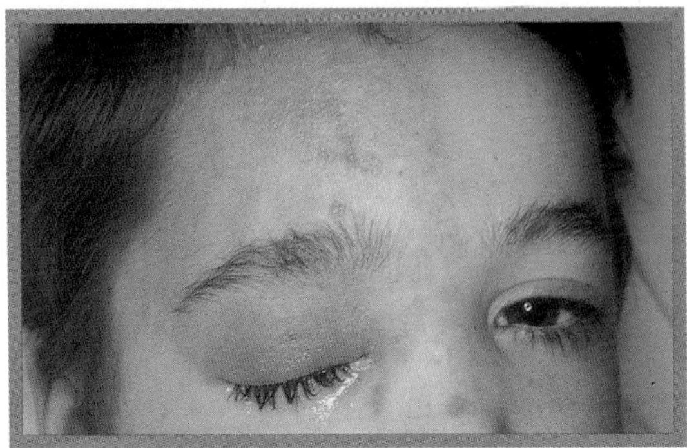

Figure 15.20 Cytomegalovirus (CMV) Retinitis. is shown in a patient who is HIV positive and who has full-blown AIDS. There are widespread areas of retinitis and haemorrhages. CMV affects 40% of adult patients with AIDS. It signifies severe immunosuppression and can also occur in other immunodeficiency states. Neonatal congenital CMV gives a similar picture. Treatment consists of administration of intravenous or intraocular antiviral agents.

Figure 15.21 Icteric Sclerae. The 18-month-old child shown here is on rifampicin, isoniazid and pyrazinamide for TB. A drug-induced hepatitis developed. In healthy infants the sclerae can often appear yellow secondary to carotenoids in infant foods and carrots.

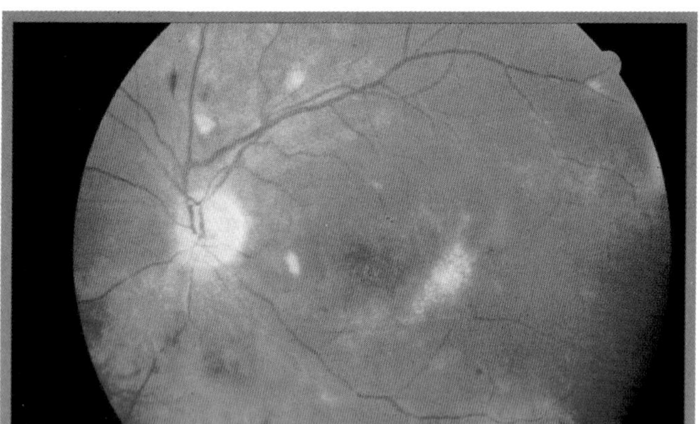

←15.20

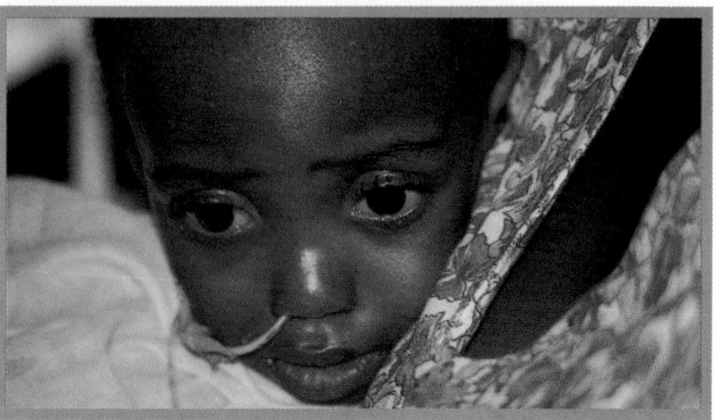

←15.21

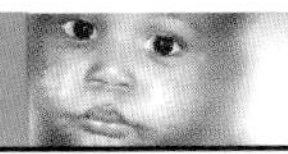

Figure 15.22 Bilateral Subconjunctival Hemorrhages. This resolves spontaneously. Usually traumatic in origin e.g. birth and non-accidental injury.
Figure 15.23 Subluxation of the Crystalline Lens. The adolescent shown here has Marfan syndrome with characteristic superior and temporal subluxationof the lens. The edge of the lens can be seen in the pupil. Subluxation and dislocation of the lens requires long-term, specialist follow up because of refractive changes and the risk of secondary glaucoma. This condition can be recognized by the edge of the lens being visible in the pupil and by iridodonesis (tremulous iris). Subluxation of the lens occurs in 80% of Marfan syndrome patients. Other ocular complications in Marfan syndrome include retinal detachment and degeneration. In homocystinuria the lens dislocates downward, whereas in Marfan dislocates upward and outward.

→15.22

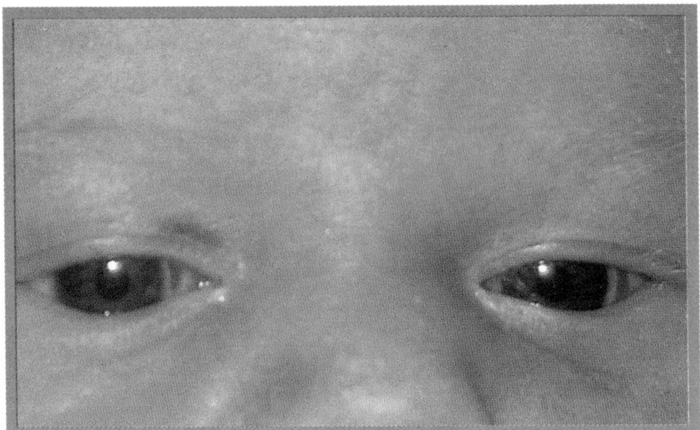

→15.23

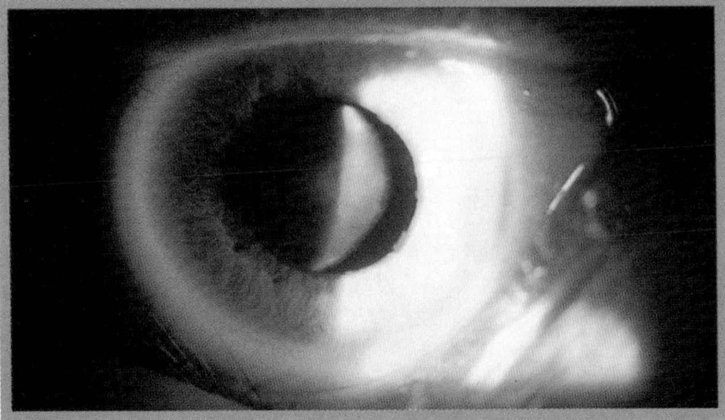

INDEX

Italic page references refer the reader to the text only.

WITHDRAWN